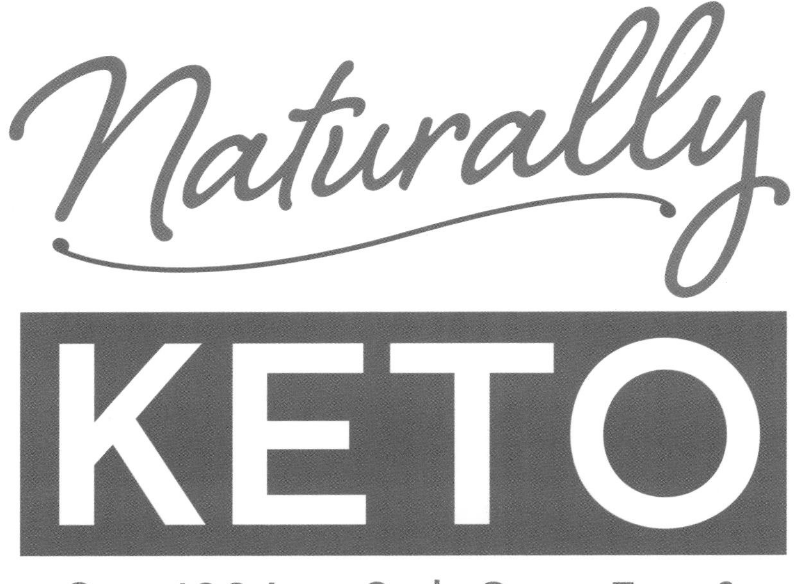

Over 100 Low-Carb, Sugar-Free &
Allergy-Friendly Recipes
The Whole Family Will Love

Brenda Bennett

Victory Belt Publishing Inc.
Las Vegas

First published in 2019 by Victory Belt Publishing Inc.

ISBN-13: 978-1-628603-73-6

Cover design by Justin-Aaron Velasco
Author photos by Shawon Davis Photography
Interior design and illustrations by Yordan Terziev and Boryana Yordanova

Printed in Canada
TC 0119

Table of Contents

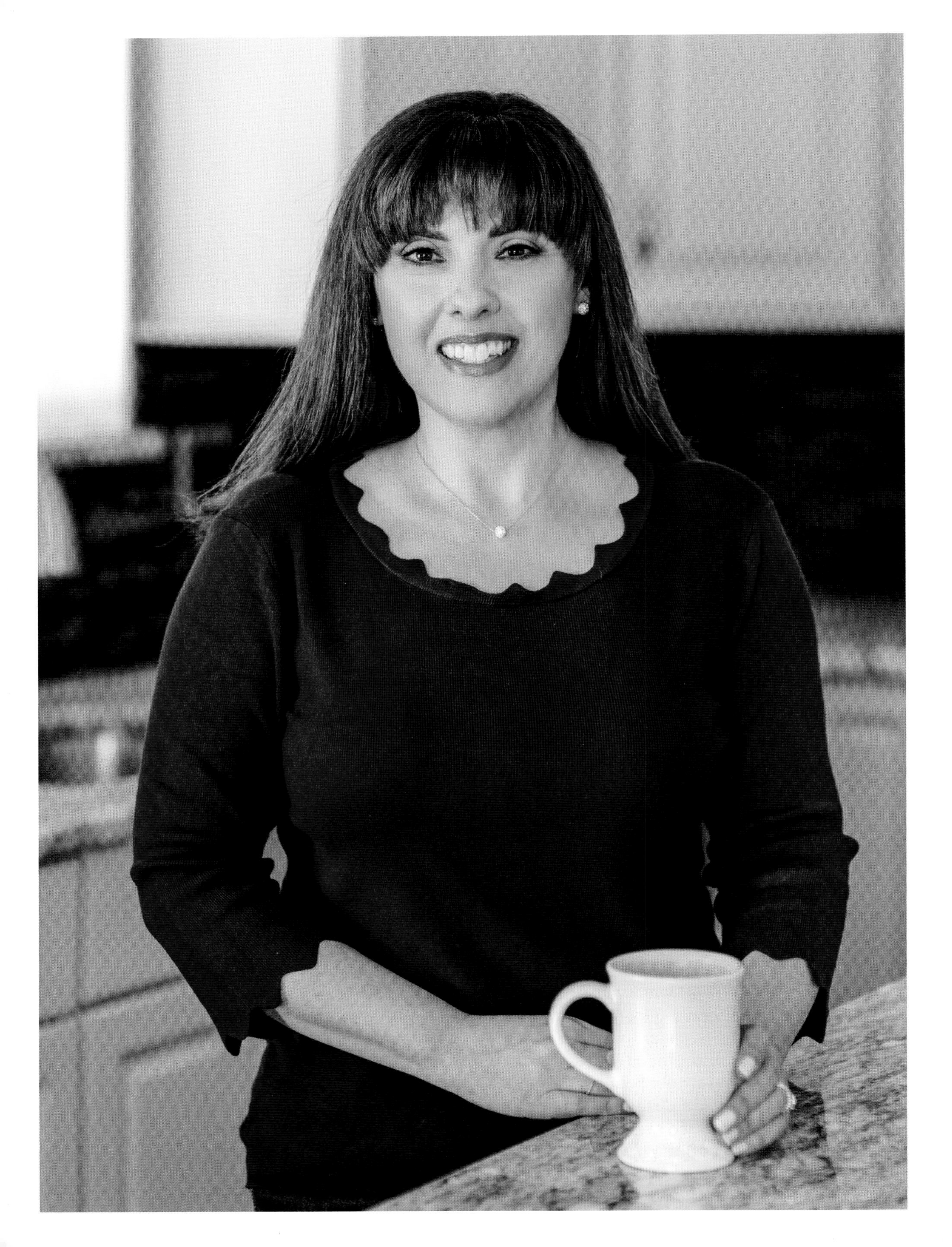

Preface:
MY JOURNEY TO KETO

My love affair with sugar began at the young age of twelve. I'm not completely sure what triggered it. Maybe it was being the oldest child in my family, feeling responsible for my younger siblings. Maybe it was having a type-A perfectionist personality and wanting to control my surroundings. Maybe it was the pediatrician who told me I needed to lose 10 pounds. I had been a dancer and an ice skater since the age of four, and as I got older, I became aware that other teens were growing taller and leaner than I was. That observation might have triggered my obsession, at least a bit. I chose to seek comfort in sugar and carbs.

By age fifteen, I had quit dance and skating and become bulimic. It's difficult to think about today, but at the time, I wanted to control something, and I chose my body. I was able to eat everything I wanted and then get rid of it to keep my weight down and avoid the consequences of my binges. My period stopped for a year. I had popped blood vessels around my eyes, but I was thin and received accolades from my family and friends, which spurred me on.

I don't know how my parents discovered my secret. I was a pro—or so I thought—at muffling the sounds by saying I was in the shower or brushing my teeth. They found me a support group, and I did eventually stop purging, but the bingeing and obsessing about my weight continued.

At my highest weight, I was 159 pounds. Being just 5-foot-2, I thought that was enormous. I hated being in my own skin. I hated how much I needed sugar to kick-start my day. I remember running to the vending machine in my college dorm—in the early mornings, of course, when everyone else was sleeping—so I could get my fix: a packaged cinnamon bun.

After graduating from college, I started attending Overeaters Anonymous meetings. I learned to manage my weight by abstaining from eating between meals. After about six months, my weight stabilized at 124 pounds, and I was content with that. I didn't have to struggle

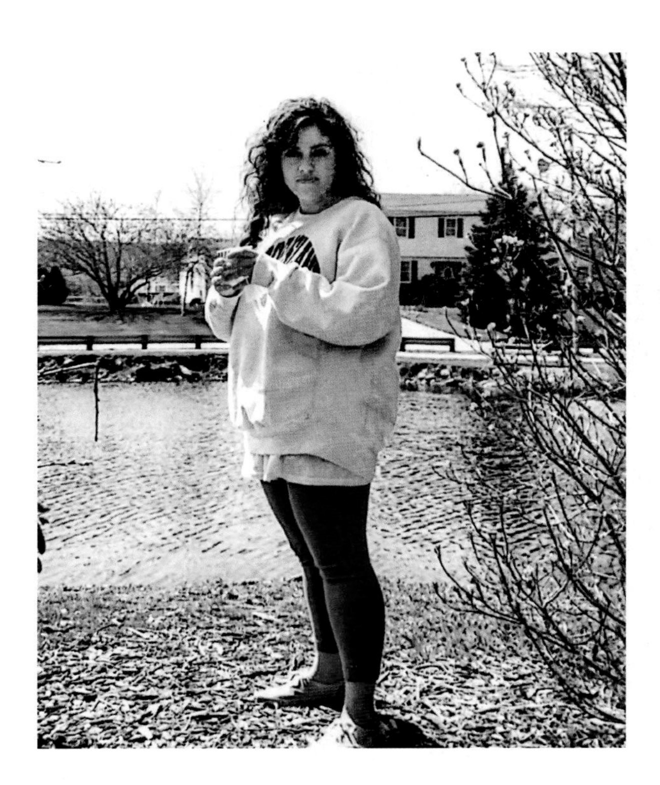

to maintain that weight. I no longer felt that I had to work out for two hours every day. Plus, I got to enjoy the foods I loved; nothing was off-limits as long as I fasted between planned meals.

This approach worked for me for quite a few years. I got married and stopped going to OA because I was "fixed." While I was pregnant with my first child, I gained 70 pounds, but I was able to lose it all within six months.

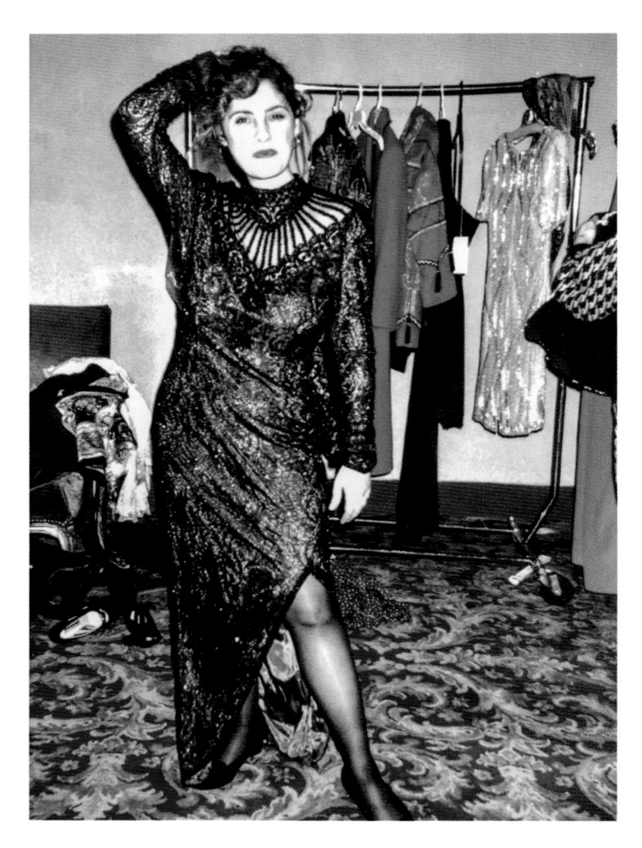

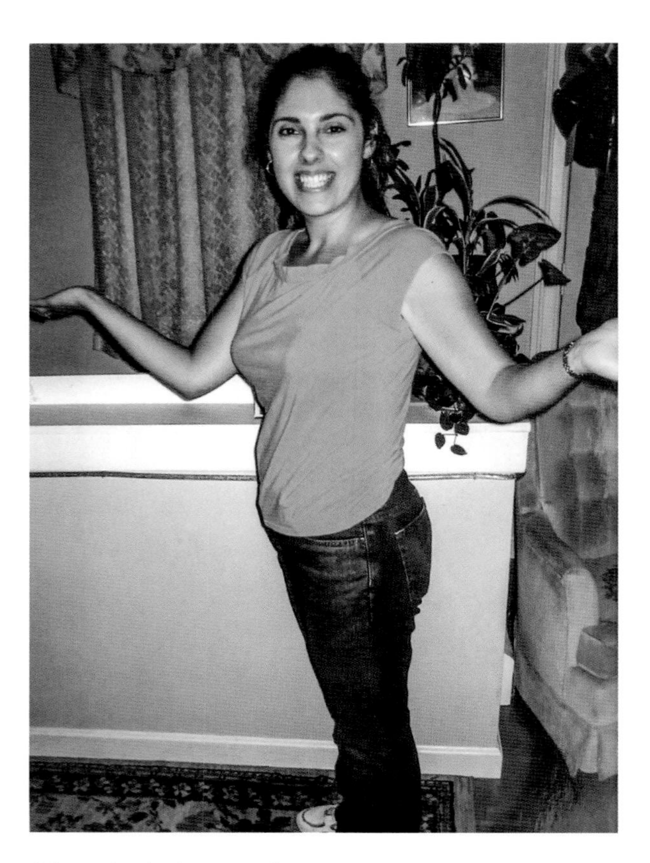

Unfortunately, after I had my second child in 2003, the last 20 pounds of weight gain would not come off no matter what I did. In 2004, I started following a Christian weight loss program called Prism that included food journaling, calorie counting, and one-on-one weekly support calls for six weeks. It also eliminated all white sugar, white flour, white rice, and white potatoes. It was my worst nightmare. I never thought I could do it, let alone be happy about it, even if the weight was coming off. I thought, "How in the world could anyone live a happy life without enjoying cake or chocolate ever again?" Inconceivable! But the weight came off, and my sugar cravings subsided. I began creating sugar-free recipes and teaching classes at my church, sharing my breakthrough with everyone who would listen. I felt I had finally overcome my cravings; sugar wasn't an obsession anymore.

Then I got pregnant again, once more eating for two. I took just one bite of a sugary treat at a party, and my obsession came back with a vengeance. I wasn't too concerned, though, because I knew what I needed to do this time. After the baby was born, I thought, I'd cut out sugar again and everything would be fine.

I was wrong. To say that the struggle to lose the baby weight was worse than any I had ever known is an understatement. After my third child was born in 2006, I was like a ravenous lion. I could not go even one day without sugar. I prayed and prayed to God to help me get back to the joy and freedom I had known before. I begged and pleaded for Him to help me regain my strength. It took me two years to break free, but I did it, and my lips have not touched white sugar since 2008.

But I wasn't on the road to keto yet. Until 2012, I cooked with honey and maple syrup and enjoyed sweet potatoes and brown rice. I followed a Paleo-type approach, which helped me maintain my weight until the age of forty-two. After starting my blog, Sugar-Free Mom, in 2011 and creating and taste-testing all those recipes, my weight began to creep up, and I knew I needed to try something different. I began using a lower-carb approach and saw some success from keeping my carb intake between 50 and 70 grams a day, mostly from vegetables.

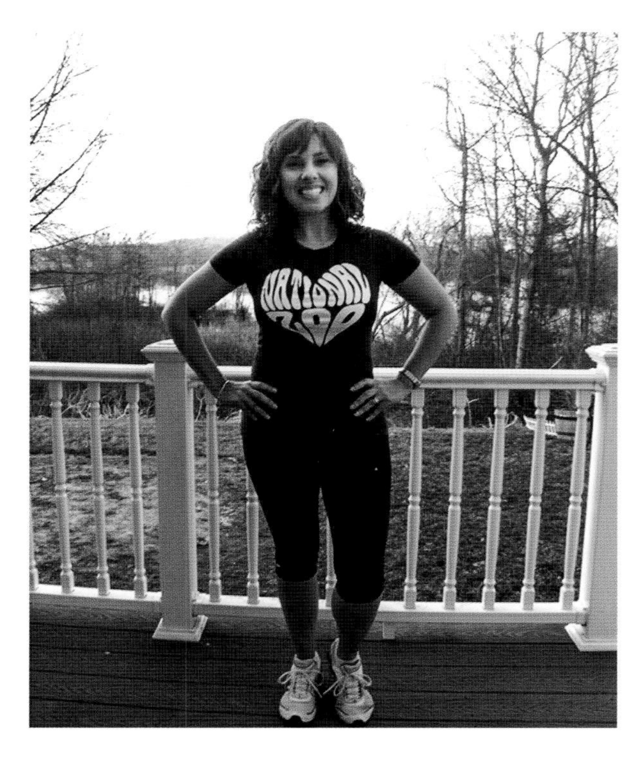

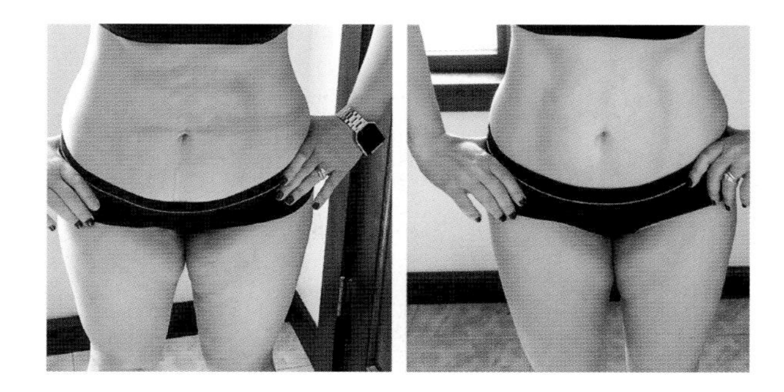

Even so, it took me another few years to try keto. Ten pounds had crept back on, but worse, I started losing some hair on the back of my head, and my eyebrows seemed to be thinning. My primary care doctor shrugged off these symptoms, saying they were probably nothing to worry about—perhaps just hormones. He told me to "eat less and exercise more." I thought I could do a little better than that, so I began eating keto, but with a very loose approach. I did not track my macros, but I thought I could eat as much fat as I wanted. I did not lose weight, but my hair started to grow back, and I felt better because I was no longer depriving myself of fat. In 2016, with no weight loss to show from what I thought was a keto diet, I hired a trainer for strength training twice a week.

I did lose those 10 pounds, but I wasn't seeing the body composition changes I wanted. I thought I just wasn't being diligent enough, so I continued to muddle along until January 2018, when I decided to go strict keto. I cut out all dairy and nuts and tracked my macros for six weeks. I shared this experience on my blog, complete with photos. The decision to share that personal information was a difficult one, but without photographic evidence, I would have missed the changes that were occurring. I lost only 3 pounds during those six weeks, but the pictures show the true fat loss.

In the spring of 2018, I broke out in horrible itchy hives on my face, chin, and neck. I didn't know the cause, but I thought it might be because I'd added back dairy and nuts. So I went on an Autoimmune Protocol Diet for three months with no improvement. I had already seen my primary care doctor multiple times, and he just wanted to prescribe prednisone, a harsh steroid I chose not to use. I also started experiencing such terrible brain fog that I was forgetting friends' names and missing familiar turns on the way home. To add insult to injury, I was so lethargic that I almost fell asleep driving in the middle of the day. Other symptoms included itchy inner ears and extremely dry skin and hair that no amount of moisturizer helped.

Because my doctor was not truly interested in helping me figure out what was going on, I sent my records to an endocrinologist, who diagnosed me with chronic Epstein-Barr virus and hypothyroidism. My free T3 number was extremely low. Your thyroid makes hormones that regulate how your body uses energy. Most doctors test only thyroid-stimulating hormone (TSH), which acts as a messenger to your thyroid gland; a normal range indicates that the thyroid is functioning properly. However, the TSH test alone is not enough; thyroxine (T4) and triiodothyronine (T3) are just as important. T4 is a "storage" hormone, but it needs T3, which is the active hormone that your body needs for many basic functions. T3 and T4 help regulate metabolism, heart rate, and body temperature and help the brain function properly. No wonder it was so hard for me to maintain my weight!

I was so relieved to finally have confirmation that the problem wasn't all in my head. With the help of thyroid medication and nutritional diligence, I stayed in ketosis and started to see results almost immediately. After starting my new medication, it took about six weeks to see 99 percent improvement in my brain fog. My tiredness improved so dramatically that I no longer needed caffeine to make it through the day. Still, the hives didn't seem to get any better, so I stayed away from nuts and dairy and kept working out with my trainer. I was being so careful, but my weight crept up and wouldn't budge. Frustrated by that and in desperate need of relief from my itchy hives, my next step was a Mediator Release Test (MRT) food sensitivities test.

I received a pretty lengthy list of food sensitivities. Honestly, the results were disheartening—I was eating these foods on a daily basis. The test showed that I react to solanine, which occurs naturally in nightshades like bell peppers, eggplant, and tomatoes. I'm also highly sensitive to salicylic acid, found in foods like almonds, apples (including apple cider vinegar), blackberries, grapes (including red wine vinegar), cloves, cucumbers, olives, pickles, raspberries, strawberries, and tomatoes. But even after I removed all of these foods from my diet, the hives didn't improve. I already knew I was highly sensitive to gluten and had been gluten-free for six years. Thankfully, I'd eliminated corn when I went low-carb—turns out I'm very sensitive to that as well. When I went back to the endocrinologist, I told her about my newly confirmed food sensitivities and discovered that the medication I was on used corn and gluten as additives. We switched to Tirosint, which has just four ingredients—and no gluten or corn.

Sadly, after six weeks on that medication, I was declining again. The brain fog and fatigue returned. I read the book *The Paleo Thyroid Solution* by Elle Russ, and I knew I needed a medication that included T3. After getting blood test results showing that my T3 number was still the lowest in the range, I begged my endocrinologist to give me the smallest dose of T3 that she was comfortable giving.

After just one month, I felt incredible! Eight pounds came off easily. The brain fog disappeared. I'm not lethargic when I wake, and I don't need caffeine to survive the day. After just six weeks on that medication, my blood work showed my T3 level to be optimal at 3.8—on the high end of the normal range.

The point of the story is that even if your test results show that your number is considered "in the range," it doesn't mean that the number is optimal for you. Some women have no issues or symptoms with a low T3 number, but others, like myself, truly need to be on the higher end of the range to feel their best. I'm currently seeing a functional medicine doctor for help in unraveling the cause of these mysterious hives.

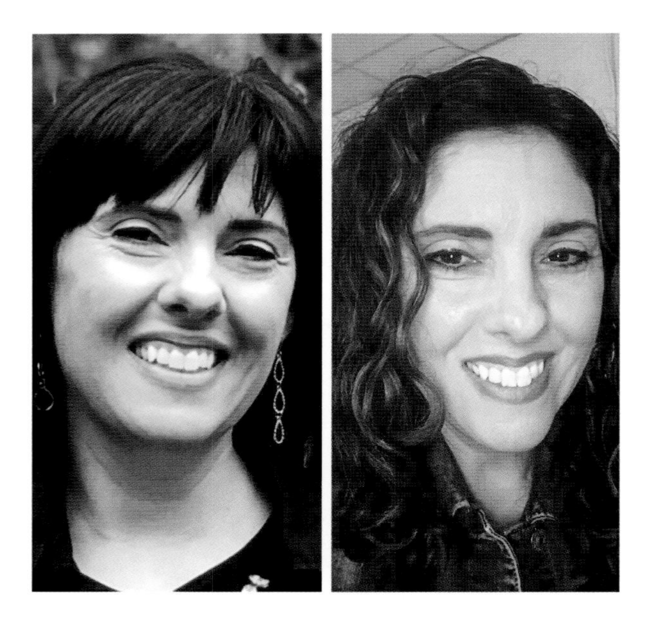

Despite all the frustration and woe with the length of time it's taken for me to start feeling better, and despite the issue of chronic hives that remains, I have faith that I'm going through this for a higher purpose: to share with and help others. For me, it's about doing all I can and letting God take care of the rest. I am on the road to recovery. I'm feeling better each day. I believe I will see an end to my symptoms, and once I do, you'd better believe I'll be sharing all about it on my blog.

Every bit of progress is something to celebrate. If you're new to the keto diet or struggling to eliminate certain foods from your diet, keep your goals in mind and give yourself time to adjust. All those years on my low-carb diet helped me stop craving sugar, but I still couldn't control my cravings for salty potato chips. After just a few months on keto, I could be around others eating potato chips and not want one. That is a complete miracle to me!

In my experience, that transitional period is well worth it, because the keto diet helps not only with weight loss but also with many autoimmune diseases. Sugar feeds disease and illness. Removing it from my life in 2008 was one of the best decisions I've ever made, and I don't regret it for a minute. Today, I don't crave sugar. I don't crave carbs. I have food freedom, and you can, too! I encourage you to start today and focus on one day at a time. You can do anything for one day. The next thing you know, it will be one week, one month, and then one year. The longer you resist the temptations, the easier it becomes.

I hope and pray that I've encouraged you to begin a ketogenic lifestyle. You can lead your best life yet.

We are all works in progress!

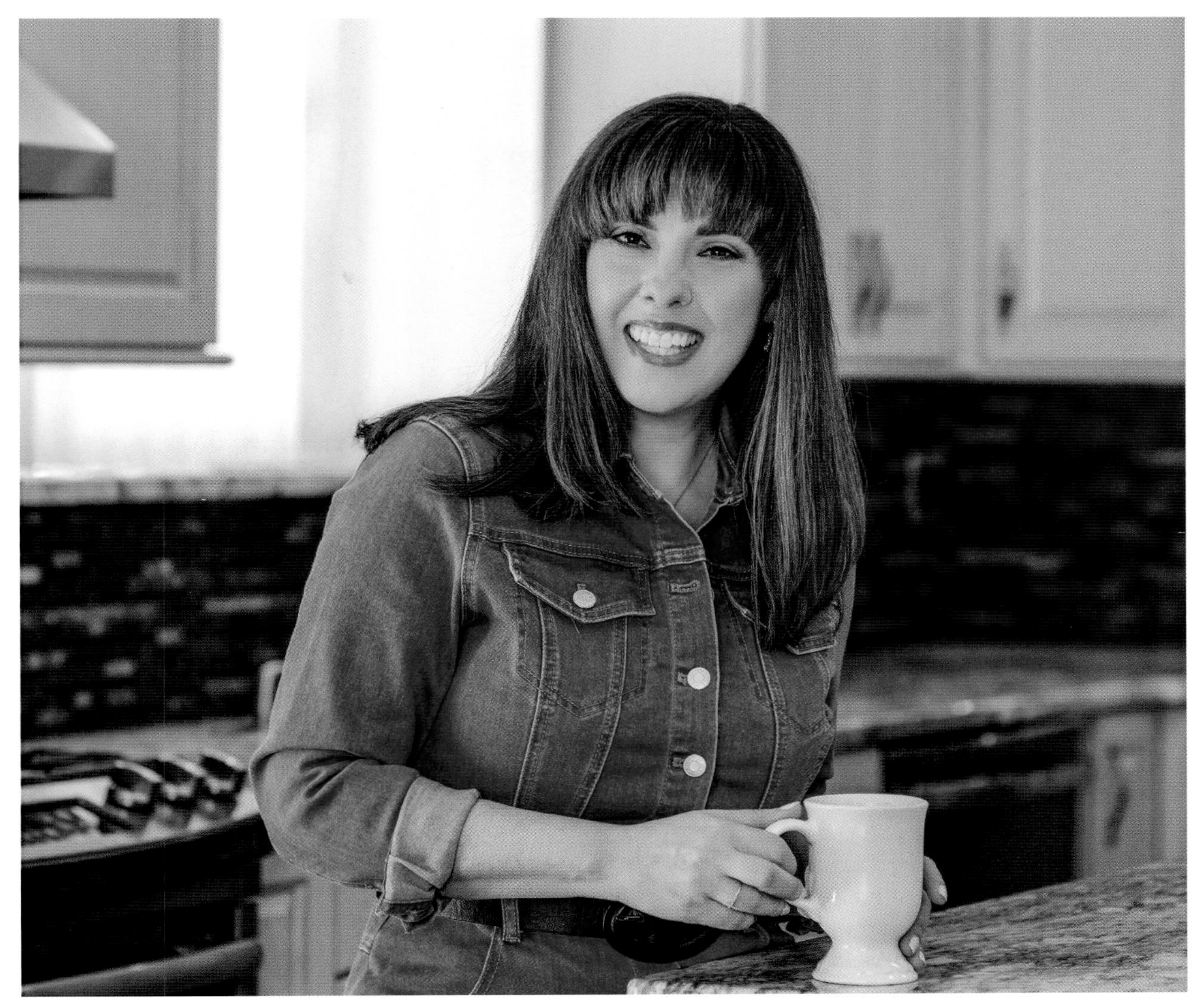

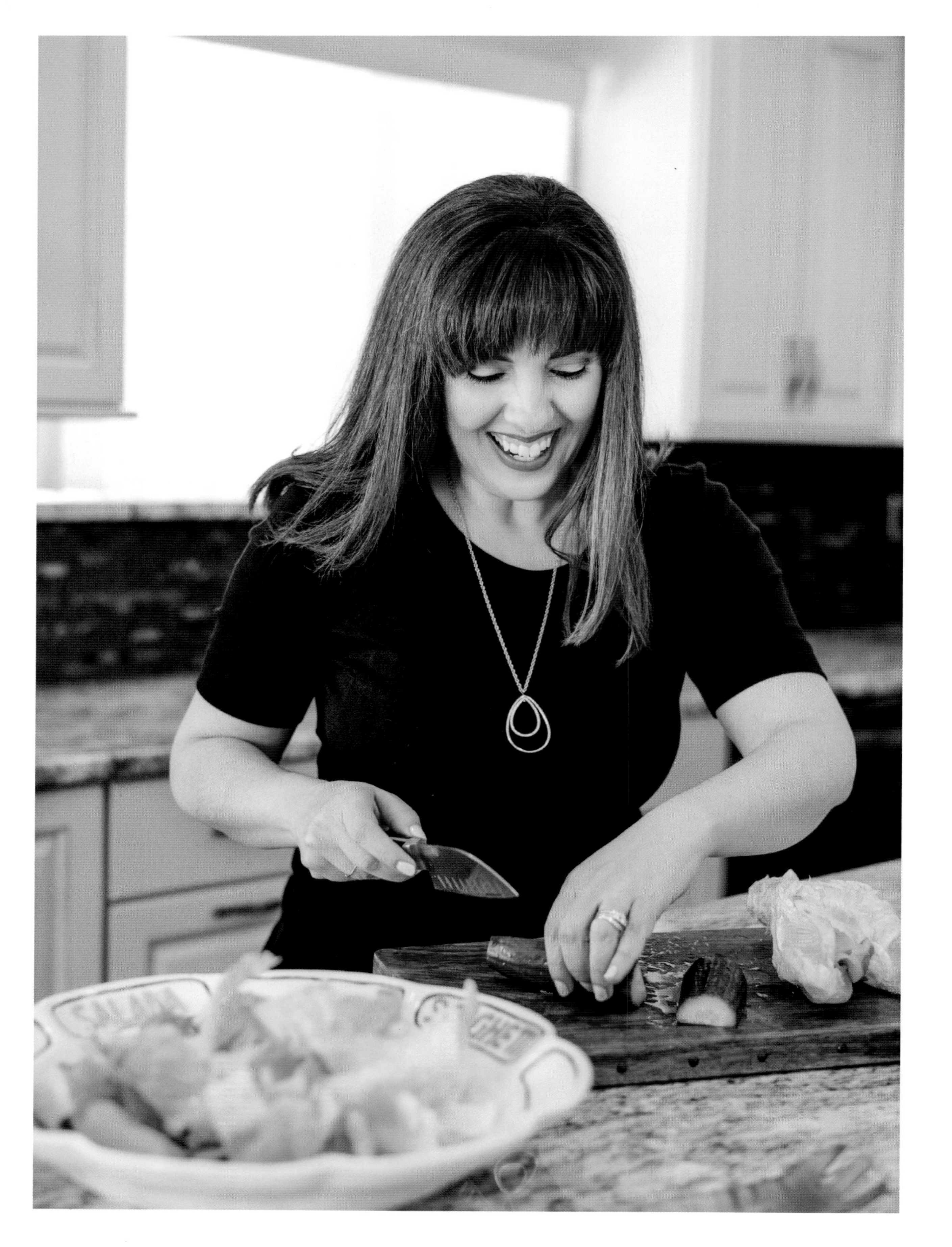

INTRODUCTION

I grew up in an Italian family, so food was and will always be an expression of love for me. Every holiday, every birthday, every time a baby was born, during times of sickness or crisis, my mother and grandmother taught me that preparing food for others showed how deeply we cared.

For as long as I can remember, I've enjoyed being in the kitchen. Even as a child, I helped roll gnocchi, prep chicken parmigiana, bake biscotti, and fill cannoli. Cooking was never seen as a chore—it was a joy to nourish the ones we loved.

This natural love for cooking and baking has lasted throughout my life; now, at age forty-seven, I still feel the same joy in the kitchen. Reimagining the traditional family favorites I grew up enjoying as low-carb, ketogenic versions brings me even more happiness. In *Naturally Keto,* you'll find classic Italian desserts like pizzelle, cannoli, tiramisù, and cream puffs. Better still, you'll find meals that you can serve even to a non-keto crowd, such as Italian meatballs in marinara sauce, lasagna, and zuppa toscana with focaccia.

If you had told me fifteen years ago that I would have a successful career as the Sugar-Free Mom, a full-time blogger creating sugar-free recipes, I would have laughed in your face. I didn't even know what a blog was! And sugar-free? Well, from the time I was twelve until 2004, I was hiding a secret: I had an uncontrollable addiction to sugar. Maybe it began because I dreamed of looking like other teens, who were tall and skinny—something my curvy 5-foot-2-inch frame would never allow.

I don't know why my struggle with sugar began, but I do know that without those deep struggles and inner turmoil, I most definitely would not be writing this cookbook today. Now, well along my path to healthy living, I am grateful for where I've been because I can show you how rewarding and sustainable this low-carb, ketogenic lifestyle truly is.

Before going keto, I believed far too many myths about food. I believed fat was to be feared. I believed you had to eat every two to three hours to keep your metabolism healthy. I believed you could eat everything in moderation and maintain a healthy weight. I believed breakfast was the most important meal of the day and whole grains were part of a healthy diet.

Are you with me? Have you fallen for these myths, too?

Just like I did, you must have some doubts about them now, or you wouldn't have picked up this book. You're hoping to lose weight, heal your gut, stop your cravings for sugar and carbs . . . the list goes on and on.

Whether you've been happily low-carb for years or you're just getting ready to dip your toe into the ketogenic waters, you'll love this cookbook if you love good food. *Naturally Keto* will make a great addition to your repertoire. It's full of delicious recipes that will please picky palates, as well as recipes that even carb lovers will enjoy. Let me show you how easy and sustainable keto living can be, one amazing recipe at a time.

Step into my kitchen, pull up a chair, enjoy a cup of coffee, and let's get cooking keto.

Welcome to Naturally Keto.

HOW TO USE THIS BOOK

Naturally Keto provides all of the recipes you will need to sustain and enjoy a healthy ketogenic lifestyle. Whether or not you've chosen to start keto alone, you can use these recipes to delight everyone in your family, even the carb-loving skeptics. I can say with complete confidence that all of the recipes in this cookbook are kid approved, as well as picky hubby approved. Better still, when you need an appetizer, side dish, or dessert to take to a party, you'll find plenty of options here that the non-keto crowd will enjoy.

PART 1: A Beginner's Guide to Keto

In Part 1, you'll find a range of helpful information, including a beginner's guide to keto, a guide to stocking your pantry with staples I use often in my kitchen, and a list of kitchen tools and equipment to make the recipes easier to prepare. You'll also find bonus sections like Allergy-Friendly Substitutions, How to Break a Stall, and Dealing with a Reluctant Spouse and Family.

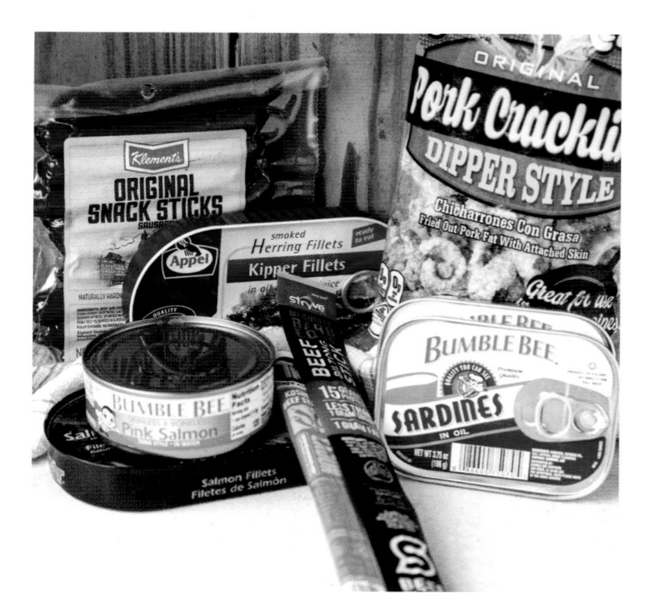

PART 2: Recipes

This section includes 134 amazing gluten-free, grain-free, keto recipes.

Quick Reference Icons

To make the recipes easier to navigate, I've included icons to make it clear when a recipe is dairy-free, egg-free, nut-free, and/or vegetarian.

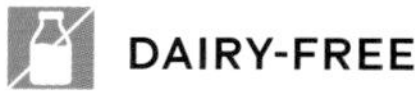

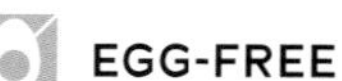

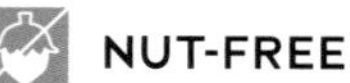

VEGETARIAN

To clarify, if a recipe uses coconut flour, I consider it nut-free; coconut is technically a fruit, and many who have tree nut allergies do not react to coconut flour. Please refer to "Allergy-Friendly Substitutions" on page 34 for more information.

I've also used icons to note some key prep details, such as whether a recipe can be made in a slow cooker or air fryer, can be prepared in thirty minutes or less, or requires just one pan or pot.

- SLOW COOKER
- AIR FRYER
- 30 MINUTES OR LESS
- ONE PAN/POT

Nutritional Information

At the end of each recipe, you'll find a breakdown of the calories, fat, protein, total carbs, dietary fiber, and net carbs per serving of the recipe, not including any optional ingredients or suggested serving items. (See page 22 for details on total versus net carbohydrates.) I've done my best to be as accurate as possible, but please note that any changes you make to the ingredients will change the nutritional information. If you do make a substitution, it's always best to calculate your own nutritional information. Note, too, that I did not include sugar alcohols in the nutritional information, as the erythritol used in these recipes does not raise blood sugar levels or spike insulin.

Weight Measurements

For the sake of accuracy and to help you achieve the best possible outcomes with the recipes in this book, especially the baked goods, I've included weights in grams as well as volume measurements for certain ingredients. Weighing your flours, protein powders, and sweeteners will give you the best results when baking.

PART 3: Meal Plans

Meal plans make sticking to any new diet much easier—and can help busy folks make the most of their time in the kitchen. With that in mind, I've included four weeks of meal plans in this book. The first two weeks feature meals with a limit of 25 grams of net carbs per day, while the second two weeks switch to a limit of 25 grams of total carbs per day. The final week is also dairy-free. This way, you can see which approach works best for you and gets you the results you want. A shopping list is included with each week's meal plan.

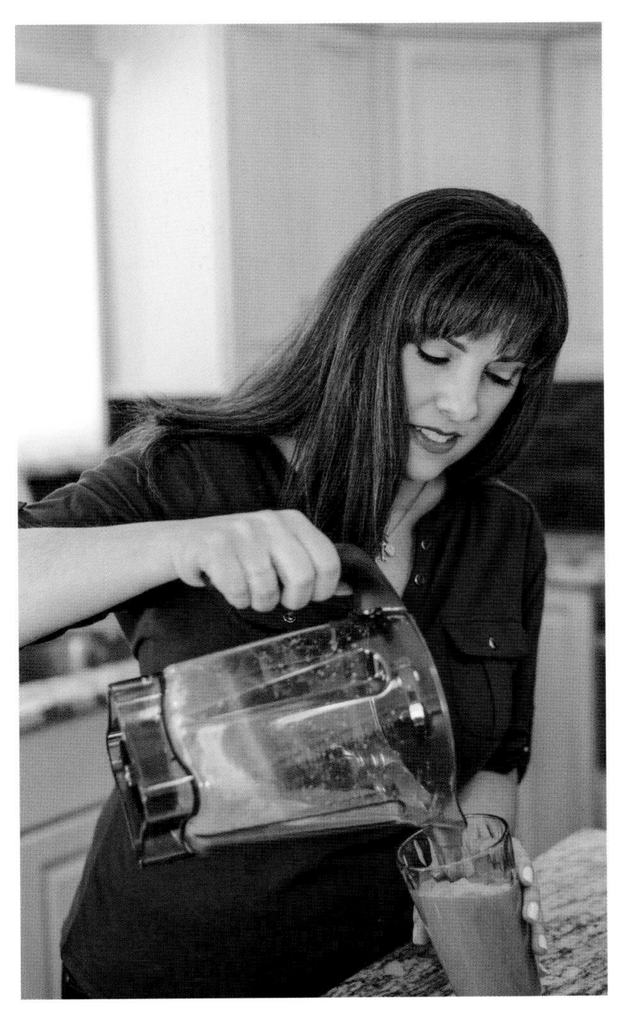

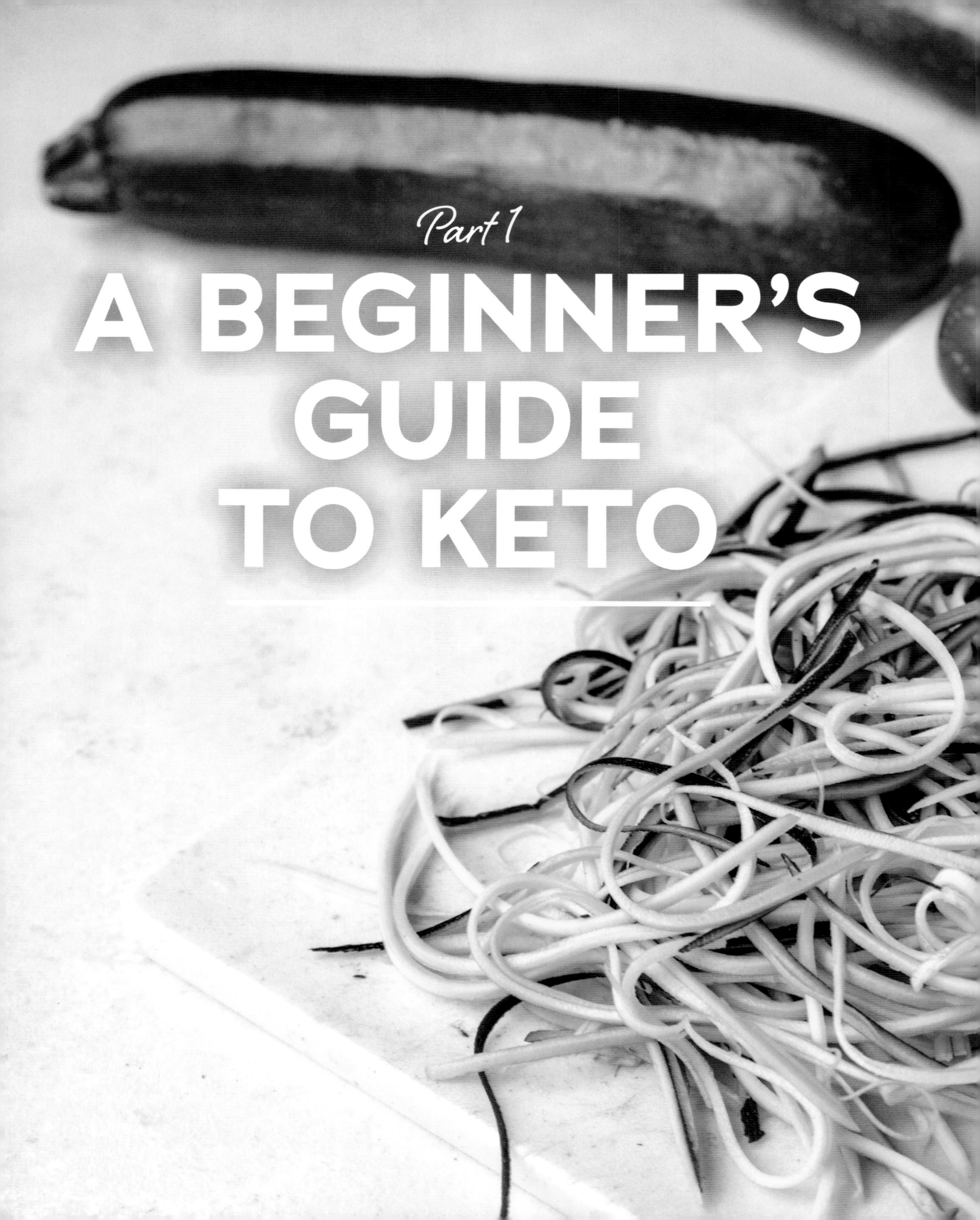

Part 1

A BEGINNER'S GUIDE TO KETO

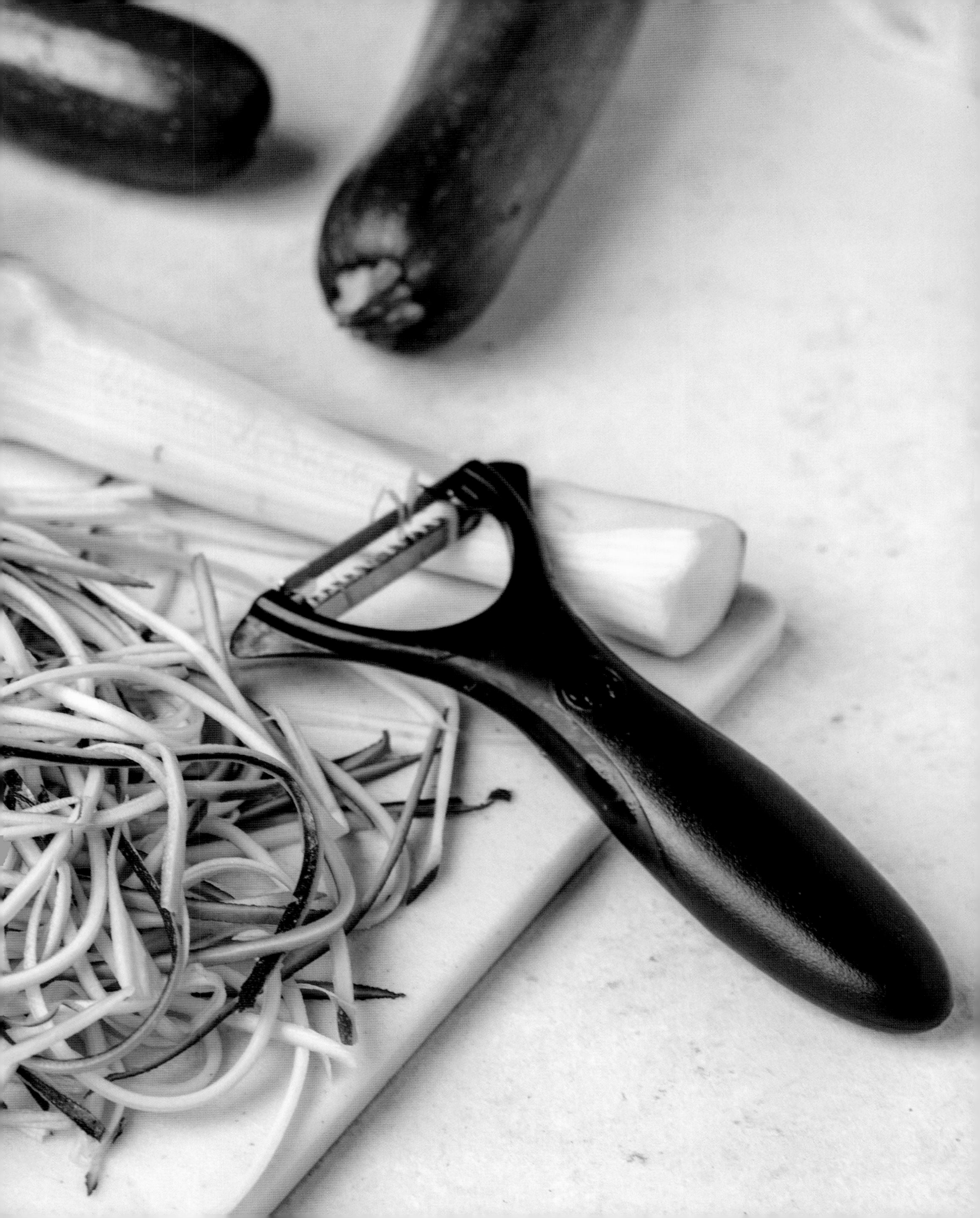

UNDERSTANDING THE DIFFERENCES BETWEEN SUGAR-FREE, LOW-CARB, AND KETO

If you're just beginning to consider the keto diet, you may be a little confused about how it differs from a low-carb or sugar-free diet. Here's what all of the terms actually mean.

Sugar-Free Versus Low-Carb

KEY POINT: The added sugar isn't the main difference between a sugar-free recipe and a recipe that is low-carb—the real difference is the total amount of carbs. If a recipe is low-carb, it is sugar-free; there's no other way around that. But sugar-free does not always mean low-carb!

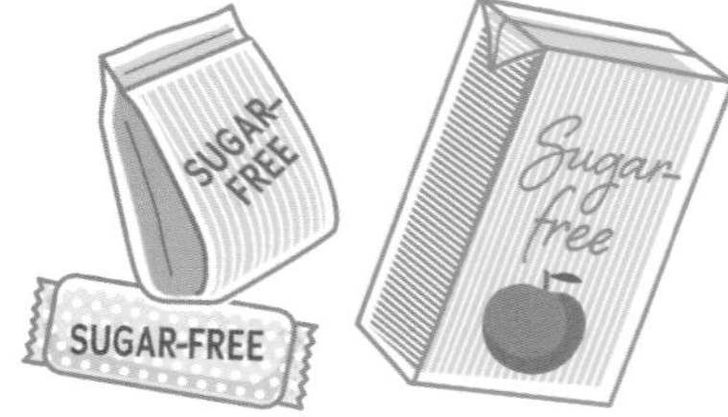

A food that has no added sugar but includes high-carbohydrate ingredients like whole wheat flour may be deceptive. Although no sugar is listed on the nutrition label, that label doesn't take into account that all carbohydrates, from simple sugars to complex carbohydrates like whole grains, are broken down into sugar in your blood. So, while checking the grams of sugar on a food label might seem good enough, that high-carb item will still spike your blood sugar.

When your blood sugar spikes, your insulin rises, and when you have high insulin, you can't lose weight, whether you're diabetic or not.

I went "sugar-free" in 2004 because I still couldn't lose the baby weight a year after giving birth to my daughter. I was still using whole wheat flour and "natural" sweeteners like fruits and honey because I was convinced that my sugar addiction was only to added and refined sugars. I followed what is now known as the "no-white approach": no white sugar, no white flour, no white rice, and no white potatoes, though I still ate dairy. Simply eliminating those ingredients was enough to maintain my weight loss for many years, even after my third child was born in 2005.

In 2013, I had been blogging for two years and was deep into writing my first cookbook. Over ten months of recipe testing, I put on about 10 pounds. I struggled desperately to lose the weight using the same methods I had successfully used for years. Nothing budged. Could I blame it on being over forty? Maybe, or perhaps my body just needed a new tactic to shock it into change; perhaps clean, low-fat, sugar-free eating wasn't enough to get the weight off. I decided I needed to give low-carb a try.

What "low-carb" means differs depending on whom you talk to. Some people say that a low-carb diet limits total carbohydrate intake to 150 grams per day, while others maintain that less than 100 grams is better. My low-carb approach consisted mostly of carbs from veggies and fruits, and my target range was 50 to 70 grams per day, which was enough for me to lose the weight and maintain that loss. Every person's body responds differently, so you may need to experiment to find the right amount of carbs for you.

Remember: You certainly can lose weight by following a low-carb diet, but you are still using glucose (sugar) from the carbs you are eating to fuel your body. This means you'll often have to eat every three to four hours to help keep yourself satiated and full of energy.

Low-Carb Versus Keto

KEY POINT: When eating a low-carb diet, you are still using glucose to fuel your body. When eating a ketogenic diet, you become fat adapted and use your own body fat to fuel your body.

The keto diet may seem extreme to some people, but maybe that's precisely why you've decided to try it. Maybe your body needs a change, and nothing else has really worked.

Most people who follow a ketogenic diet stay at around 20 grams of net carbs (total carbs minus dietary fiber and any sugar alcohols) per day, which is about 5 percent of your daily food intake. Some people limit carbs even further. Protein consumption tends to be moderate, at around 15 to 25 percent of your daily food intake. If you are active like I am, doing weight training or other exercise, 20 to 25 percent protein may be appropriate. If you lead a more sedentary lifestyle, you don't need as much protein—more like 15 to 20 percent.

The biggest difference is in the amount of fat you eat! Moving from a low-carb diet to a ketogenic diet means getting past the myth that dietary fat is evil and should be avoided. Learning to embrace healthy fats like avocados, coconut oil, olive oil, and, yes, even butter, is imperative to your success on keto. Healthy fats keep you satiated. Eat the right amounts of the right kinds of fat and you'll be less likely to fall off the wagon and binge on junk food and carbs.

Your fat intake should be around 70 to 75 percent of your daily food intake. When I first heard those numbers, I was shocked. I thought, "Are you kidding? That's a surefire way to pack on the pounds!" But I was misguided, to say the least. I think we've all bought into the longstanding myth that fat makes you fat. That couldn't be further from the truth. Let's not blame the butter for what the bread did. Sugar and carbs are the real culprits behind weight gain and many other health issues.

I stayed low-carb for three years. I was eating a moderate amount of protein, a small amount of fat, and less than 50 grams of net carbs a day. It seemed right, as I was maintaining my weight, yet it just wasn't enough for me to achieve the changes I wanted. I couldn't firm or tone my body, even while working with a trainer twice a week. I also still gave in to potato chips at parties—I couldn't seem to resist. In the end, I simply wasn't satisfied with how my body was responding to my low-carb diet. That's when I became curious about keto. I was slightly reluctant to try it, though, because I didn't think I could go so low in carbs considering how much I love vegetables.

Once you start eating such a low amount of carbs, your body becomes keto adapted. That means you're depriving it of the easy carbs it previously relied on. Now it needs to find a new source of fuel, and that source is your own body fat. Thus, in nutritional ketosis, as your body starts burning fat for energy, you shed body fat and enjoy many other benefits. How amazing is that?

It could take a few days, a few weeks, or a few months to get into ketosis—everyone is different, but it will happen eventually. Be patient. Because I had been eating low-carb for a few years, I thought it would take me just a few days, but that wasn't the case. It took a whole week until I saw consistent ketone readings. (See page 20 for more on testing your blood for ketones.) Trust me, though: it's worth the diligence!

The Benefits of a Keto Diet Versus a Low-Carb Diet

- *You're not hungry between meals. You can go anywhere from six to twelve or even sixteen hours without eating without feeling like you're starving!*
- *You no longer crave sugar. Instead, you start craving healthy fat!*
- *Your hormones are balanced: no crazy mood swings or irritability.*
- *You have great mental clarity: no more brain fog.*
- *You have a ton of energy without the need for caffeine.*
- *You lose body fat and see the differences reflected in your shape and muscle tone, not just the number on the scale!*

SIX TIPS FOR GETTING STARTED ON KETO

For many people, the early days of keto are the hardest, and they give up before they can enjoy the many benefits of eating this way. To help you get over the hump, here are six useful tips.

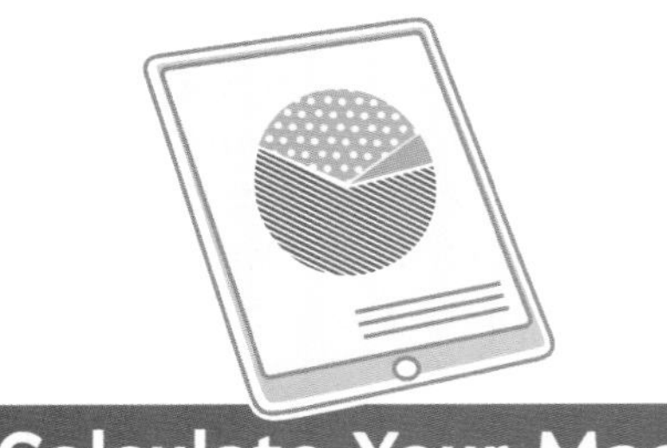

Calculate Your Macros

Macros is short for macronutrients, which refers to carbohydrates, protein, and fat. Whether you are coming to keto from a standard American diet (high in carbs, sugars, and processed foods) or you are already eating low-carb, figuring out the appropriate carb, protein, and fat intake for your current weight and height is helpful. Do you need to stick to these exact targets every day? No! Really, the only thing you have to pay super close attention to is the amount of carbohydrates you are eating. Don't exceed 20 grams per day if you are trying to lose weight. If you aren't doing the keto diet for weight loss and are mainly seeking the other benefits of ketosis, you may be able to go a bit higher and remain in ketosis. There is no way to know other than through experimentation, as every person has a unique carb tolerance.

The biggest mistake I made in the beginning was eating too much fat. I thought I could eat as much as I wanted. At the start of my keto journey in 2015, I did not lose weight; in fact, I think I gained some. That's because you should eat fat only to satiety. You do not need to eat copious amounts of fat to hit your macros each day. If you're completely satisfied before you hit your target number of fat grams, do not eat more fat just to hit that number! Remember, you want to burn your own body fat—and if you're eating more fat than your body needs, then it will use that fat rather than the fat on your body, and you won't lose weight.

I used three online calculators to come up with rough macro ranges for myself. My fellow cookbook author and friend Maria Emmerich has a great keto calculator on her website, mariamindbodyhealth.com; ketogains.com also has a good one, and the KetoDiet app includes a calculator with your purchase of the app.

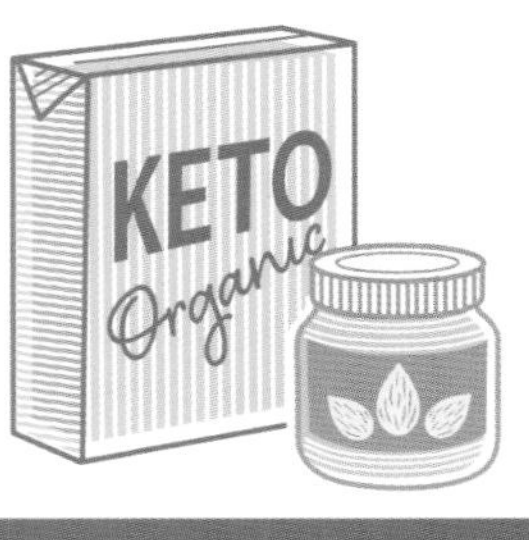

Eat Real Food

There are many keto products on the market now, with more coming out every day. Meal bars, fat bombs, shakes—the list goes on and on. It can be quite tempting to fill your shopping cart with convenience foods if you're busy (and who isn't?) or you don't like to cook, but relying too heavily on these products may not help you reach your goals. Of course, there will be times when you do need convenience, especially when traveling. I thank God for all of the keto products that have been created for just that reason. On a daily basis, however, eating real, whole foods is the key to lasting health.

Remember, the ketogenic diet isn't just for weight loss. The health benefits of ketosis go far beyond maintaining a healthy weight. I won't ever go back to my old ways of eating because I feel my very best on keto. Real foods made from just a few ingredients that aren't processed or man-made—organic grass-fed or pastured meats, healthy fats, fresh low-carb vegetables—should be the focus of a sustainable ketogenic lifestyle.

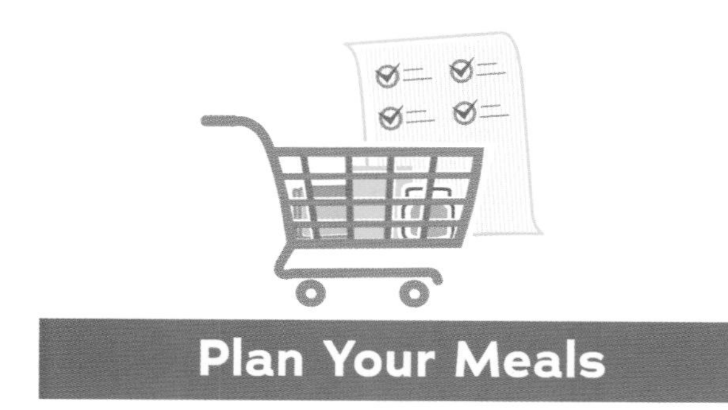

Plan Your Meals

I know you've heard it before, but I'm going to say it anyway: "If you fail to plan, you plan to fail." There is just no way around it: you must plan ahead. You've got to look at the coming week and see which days will be hectic and which days will leave you with more time for shopping and cooking. Prepping easy grab-and-go breakfasts and lunches on the weekend is a huge time-saver. Opting for slow cooker or Instant Pot recipes on busy days is smart, too. (Look for the slow cooker icon to see which recipes make use of this handy tool.) You'll be less stressed, your family will be happy, and you won't be tempted to resort to a drive-through!

Meal planning doesn't have to be a chore. Part 3 of this book includes four weekly meal plans with grocery shopping lists. To help you make keto-friendly dinners without stress, I also have a meal planning membership option on my website at www.mealplans.sugarfreemom.com. You get shopping lists with these plans, too. The best part is that you can make modifications to the plans. If you don't like a particular meal, you can swap it for something else, and the shopping list will automatically adjust accordingly. If meal planning is a challenge for you, I encourage you to check it out!

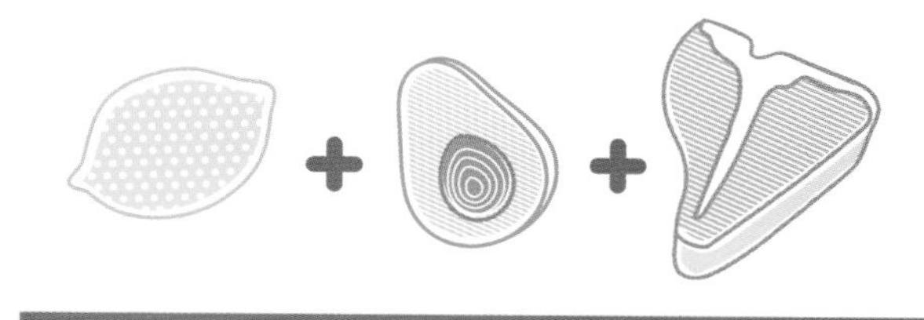

Track Your Food

If you're trying keto for the first time and you've never counted how many carbs you're eating on a daily basis, you need a baseline to work from. You probably won't need to track your food forever, but I highly recommend starting out this way to create some accountability and learn what is and is not working for you. Tracking is also helpful if you're dealing with health conditions other than excess weight, like my hives. Observing which foods, after eating them, trigger a reaction like stomach upset, gas, or bloating gives you really useful information.

You can use any kind of tracking system you like. There are plenty of great apps to help with this task. If you're more of a paper and pencil person, simply grab a notebook and write down everything you consume and how you feel each day. Then you'll need some sort of tracker to look up the carbs, protein, and fat counts in those foods (or keep it simple and just count net carbs, and try to stick to no more than 20 grams per day). I actually use both: a notebook so I can easily see which foods did or did not agree with me, plus an app for looking up the macros in those foods. MyFitnessPal has a free tracking app, but I find that it isn't entirely reliable. I use the KetoDiet app instead, which charges a one-time fee but is extremely accurate. I've also heard that Carb Manager works well.

No matter which tools you choose, tracking is important for making sure you stay on target. My eyes deceive me every time—I always think I'm eating much less than I am. When I track my portions, I find that the carbs add up quickly! Armed with that knowledge, I can adjust accordingly and stay in ketosis.

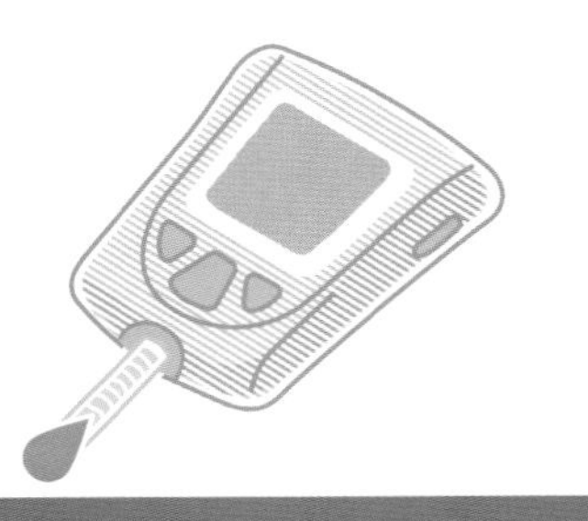

Evaluate Your Progress

As helpful as food tracking is, if you really want to make sure you are in ketosis, then I suggest buying a glucometer. This testing device uses a simple prick of your finger and a drop of your blood to measure your ketone level. A reading of 0.5 mmol/l or higher means that you are likely in ketosis. I often don't register ketones at all in the morning.

I use a Precision Xtra glucometer, which tests both blood glucose and ketones. If you test first thing in the morning in a fasted state (before eating), you can get a good idea of how much sugar is in your blood. Testing one hour after a meal is a good way to see if what you just ate spiked your blood sugar and/or kicked you out of ketosis. For example, if your blood glucose number in a fasted state is 85, and after a meal it rises to over 100, that is a definite spike, and what you ate may have kicked you out of ketosis. You certainly don't need to test yourself three or four times a day, but in the beginning it's helpful to see the correlation between the food you eat, the ketones you produce, and the wonderful feeling of being in ketosis.

A glucometer is not cheap, but it gives you the most accurate measurements. Using urine ketone strips is fine in the beginning stages, but once you are fat adapted, you won't see accurate results because your body will essentially be using the ketones as fuel, and they won't make it into your urine. If you can't stand the idea of a finger stick or the sight of blood, you can opt for a breath ketone meter instead.

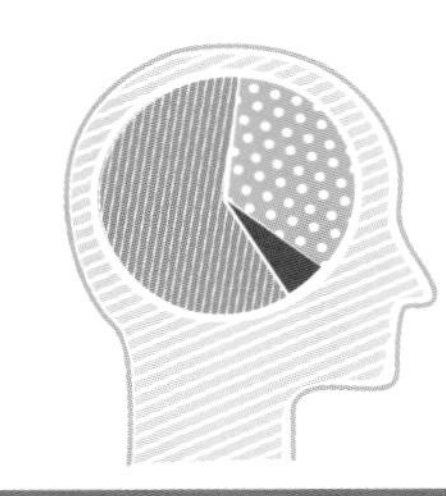

Adjust as Needed

If you're diligent about eating no more than 20 grams of net carbs a day, yet you aren't seeing results after a month, you may need to make some tweaks. Maybe you need to eat more protein and reduce your fat intake a bit. Maybe you need to start counting total carbs instead of net carbs. If you're happily losing weight and feeling wonderful, don't change a thing! But know that there's no one right way to do keto. Someone else's "proven" method won't necessarily be right for you or your body.

Plus, our bodies' needs change over time. I'm a big proponent of listening to your body and making adjustments as needed. I've experienced more stalls than I can count, so I know how frustrating it can be. I also know that I waited too long to change anything because I thought I should see the same results others were seeing. Don't do what I did and wait a year before you adjust! Check out the tips in the next section if you find that you need to change things up in order to get the results you're looking for.

BREAKING A STALL

If there's one thing I know a whole lot about, it's the feeling you get when your weight won't budge. You seem to be doing everything right down to the letter on your keto diet, but nothing is working. I've been stalled quite a few times, both before and after I was diagnosed with hypothyroidism, so I know how frustrating it is to struggle. I was so down on myself—I felt like I wasn't being diligent enough or was surely doing something wrong, all because I wasn't seeing the results that others seemed to be attaining so easily.

If you are facing a stall, some of these tips might help get the scale moving. I'm sharing what has worked for me in the hopes that this information will inspire you to change things that are not working for you, even if they seem to work wonderfully for someone else. Bear in mind these words of wisdom: "The definition of insanity is doing the same thing over and over again and expecting a different result."

Remember That Calories Count

Despite popular belief in the keto world, calories do count. How much fat you eat counts, too, especially if you're someone like me who wanted to lose only 10 or 15 pounds. If you've been winging it, just trying to stick to high fat, moderate protein, and low carbs, and you're not losing weight, there's a good chance that you're simply eating too much of everything!

Just because you're eating keto foods doesn't mean you can eat as much as you want—you may even gain weight if you do. The first time I started keto, I thought I could eat copious amounts of fat as long as I kept my carbs low. But guess what? That approach didn't work for me. I wasn't tracking my macros each day, either; I was merely estimating how many grams of carbs, protein, and fat I was eating. If you aren't using a good keto tracker, you may be deceiving yourself. I use the KetoDiet app. If I'm not diligent about tracking my food, my portions get out of control and I gain weight. You may not need to track for the rest of your life, but if you've been trying to lose weight without success, this may be the only thing you need to do to get the weight off.

Watch Your Intake of Nuts and Dairy

After I started tracking, my weight stalled again. This time, the issue was that I was overconsuming nuts, nut butters, and dairy products. I was counting just 2 tablespoons of natural, no-sugar-added nut butter for a recipe, but in reality I was sneaking a few extra spoonfuls from the jar. Or I would measure out some almonds and then pop a few more from the bag. I would add cheese to just about everything without measuring how much I added. And let's not even talk about cream cheese! That was my favorite; I could easily eat 4 ounces a day. Once I decided to remove nuts and dairy altogether for about three months, the weight slowly started coming off again.

Dairy and nuts may not be an issue for you, but they are inflammatory for many people, if not outright allergens. I didn't have a nut or dairy allergy per se, but I certainly overate those foods, causing my weight loss to stall. You may not need to eliminate them forever, but removing nuts and dairy for a short time may be just what you need to get your progress going again.

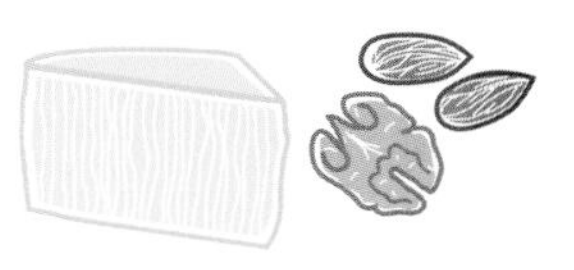

Try Weight Training

Even if the number on the scale isn't moving the direction you'd like it to, you can still change your body composition through weight training. One of the best things I've done was to start working with a trainer twice a week to help me build muscle. He showed me how to use the weights in the gym properly so I wouldn't hurt myself, then kept me on task. There's plenty of free information on the internet, of course, but make sure you're getting your info from a reputable source. The last thing you want to do is injure yourself. My trainer is also a physical therapist, so he was able to modify my exercises to account for any injuries or other difficulties.

Why weight training? Remember, the goal of keto is fat loss. One of the best ways to burn fat is to have more lean muscle mass on your body. Muscle tissue burns more calories than fat tissue, even in a resting state. Strengthening your muscles is also important for stronger bones—which are especially crucial as we age. You can do all the cardio you want, but cardio will not change your physique or strengthen your core.

Focus on how your body is changing and how your clothes are fitting; those things are more important than the number on the scale. The photos of me in the "My Journey to Keto" section show that I lost only 3 pounds over six weeks of strict keto, with diligent tracking and weight training, but look at the obvious fat loss! Measure your waist, chest, hips, and even upper arms and thighs before starting a weight training program, and then check your progress regularly. For the best results, get sound advice from an expert in the field—it's worth every penny.

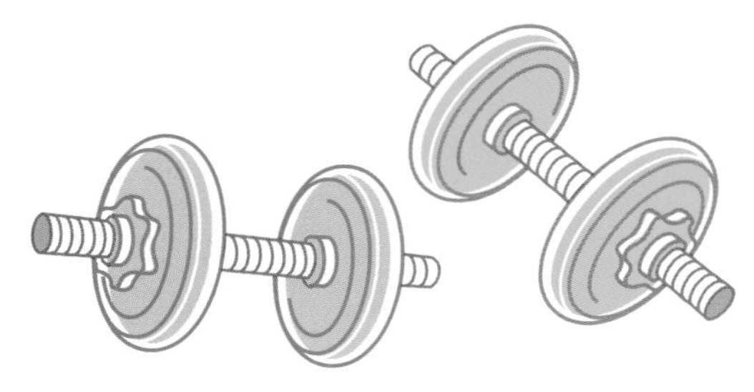

Count Total Carbs Instead of Net Carbs

When I first started eating keto, I thought counting 20 grams of net carbs a day was going to be hard enough. I didn't even want to think about limiting myself to just 20 grams of total carbs! If you're unfamiliar with these concepts, you tally net carbs by subtracting dietary fiber and any sugar alcohols from the total carbohydrates you consume. Many people who follow a ketogenic diet count net carbs.

When I lost weight after eliminating nuts and dairy, I did so while enjoying 20 grams of net carbs a day. But bodies change. Before I was diagnosed with chronic Epstein-Barr and hypothyroidism, I had trouble maintaining that weight loss on the same 20 grams of net carbs a day. When I made the switch to total carbs, I was better able to maintain my weight loss. While it may not be the case for everyone, counting total carbs instead of net carbs might help you achieve your goals.

Practice Intermittent Fasting

Intermittent fasting is basically having specified time frames in which to eat and not eat. We all fast each night while we sleep, but with intermittent fasting, you create a set window for eating during the day. Fasting can help your body repair itself, giving it a break from digesting and processing the foods you've eaten. Allowing your body to enter a fasted state has many health benefits beyond weight loss. Intermittent fasting can help reduce insulin resistance, improve energy and memory, and even help your body fight various diseases.

There are quite a few different ways to incorporate intermittent fasting into your day. I've tried many of them but will talk about three in particular, as these approaches are the ones that truly worked to break the vicious cycle of weight gain that I experienced while taking a medication for hypothyroidism.

An intermittent fast can consist of anywhere from fourteen to forty-eight hours or more of not eating. The most common variety is a 16/8 fast, in which you fast for about sixteen hours and eat within an eight-hour window (although you can flex this plan to use windows of fourteen to sixteen hours of fasting and six to eight hours of eating). You can fast daily if you like or just a few days a week. You can also set your own time to stop eating. For example, you could stop eating at 6 p.m. and not eat until 10 a.m. the next day—that's considered a sixteen-hour fast. This type of fast came the most naturally for me, as I was never a big breakfast eater and never woke up hungry even before I went keto. I also like to exercise first thing in the morning on an empty stomach. So for me, waiting until mid-morning to eat was pretty easy to do. Although this type of fast was not enough for me to achieve weight loss, it worked to maintain my weight.

Another option is to eat breakfast and lunch but skip dinner. For example, you might eat between 8 a.m. and 4 p.m. and then consume no food until 8 a.m. the next day. This is also a sixteen-hour fast. I tried this approach a couple of times a week, but it was quite difficult when I still had to feed my family and refrain from eating while they enjoyed dinner together. I didn't like having to make the meal and not join my husband and kids at the dinner table. I used this method only when everyone was out of the house for an activity and eating separately.

A third type of intermittent fasting is to not eat for a full twenty-four hours once or twice a week. I used this method to maintain my weight for a long time, and I needed to do it only once a week for success.

If you'd like to learn more about fasting, a fantastic book is *The Complete Guide to Fasting: Heal Your Body Through Intermittent, Alternate Day, and Extended Fasting* by Dr. Jason Fung and Jimmy Moore.

Try a Protein-Sparing Modified Fast

I learned about this type of fasting from my friend Maria Emmerich. She has a ton of resources on her website and in her many books. In her book *Keto: The Complete Guide to Success on the Keto Diet*, she goes into detail about protein-sparing modified fasting. She recommends doing this only to break a stall. I thought I could never make it through even one day on this super-low-calorie diet. In fact, that was my plan: to try it for just one day.

I was shocked by how well my body responded. This type of fast requires you to increase your protein intake and reduce your total carbs to 20 grams or less per day, but that's not all; you also reduce your daily fat intake to just 40 to 50 grams. Thus, you are preserving your lean muscle mass and using stored body fat to fuel your body. I worried I'd be hungry after reducing my fat intake so steeply. Surprisingly, the extra protein I ate was enough to keep me satiated even though I was eating 10 grams or less of total carbs on some days and only about 1,000 total calories a day! In the first week, I lost 3 pounds. That doesn't sound like much, but after having been stalled for months, I was ecstatic! I highly recommend trying this technique if you've been stalled and other methods haven't worked.

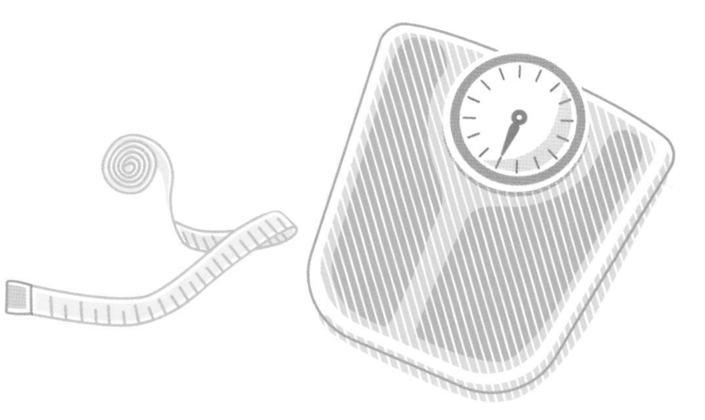

DEALING WITH A RELUCTANT SPOUSE AND FAMILY

As a woman who has been married for twenty-two years and has spent the last fifteen years living a sugar-free lifestyle, I totally understand if you choose to adopt the keto lifestyle on your own. Only in the past year, as I was writing this cookbook, did my husband finally choose to adopt a keto diet as well. He's had great success, losing about 30 pounds, and plans to continue in the hope of losing a bit more. But we haven't always eaten the same way.

It's not that my husband was against eating this way; he just didn't think he could do what I was doing. He was always supportive and always ate whatever I cooked for dinner, but throughout the rest of the day, he chose carbs. I knew that, given his personality, any nagging on my part would only push him away from keto. I chose to set an example instead. I knew that as long as he liked the food I was making, there wouldn't be any complaining. I wasn't able to control what he ate outside of our home, but at least he would enjoy a delicious keto meal for dinner.

Here are my top tips for dealing with a reluctant spouse or family:

Be an example.

You can't make anyone do anything until they're ready. If you remember that, you can eliminate the stress of trying to convert everyone in your family to keto. I learned this early on. No amount of nagging would really do anything. My husband didn't decide to go keto until his fiftieth birthday was looming. Something must have clicked; maybe he wanted to be healthy for our kids and our future. I'm not sure what triggered his desire, but when he was ready, he made it happen. The best thing you can do is to have patience. Wait it out. Do your own thing. Make the recipes. Revel in your success. The rest of your family will watch you lose weight, become free from sugar cravings, and stop bingeing. They will observe your success, even if they say nothing. Remain confident that you have planted a seed and that each day, they will get closer to wanting for themselves the benefits they see you enjoying.

Don't deprive anyone.

When your family members see that you are not deprived and can enjoy pretty much anything you want simply by making a few clever keto adaptations, they will be curious and wonder if they might be able to do it, too. They'll see that you don't feel hungry or like you can never enjoy dessert again. Make recipes that are so satisfying your whole family will be shocked that they are eating keto. It's one of the best things you can do to change their minds and hopefully get them to join you. One of the most important factors in changing my husband's mind was changing our meats. When I was just doing low-carb, I chose leaner meats. But when I made the switch to keto, my body craved steak, ground beef, ribs—luscious meats that my husband loves. He realized that this "diet" couldn't be so bad if we got to eat all of these delicious meats and still lose weight!

Stock up on keto snacks.

It will be much easier for your family to choose healthy snack options if you've got a fully stocked pantry and refrigerator for them to pick from. If junk food is available, they will naturally choose those items over keto options. But if high-carb foods aren't available because you do not bring them into the house, it will be much easier for them to make better choices. Check out my "Stocking Your Keto Pantry" section on pages 27 to 33 for help in making good selections.

Support the little changes.

Some people just can't go all-in with keto. My husband was like that for years; only his dinner was low-carb. Be supportive no matter how small the changes your family members are making. If they eat keto only at dinner and munch on carbs the rest of the day, encourage them anyway. Some folks require a more gradual approach. Start small with one meal at a time. Make a keto breakfast they like, and they will want to continue eating that way throughout the day. I always kept keto breakfast options like keto waffles, pancakes, muffins, and egg dishes on hand. That makes it easier for my husband and kids to choose the healthy, delicious meal over other options. Encourage every positive choice they make along the way. Before you know it, they may be fully keto right alongside you.

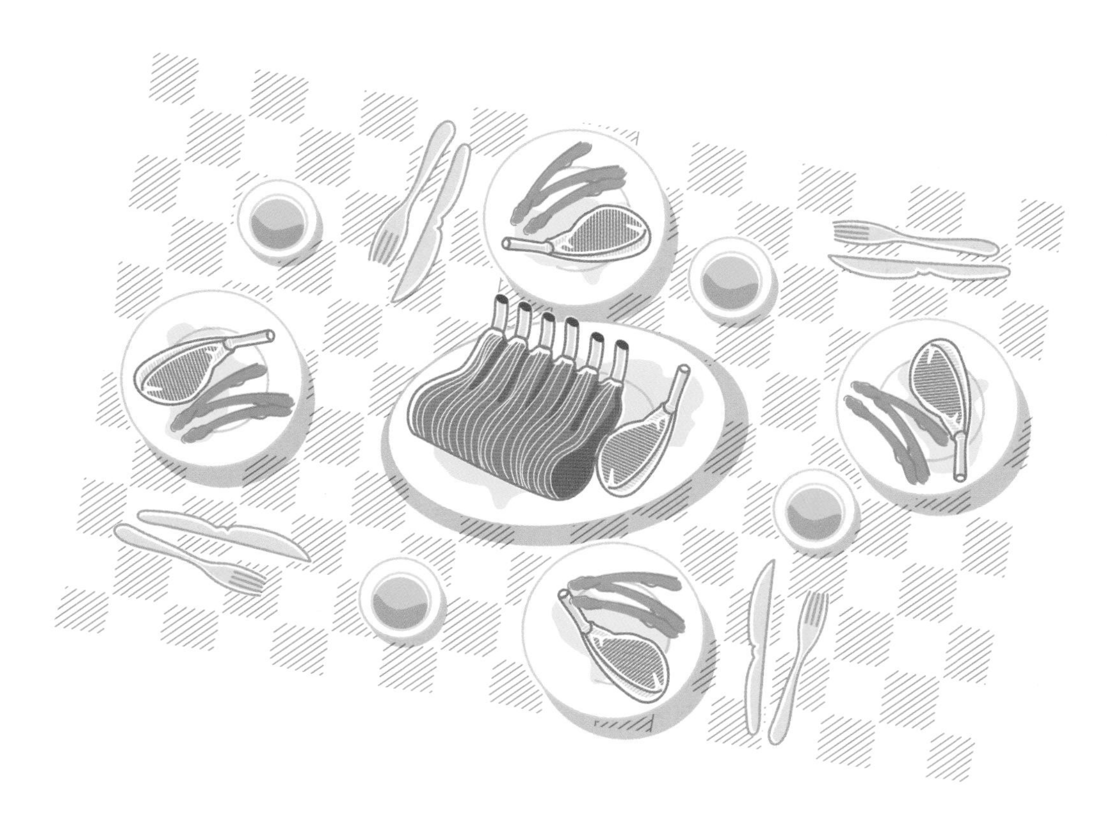

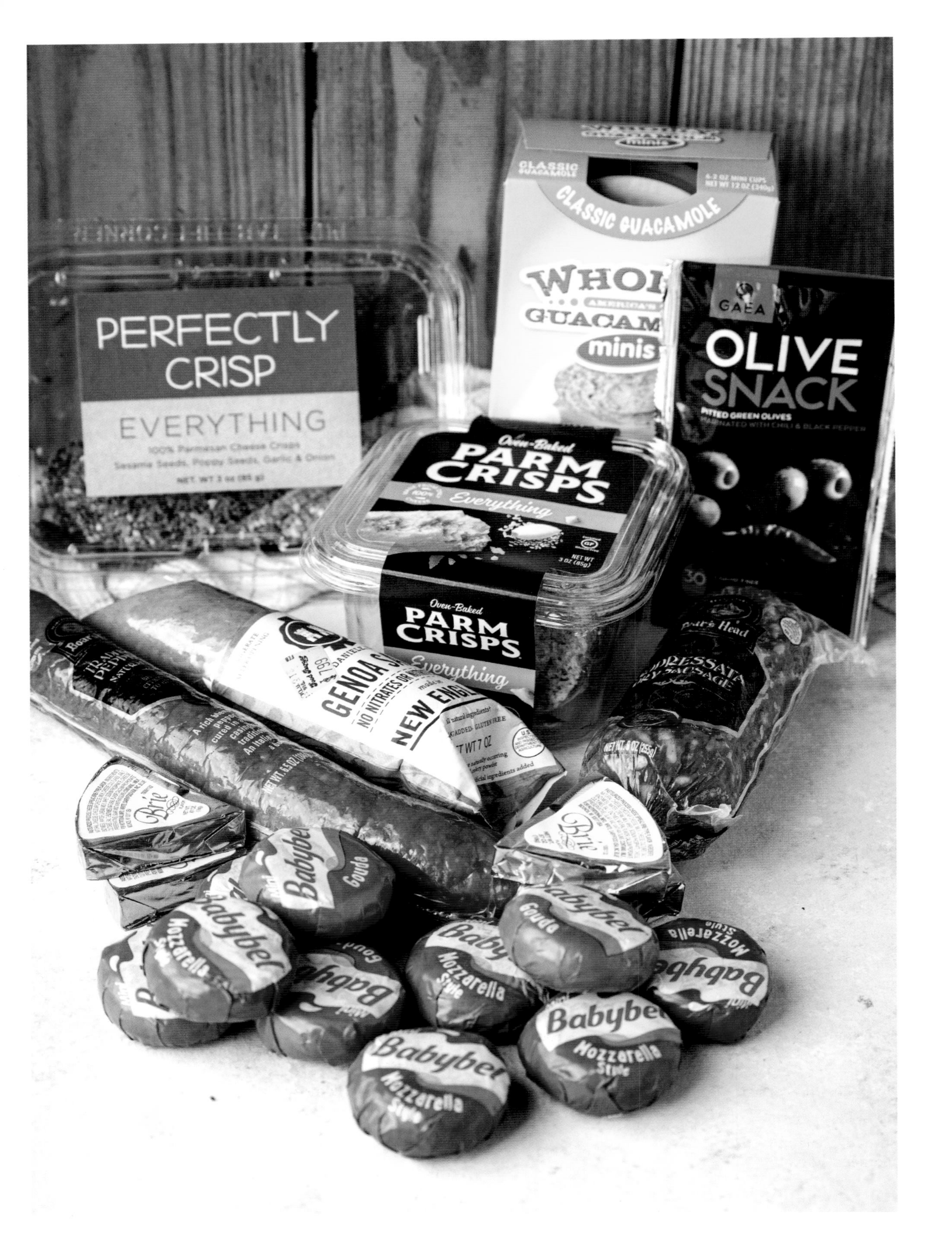

PERFECTLY CRISP
EVERYTHING
100% Parmesan Cheese Crisps
Sesame Seeds, Poppy Seeds, Garlic & Onion
NET WT 3 oz (85 g)
CLASSIC GUACAMOLE
CLASSIC GUACAMOLE
GAEA
OLIVE SNACK
PITTED GREEN OLIVES
MARINATED WITH CHILI & BLACK PEPPER
Oven-Baked
PARM CRISPS
Everything
NET WT 3 OZ (85g)
Oven-Baked
PARM CRISPS
Everything
GENOA
NET WT 7 OZ
Brie
Brie
Babybel
Gouda
Babybel
Mozzarella Style
Babybel
Mozzarella Style

STOCKING YOUR KETO PANTRY

Stocking a keto pantry doesn't have to be hard. In fact, you may already have a bunch of the items you need. If not, stocking your pantry with low-carb and keto essentials may take a little time and effort, but with a few great items, you will be well on your way. Keep in mind that you can do it over time! Try adding one new ingredient each week.

You'll need three things to be successful on a keto diet: good-quality proteins, healthy fats, and keto snacks for when you are on the go and don't have time for a meal at home. And a good supply of flavorings and other pantry staples will help you prepare tasty dishes. (I cover keto baking ingredients and sweeteners separately following these lists.)

Good-Quality Proteins

- Beef
- Bison
- Chicken
- Eggs
- Fish
- Pork
- Shellfish
- Turkey
- Venison

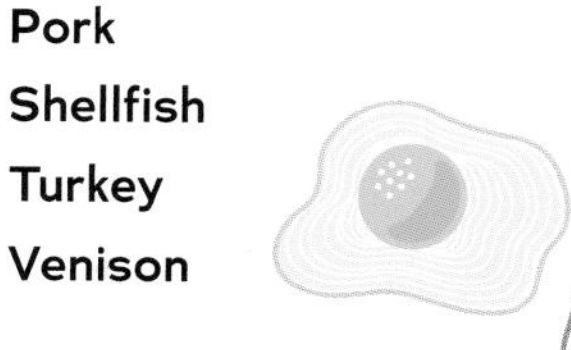

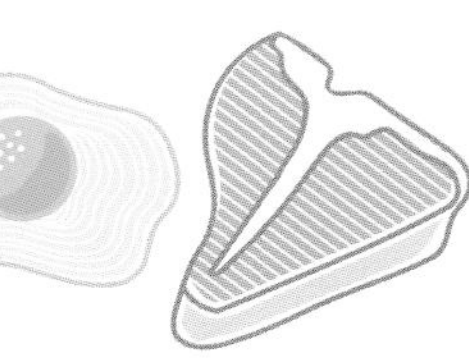

Healthy Fats

- Avocado oil
- Coconut oil
- Extra-virgin olive oil
- Ghee
- Grass-fed butter

Keto Snacks on the Go

- Almonds
- Avocados
- Bacon strips
- Beef sticks
- Canned salmon
- Canned sardines
- Canned tuna
- Cheese
- Cheese crisps
- Dark chocolate (85% cacao)
- Hard-boiled eggs
- Jerky
- Lily's chocolate bars
- Macadamia nuts
- NuttZo (a blend of nut and seed butters)
- Olives
- Pecans
- Pepperoni
- Pili nuts
- Pork rinds
- Pumpkin seeds
- Salami
- Smoked oysters
- Sunflower seeds
- Unsweetened almond butter
- Unsweetened coconut butter
- Unsweetened peanut butter
- Walnuts

Other Pantry Items

- Apple cider vinegar
- Avocado oil mayonnaise
- Avocado oil–based salad dressings
- Balsamic vinegar
- Black pepper
- Bone broth
- Canned coconut milk
- Chili powder
- Coconut aminos
- Collagen peptides
- Dill relish
- Dried basil
- Dried oregano leaves
- Dried parsley
- Ground cumin
- Italian seasoning
- Mustard
- No-sugar-added tomato sauce
- Pink Himalayan salt, in fine and coarse grinds
- Red wine vinegar
- Smoked paprika
- Sugar-free imitation maple syrup
- Sugar-free ketchup

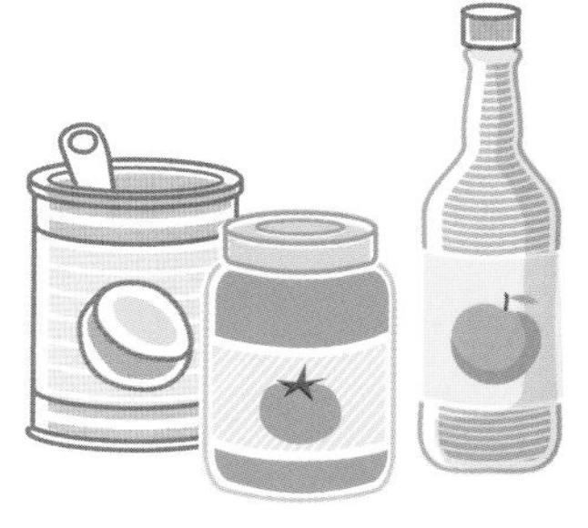

Keto Baking Essentials

Keto baking involves replacing regular wheat flour with low-carb alternatives that you may not be familiar with. I use all of the following ingredients regularly in my cooking, and you will need them for the recipes in this book.

Almond flour is made by processing raw, blanched almonds that have had their skins removed. Almond meal is made from ground almonds with the skins left on. The coarser almond meal can be used in place of breading in dishes like meatballs, but baking is a different story. There, you want very finely milled almond flour to yield the best texture. I don't have many recipes that use almond flour because my youngest son has tree nut and peanut allergies, but when I make a recipe just for myself and/or my husband, I like using blanched super-fine almond flour. Brands I like are Bob's Red Mill and Anthony's.

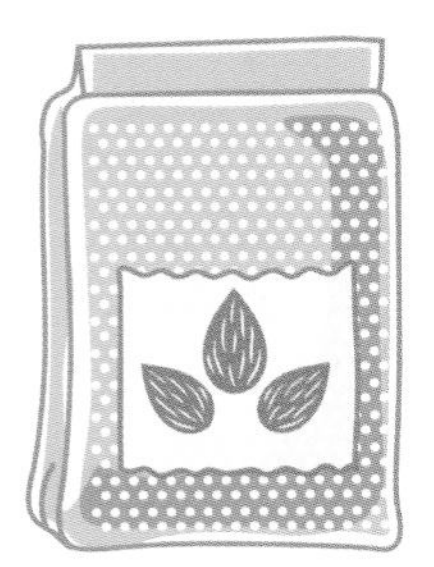

Baking powder is a leavening agent. It is a mixture of sodium bicarbonate and cream of tartar that's used instead of yeast in baking. Especially helpful in low-carb baking, it gives a nice lift to many baked goods. If you have run out of baking powder, you can substitute a mixture of baking soda and cream of tartar: use 1/4 teaspoon of baking soda plus 1/2 teaspoon of cream of tartar to replace 1 teaspoon of baking powder.

You have a bit more flexibility when using baking powder instead of baking soda. That's because baking powder has a double acting reaction. It reacts first and most powerfully when combined with other ingredients, then reactivates a bit more gently when heated. That means you don't have to worry about rushing your baked good into the oven; you'll still get a good rise.

Baking soda is also a leavening agent, but it has four times the power of baking powder. In other words, 1/4 teaspoon of baking soda is equal to 1 teaspoon of baking powder. Once the baking soda is mixed with wet ingredients, it starts giving lift immediately. That's why you need to get the batter into the oven as soon as possible, before the reaction starts petering out. I like to use both baking soda and baking powder in my recipes because the combination can give baked goods a nice airiness. Baking soda also enhances browning, giving baked goods a nice golden hue.

Chocolate is used in three different forms in the recipes in this book and on my blog. Sugar-free chocolate chips and dark chocolate (85% cacao) are interchangeable in my recipes, so it really depends on your personal preference. But do not swap either of these forms for unsweetened chocolate! I stay away from sugar-free chocolate that contains maltitol, as it can cause severe stomach upset. Personally, I love Lily's Sweets chocolate, which is sweetened with stevia and erythritol.

When choosing chocolate, remember that 85% dark chocolate is quite bitter. If you dislike the bitter taste, you might prefer 80%. The percentage tells you how much of the bar is made from pure cacao beans and how much involves added sugar. So if the label says 70% cacao, the remaining 30% is coming from sugar. That's why I opt for 85%—it has a very small amount of added sugar and an intense chocolate flavor, far beyond what you get from sugar-free chocolate. Unsweetened chocolate is pure chocolate made with 100% cacao, with no added sugar or sweetener. It should not be used in place of sugar-free chocolate chips or 85% dark chocolate in a recipe without adding other sweeteners to the recipe.

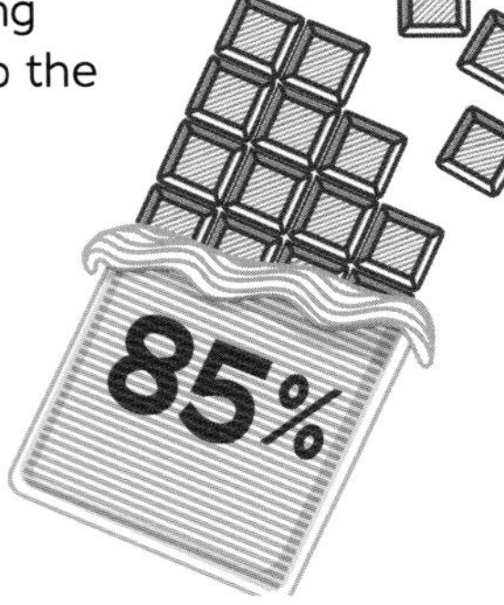

Cocoa powder (unsweetened) is raw cacao that has been roasted at a high temperature. Raw cacao is made by cold-pressing unroasted cacao beans. That process removes the fat, known as cacao butter. I use cocoa powder in many recipes to add a deep chocolate flavor. Cacao butter is great when melted and mixed with other ingredients to make your own chocolate bars. These ingredients cannot be swapped in recipes because cocoa powder is just that, a powder, and does not have the fat content of cacao butter.

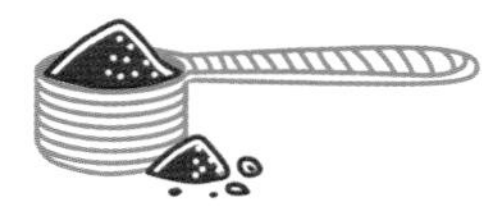

Coconut flour is my recommendation for anyone trying to consume fewer nuts or who has a nut allergy. I had a love-hate relationship with coconut flour for a long time. You might have a similar bias because of a few bad experiences; this super absorbent ingredient can be finicky. But once you get the correct ratio of flour to liquid and eggs, you'll wonder why you didn't fall in love with coconut flour sooner! Unfortunately, because of its absorbency, it can't easily replace almond flour or any other flour one-for-one—and there is no foolproof formula. I've found that about ¼ cup to ⅓ cup of coconut flour can sometimes replace 1 cup of almond flour. Plus, you often have to double the number of eggs and increase the amount of liquid called for in the recipe. I use Bob's Red Mill and Anthony's brands.

Cream of tartar is a leavening agent. When combined with baking soda, it produces carbon dioxide gas, the same gas that yeast produces when bread bakes. Cream of tartar is especially helpful in making my Cloud Bread Loaf (page 112), as it helps reinforce the air bubbles in the egg whites and slows their tendency to deflate.

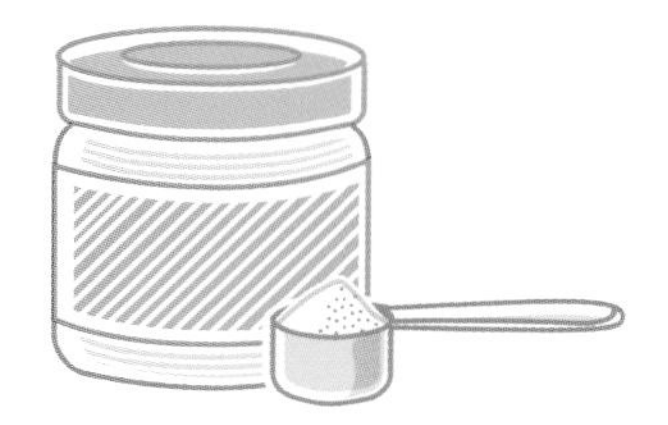

Flavored extracts, while not completely necessary, can add tons of flavor to recipes. I love them all! You definitely need apple extract if you plan to make my Apple Crisp (page 222), and you'll need banana extract for my Banana Bread (page 108). My maple syrup recipe (page 70) requires maple extract, so I say, start stocking up! I always have almond, apple, banana, caramel, coffee, corn, lemon, maple, peppermint, raspberry, and of course vanilla extract on hand.

Gelatin is a tasteless water-soluble protein prepared from collagen, which usually comes from boiling the bones and cartilage of cows or pigs. For the best quality, I recommend choosing a grass-fed powdered gelatin, like the one made by Vital Proteins. Gelatin acts like glue in recipes and gives baked goods some of the chewiness that gluten otherwise would have provided. Collagen peptides cannot be substituted for gelatin in recipes, as it will not gel up like gelatin does when combined with cold water.

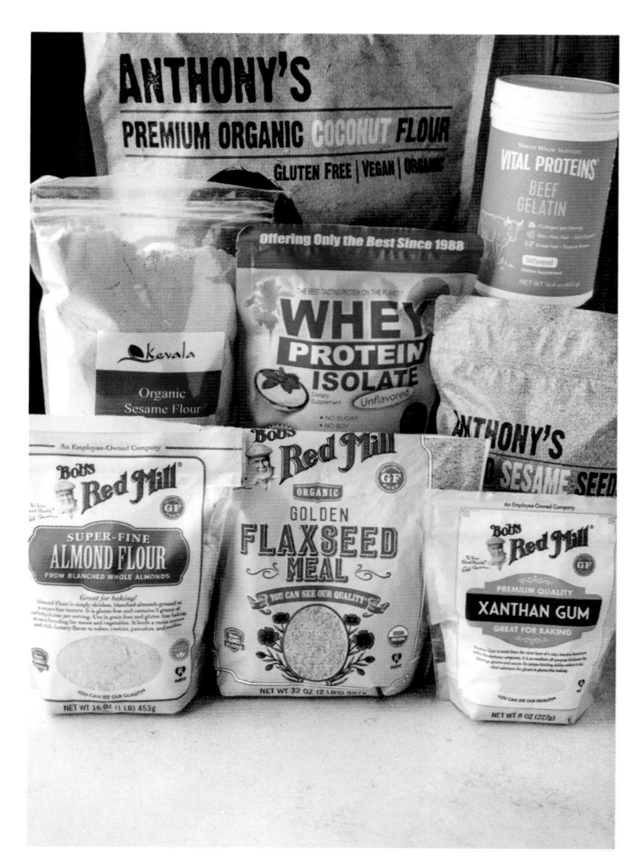

Ground flaxseed is useful for adding fiber to recipes. Plus, it gives my Coconut Flour Bread (page 114) an amazing texture and the satisfying chew of wheat bread. I like ground flaxseed as opposed to whole flaxseeds because it eliminates a preparation step. Plus, whole flaxseeds pass through your intestines without being digested and therefore offer none of the health benefits you get when using ground.

Hemp hearts are hulled seeds of the hemp plant. They have a mild, nutty flavor and boast more protein than chia or flax seeds. They are also high in healthy fats. They are delicious in my Prep-Ahead Hot Cinnamon Cereal (page 94).

Pork rinds are great not only as a snack but also as an ingredient. Finely ground, they're a useful low-carb swap for panko and breadcrumbs. Just pulse the pork rinds in a food processor until they become fine crumbs. You can also save time by buying preground pork rind crumbs. I like Bacon Heir and Pork King, both of which can be found on Amazon.

Protein powder is added to many of my baking recipes, like my Cloud Bread Loaf (page 112). I usually use unflavored whey protein powder because it won't affect the sweetener I've already included in the recipe and because flavored protein powders tend to contain a lot more fillers. On occasion, you might want to add flavored whey protein powder to smoothies. Protein powder adds bulk to baked goods in addition to helping with the texture. I don't recommend leaving it out when a recipe calls for it; I often test recipes both with and without the protein powder, and the texture is usually better when it's included.

If you are allergic to whey protein powder (which contains milk proteins), you might prefer egg white protein powder. The brand I use most often is Jay Robb; I also like Isopure. They have some delicious flavored options that are made with keto-friendly sweeteners.

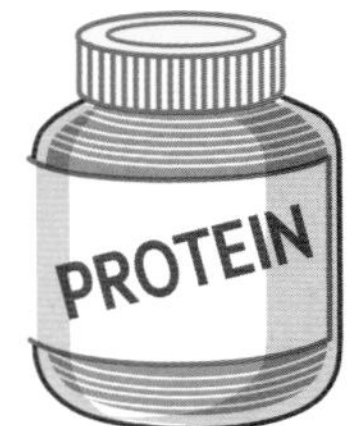

Sesame flour is a fantastic alternative to almond flour for those with nut allergies. This gluten-free flour is made from finely ground white or brown sesame seeds. It's high in fiber, calcium, magnesium, and zinc and has a mild and nutty aroma. My favorite brands are Sukrin and Kevala, both of which can be found on Amazon.

Shredded coconut starts with the shredding of the flesh of a ripe coconut. The sweetened version is partially dried and has sugar added to it, so it's best avoided. Unsweetened shredded coconut is completely dried and more finely shredded than its sweetened cousin; it has a long shelf life. I love to use unsweetened shredded coconut in my Slow Cooker Granola (page 92) and in no-bake pie crusts.

Sunflower seeds are another great replacement for almond flour for those with nut allergies. I have not found it preground and sold as flour, but grinding your own is easy. Buy raw sunflower seeds and then grind them in a food processor. (I don't recommend using a blender here, as it could turn your seeds into butter.) If you want to use sunflower seeds in a recipe that also includes baking powder, be aware that the natural chlorophyll present in the seeds creates a chemical reaction with baking powder . . . it tends to turn baked goods green! The taste won't be affected, but if you don't want green cookies or biscuits, steer clear.

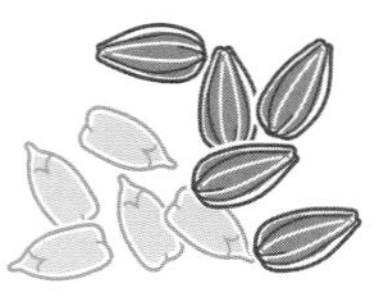

Xanthan gum is a fantastic thickening agent; a little goes a long way. I use it for thickening gravies, add it to smoothies, and even use a bit in my Vanilla Gelato (page 254). I often add it to get the elasticity that gluten would have provided in a high-carb baked good. I wouldn't leave it out of any recipe that calls for it. If you are in the middle of cooking and realize that you have run out, you can replace it with double the amount of unflavored gelatin.

You can use sesame seeds to make flour if you don't want to purchase sesame flour online. Making it at home is a little cheaper than buying it. Unhulled sesame seeds have their outer covering, or husks, intact. They have more iron and calcium than hulled sesame seeds. The label doesn't tell you whether they're hulled? Just remember: white sesame seeds are hulled and brown seeds are whole and unhulled. If you process the seeds further, you'll get a nice tahini, or sesame butter.

SESAME FLOUR

YIELD: 1¼ cups (2 tablespoons per serving)

PREP TIME: 2 minutes

Ingredients

1 cup raw, unhulled white or brown sesame seeds (see Tip)

Special Equipment: *High-powered blender*

1. Place the sesame seeds in a high-powered blender and cover with the lid.
2. Select the lowest setting and slowly increase the speed for 10 seconds. Open the lid and use a spatula to remove any seeds from the sides of the container. Secure the lid and blend again for another 5 to 10 seconds, or until you don't see any unprocessed seeds.
3. Pour the processed seeds into a mesh sieve to sift the flour over a bowl. Remove any clumps by pressing the flour against the sides of the sieve with a fork until all of the clumps are gone.
4. Store in an airtight container in the refrigerator for up to 2 months or freeze for up to 6 months.

Tip: Process only 1 cup of sesame seeds at a time for the best results. If you want more flour, make multiple batches.

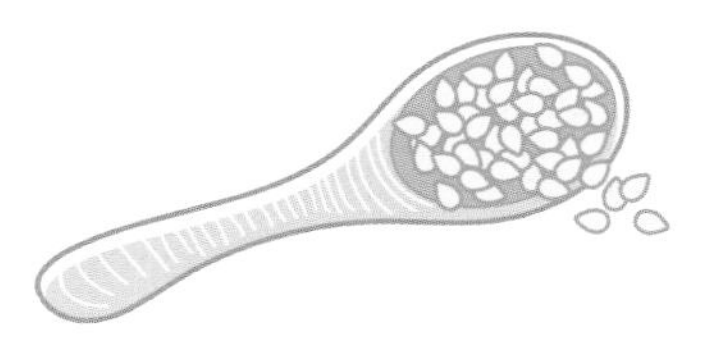

CALORIES: 85 FAT: 7g PROTEIN: 3g
TOTAL CARBS: 0g DIETARY FIBER: 0g NET CARBS: 0g

Keto Sweeteners

When you begin a keto diet, you sharply reduce your carbohydrate intake to get your body into ketosis and burn fat. Therefore, it's crucial to check every food label for sugar and carbs. There's no way around it: natural sugars like those found in honey, dates, and maple syrup produce the same effect as refined white sugar in your blood. Therefore, they should be avoided. This may seem strange if you are used to Paleo, which often incorporates natural sweeteners. That's because Paleo is not concerned with carbohydrates, but rather with eating foods in their most natural form.

Now, don't get me wrong: eating real, whole foods is important no matter which diet you're following—it's the key to healing your body. But on the keto diet, the real goal is reducing the carbs you consume. Why? All sugars and carbohydrates, whether natural or refined, raise your blood sugar. When that happens, you experience a spike in the hormone insulin. When your insulin is high, you are kicked out of ketosis and stop burning your own body fat. That's why natural sugars are not recommended on the keto diet. Instead, I recommend using sugar-free sweeteners that will not spike your blood sugar or kick you out of ketosis.

There are many sugar-free sweeteners on the market today; figuring out which is the best to use for one purpose or another can be quite confusing. Unfortunately, the product labels can be misleading, and not all sugar-free sweeteners are created equal.

When I first went sugar-free in 2004, I didn't know of any sugar-free sweeteners beyond aspartame, Splenda, and stevia. I tried several artificial sweeteners, and after two sugar-free years, my sugar cravings were still just as bad, if not worse. While stevia wasn't the most popular choice at the time, I had to start somewhere. After I switched, I quickly learned that stevia is difficult to bake with, as the liquid and concentrated forms do not provide the bulk that sugar would give. After some experimentation, I started using a combination of erythritol and stevia to yield the perfect bulk and sweetness.

Erythritol

I discovered erythritol in 2008 under the brand name Truvia. I was reluctant to use it, as the generic name sounded like a scary artificial chemical to me. I was wrong! Erythritol is a sugar alcohol that occurs naturally in fruits. Unlike most artificial sweeteners and other sugar alcohols, like maltitol, erythritol does not cause digestion problems or laxative effects. Erythritol is only about 70 percent as sweet as sugar, but in terms of volume, it can be swapped one for one in place of sugar in recipes. I usually combine erythritol with stevia to get the perfect amount of sweetness. Some people experience a cooling effect on the tongue from erythritol, while others find stevia bitter. But combine the two and the aftertaste disappears!

When looking for erythritol, watch out for fillers and bulking agents like dextrose and maltodextrin, which are known to kick some people out of ketosis. I recommend the brand Swerve. I also like Sukrin, but I have had more success using Swerve in most recipes. Swerve comes in a granulated form that's great for cookies, a confectioner's style that is perfect for my Vanilla Buttercream Frosting (page 231), and a brown sugar form that tastes just like traditional brown sugar. I use the brown sugar variety in my Cinnamon Rolls (page 86) and any time I want a deep molasses-like flavor. I do not recommend using the granulated form in any recipe that calls for confectioner's, as it may affect the result. The granulated form can give certain foods a gritty texture, especially unappealing in a no-bake recipe like my No-Bake Coffee Cheesecake (page 266).

Erythritol is calorie-free and does not raise blood sugar levels or spike insulin. For this reason, I do not include it in my calculations for the nutritional information for my recipes.

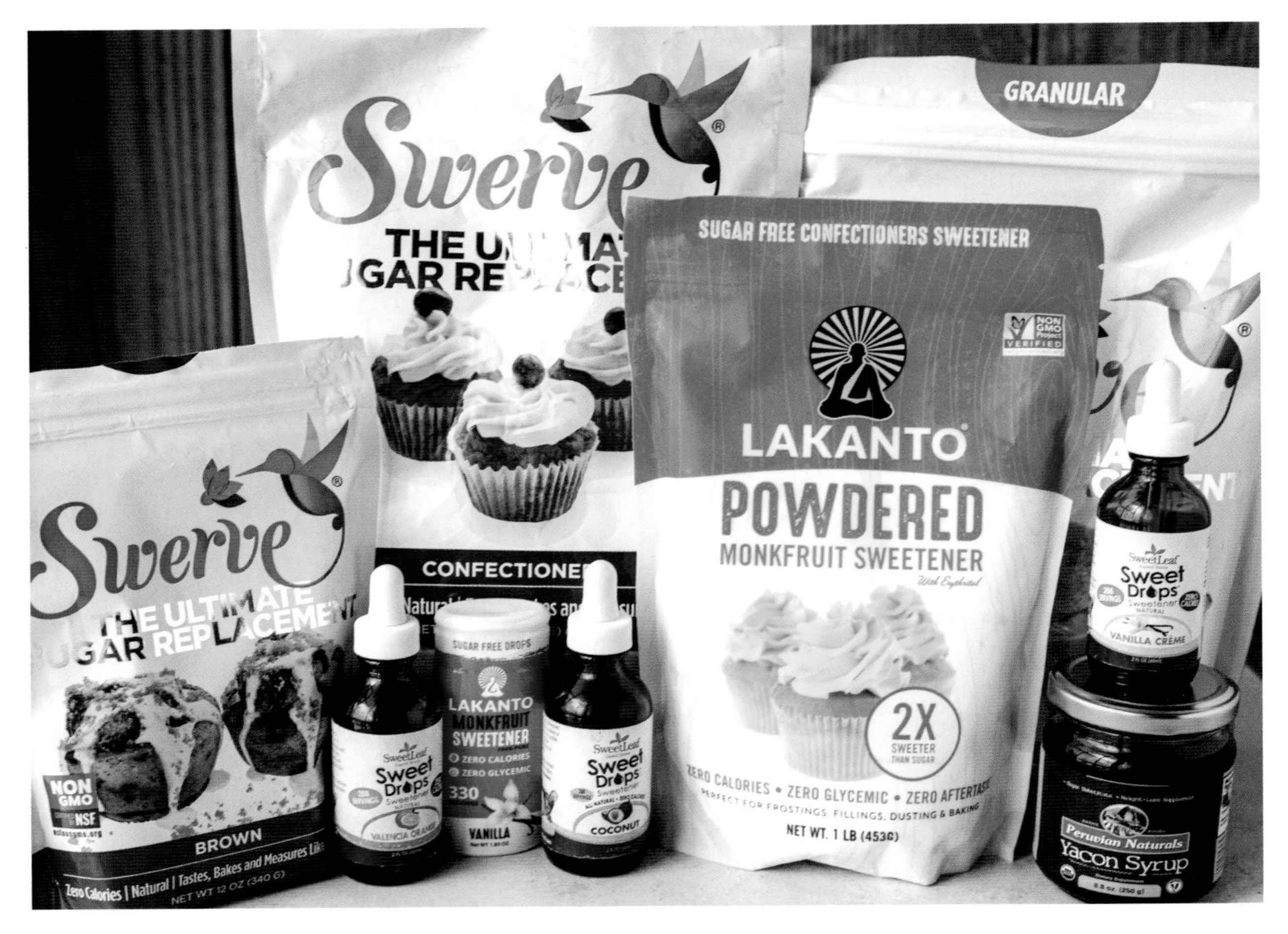

Monk Fruit

Monk fruit extract comes from the monk fruit, luo han guo, a cousin to the cucumber and melon that's native to China and Thailand. Monk fruit is rarely used fresh but more often is dried and used as a sweetener. It is 300 percent sweeter than sugar but is calorie-free and does not raise blood sugar levels. It is sold as a pure liquid concentrate and also can be found combined with erythritol to swap cup for cup with sugar. Some people find that it tastes better than stevia and has no aftertaste; some experience a cooling effect as with erythritol. You'll have to experiment to see if you like it.

Note: If a recipe calls for ½ cup Swerve and ½ teaspoon liquid stevia and you want to use granulated monk fruit instead, your best bet is to use ½ cup but leave out the stevia. The brand of monk fruit that I've had the most success with is Lakanto.

Stevia

Stevia comes from the stevia plant, typically grown in Paraguay. Its leaves are boiled down to produce the liquid form on the market today. Stevia leaves are also dried and sold as a pure concentrated extract with no added fillers. A calorie-free option, it is 300 times sweeter than sugar and does not cause digestive issues, raise blood sugar, or spike insulin. Bear in mind that if you see a stevia blend that measures one for one like sugar, it likely contains fillers such as maltodextrin, which you want to avoid. I've even seen some stevia blends that have sugar listed in the ingredients! I prefer to stay away from all baking varieties of stevia, as they are all highly processed and contain added carbohydrates.

The type of stevia I use most frequently is SweetLeaf brand flavored liquid stevia. Depending on the extraction process used, some brands may be sweeter or more bitter than others. I have tried so many, and SweetLeaf is always my favorite. The flavored varieties include a small amount of natural extracts like vanilla, lemon, and coconut to enhance their flavor. If you have only unflavored liquid stevia on hand, just use the amount called for in the recipe and then add ¼ teaspoon of your chosen extract. Liquid monk fruit can be evenly swapped with liquid stevia, as they have about the same level of sweetness.

Yacón Syrup

Yacón syrup is a thick, brown, sweet syrup that looks and tastes much like molasses. It's extracted from the yacón plant found in Peru and Brazil. A small amount makes a perfect addition to any recipe that needs that special molasses flavor, like in my BBQ Sauce (page 45), Caramel Sauce (page 63), and Maple Syrup (page 70). Yacón syrup does contain some fructose, but when used in small amounts, it should not raise your blood sugar. You can swap yacón syrup with Lakanto brand sugar-free maple syrup if you prefer.

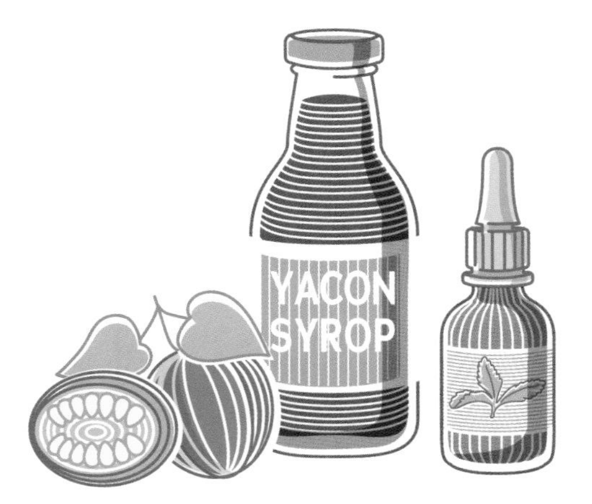

ALLERGY-FRIENDLY SUBSTITUTIONS

Having food allergies is incredibly difficult. I know this reality all too well, as my oldest child was diagnosed with a peanut and soy allergy when he was seven, and my younger son with a tree nut and peanut allergy at the age of four. Now, at fifteen, my daughter is having stomach problems, so we have removed dairy from her diet to see if it helps. (It has.) Having to scan every single label for possible allergens is scary and worrisome enough, but making low-carb, keto-friendly foods without almond flour—a common keto ingredient—is even harder. I've learned to use substitutions to create fantastic nut-free options not only for my family, but for all of the other keto families dealing with food allergies.

Here are the substitutions I use for common allergens:

Almond flour:
An equal amount of sesame or sunflower seed flour can often be substituted for almond flour. Coconut flour cannot be swapped one-for-one with almond flour but can be substituted in combination with adjustments to the amounts of egg and liquid in a recipe. (Coconut flour is very absorbent, so you need to add more liquid to compensate.)

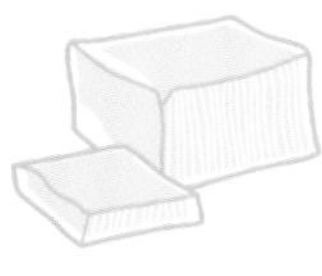

Butter:
Avocado oil, olive oil, ghee (a form of clarified butter that is 99% lactose-free)

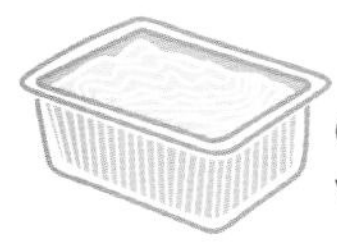

Cream cheese:
Vegan cream cheese

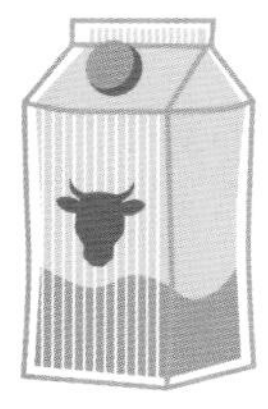

Dairy milk:
Almond milk, coconut milk, hemp milk

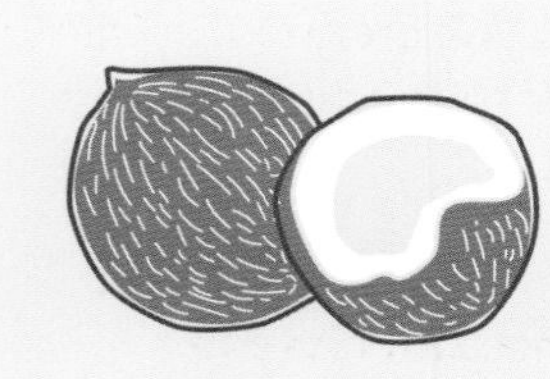

Is Coconut a Tree Nut?

I'd like to clear one thing up before going any further: While the U.S. Food and Drug Administration (FDA) claims that coconut is a tree nut because it comes from a tree, it is in fact a fruit. Yes, people who have tree nut allergies may be allergic to coconut as well, but being allergic to coconut is not the same as having a tree nut allergy.

The American College of Allergy, Asthma and Immunology says it well: "Coconut is not a botanical nut; it is classified as a fruit, even though the Food and Drug Administration recognizes coconut as a tree nut. While allergic reactions to coconut have been documented, most people who are allergic to tree nuts can safely eat coconut. If you are allergic to tree nuts, talk to your allergist before adding coconut to your diet."

With this in mind, and knowing that members of my own family have tree nut allergies, I feel very strongly that calling a recipe nut-free is acceptable when it contains coconut.

Eggs:
Gelatin or flax eggs are a fantastic option for replacing one to three eggs in a recipe; simply double or triple the ingredients below if you need two or three egg replacements. I wouldn't use gelatin or flax eggs as a replacement if the recipe calls for more than three eggs, however. I once attempted a bread that called for five eggs, and replacing them with gelatin eggs was a complete failure. If you need to substitute for more than three eggs, try Bob's Red Mill powdered vegetarian egg replacer, which can mimic the properties of egg in most recipes.

Heavy whipping cream:
Coconut cream (the thick part that rises to the top of a can of coconut milk)

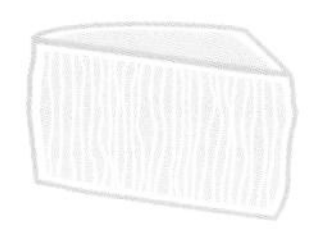

Parmesan cheese:
Nutritional yeast

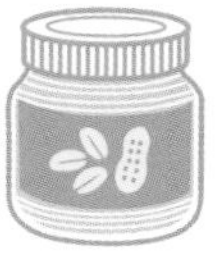

Peanut butter:
Sunflower seed butter, almond butter (if no tree nut allergy)

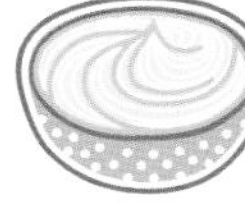

Sour cream:
Vegan sour cream

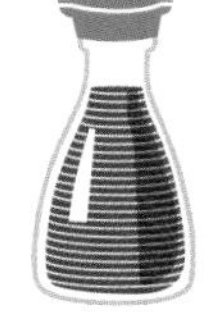

Soy sauce:
Coconut aminos

Tree nut butters:
Sunflower seed butter, tahini (ground sesame seeds), coconut butter

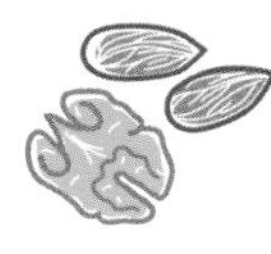

Tree nuts:
Pumpkin seeds, sunflower seeds, hemp seeds, sesame seeds

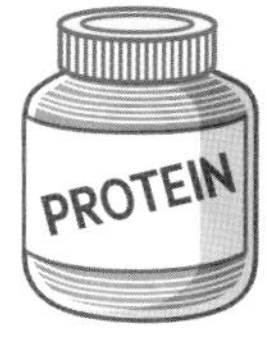

Whey protein powder:
Egg white protein powder, hemp protein

GELATIN EGG

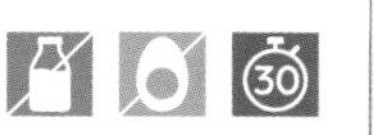

YIELD: 1 egg replacement

PREP TIME: 1 minute **COOK TIME:** 2 minutes

Ingredients

1 tablespoon unflavored gelatin

3 tablespoons water, divided

1. Place the gelatin in a small bowl and stir in 1 tablespoon of water. Mix until a thick paste forms.
2. Pour the remaining 2 tablespoons of water in a small ramekin and bring to a boil in the microwave, then pour into the gelatin mixture. Stir until dissolved. Use immediately.

CALORIES: 13 **FAT:** 0g **PROTEIN:** 3g
TOTAL CARBS: 0g **DIETARY FIBER:** 0g **NET CARBS:** 0g

FLAX EGG

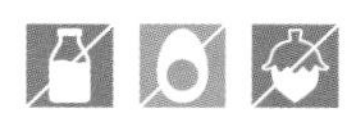

YIELD: 1 egg replacement

PREP TIME: 1 minute, plus 15 minutes to chill

Ingredients

1 tablespoon ground flaxseed

3 tablespoons water

1. Place the flaxseed in a small bowl and stir in the water until combined.
2. Place bowl in the refrigerator for 15 minutes. Stir and use as a substitute for one egg. Use immediately.

CALORIES: 35 **FAT:** 2g **PROTEIN:** 2g
TOTAL CARBS: 2g **DIETARY FIBER:** 2g **NET CARBS:** 0g

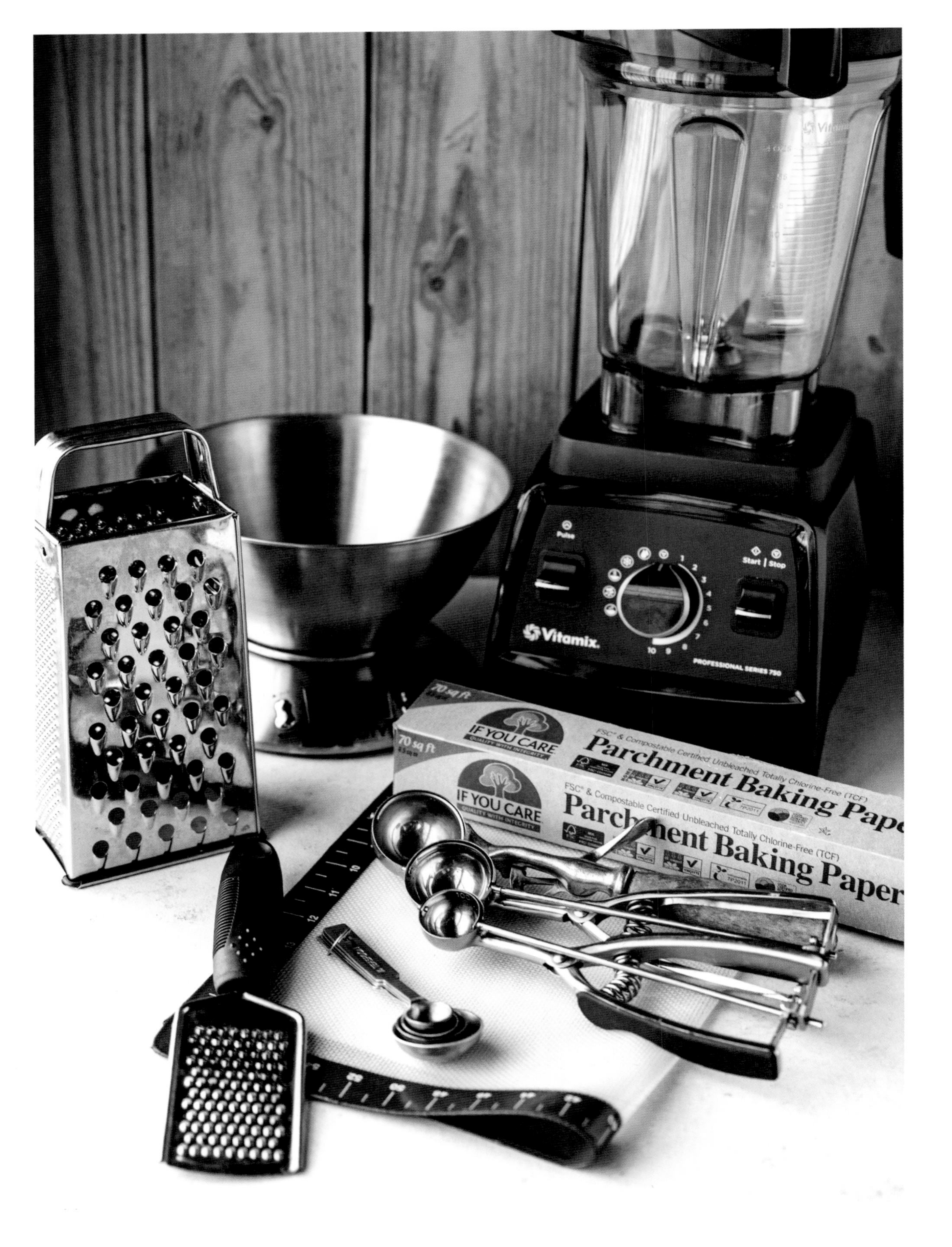
Pulse
Start | Stop
Vitamix
PROFESSIONAL SERIES 750
70 sq ft
IF YOU CARE
QUALITY WITH INTEGRITY
FSC® & Compostable Certified Unbleached Totally Chlorine-Free (TCF)
Parchment Baking Paper

MY FAVORITE KITCHEN TOOLS

In addition to the basics that you probably already have on hand—a set of pots and pans, measuring cups and spoons, a couple of sharp knives, and so on—there are some "extras" that I find are particularly handy to have in my keto kitchen.

Cookware and Bakeware

Cast-iron skillet: For the same reason I love my Dutch oven, I enjoy having cast-iron skillets in different sizes. Cast iron cooks food more evenly than regular nonstick pans. I also love being able to start cooking food on the stovetop and then easily transition the pan to the oven without worry. No other skillet will get you that nice crispy outer edge that makes my Skillet Chocolate Chip Cookie Pie (page 262) especially delicious.

Donut pan: I have two Wilton donut pans. Each pan has the capacity for six donuts or bagels. Free-forming bagels is fine, but when you really want a donut to look like a donut, this type of pan is the best. It's even dishwasher safe! Although they have a nonstick surface, I still grease my donut pans for added insurance.

Dutch oven: I have only one Dutch oven; one is all you need. These heavy-duty pots are usually made from cast iron, though some are ceramic or clay. They're all perfect for braising meats and cooking soups and stews. The reason I love it so much is that it can withstand high temperatures—you can easily brown an ingredient on the stovetop and then place the whole thing right in the oven. Because it conducts heat so well, it also keeps food warmer for much longer than a standard pot would.

Ramekins: Ramekins are great for portion-controlled recipes, as they come in a variety of sizes. The 7-ounce size is perfect for making my 2-Minute English Muffins (page 88), as well as the Quick Strawberry Shortcakes (page 248). I also use ramekins to make all of the one-minute mug cakes on my blog.

Silicone bakeware: Silicone bakeware is fabulous at preventing sticking when baking. Plus, when you're preparing a no-bake recipe like muffins, fat bombs, truffles, or candy, they make for easy removal with just a little tug. While they are stick-resistant, you should still grease them lightly whenever a recipe instructs you to grease the pan. Silicone is safe to use at high temperatures in the oven, as well as in the microwave or freezer, and is dishwasher safe.

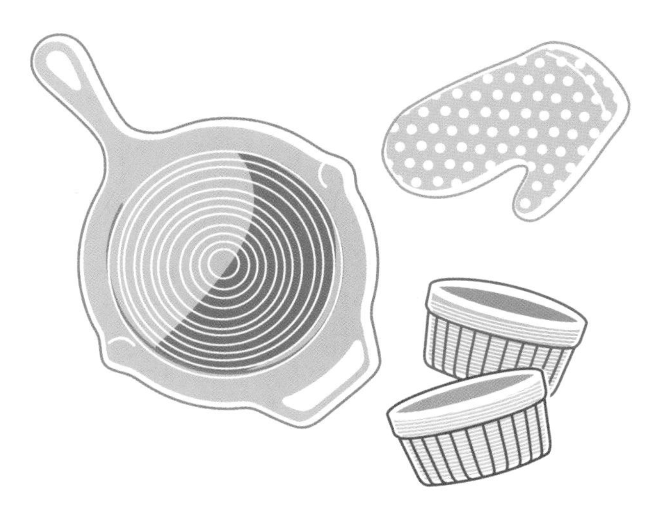

Small Appliances

Air fryer: Air fryers are all the rage these days. This countertop appliance uses convection to circulate air around food in order to cook it, thereby using far less oil than traditional frying. Now, you might be thinking that you don't often fry foods, so what's the point of this appliance? But it's not just for frying! The big selling point of an air fryer is the time it saves. It doesn't need to be preheated like a typical oven: it's hot and ready to go in seconds. It can cook foods much faster, in about half the time it would take in the oven. In my chicken wings recipe (page 160), I give instructions for using either an air fryer or the oven. I have a Philips XXL with a capacity of 3 pounds (4 quarts) because I have a family of five and most versions are written to serve two to four people.

Blender (high-powered or regular): I use my blender every day. I start the morning with coffee blended with collagen peptides and heavy cream. Of course, you could just stir everything together, but there is something about blending it that takes the experience to another level. The foaminess that blending creates is simply the best. Even if you're not a coffee drinker, a blender comes in handy for making smoothies, sauces, condiments, and dips. It's a must-have in my keto kitchen. I used to have a high-powered Blendtec, but I recently purchased a Vitamix, which seems more powerful and sturdy.

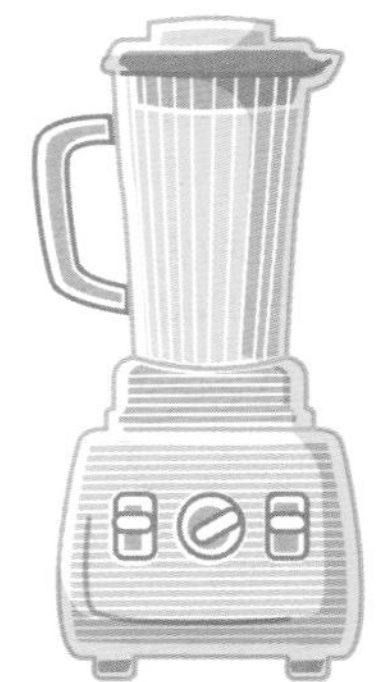

Dehydrator: This kitchen appliance isn't totally necessary, but I have come to love and use mine often. A dehydrator uses a heating coil and a small fan to circulate gently heated air, reducing the amount of water in veggies, fruits, and meats. In the oven, vegetable chips like my Salt and Vinegar Zucchini Chips (page 124) don't come out as crispy and chiplike—the dehydrator makes all the difference. I have the Nesco brand with adjustable temperature settings for veggies, fruits, and meats. It comes with five trays but can expand to twelve for big batches.

Food processor: What's not to love about this appliance? It can dice, slice, shred, knead, mix, chop, and even puree! I love it for chopping veggies, grinding nuts and seeds, making pie crusts, and even mixing dough. I have a Cuisinart with a 14-cup capacity.

Ice cream maker: I have an ice cream attachment for my KitchenAid mixer. It's just a simple bowl that stays in my freezer, ready for whenever I want to make ice cream for the family. If you are looking to purchase an ice cream maker, I would suggest purchasing a model that has a frozen bowl attachment. It's more convenient than having a model that requires using rock salt and ice to freeze the ice cream. If you have a family, find a model that can make up to 2 quarts of ice cream. Making homemade ice cream is far less expensive than buying one of the low-carb varieties on the market today and the taste can't be beat.

Immersion blender: This tool is handy when you don't want to get out the food processor (see above). I use it to make homemade mayonnaise, and you can also blend and thicken soups right in the pot. I have the Breville brand, which comes with a container for making smoothies.

Instant Pot: While this appliance is fairly new, it's a pretty fabulous tool to have on hand when slow cooking isn't an option and you need to get dinner ready in a hurry. In most cases, you can cut a recipe's cooking time in half using this type of electric pressure cooker. Some Instant Pots have a dual feature function that allows you to slow-cook as well. My Chili and Short Ribs recipes (pages 142 and 194, respectively) include instructions for both Instant Pot and slow cooker methods.

Pizzelle maker: Having a pizzelle maker might seem frivolous, but if you're into Italian desserts or you want to make homemade ice cream cones, it's really a must. I have the Chef Choice PizzellePro, which works beautifully for making my keto pizzelle (page 256).

Slow cooker: If you've not yet bought yourself a slow cooker, you need to break down and get one. If I could buy only one appliance, this would be my choice—it's ideal for stress-free dinners! It doesn't get any easier than placing ingredients in a pot and letting them slow-cook all day. Coming home to a scrumptious aroma in the kitchen after a long day of work can't be beat! I have a Hamilton Beach programmable slow cooker. Once it reaches the preset cooking time, it automatically switches to the warm setting, which is really helpful if you don't get home in time to turn it off.

Stand mixer or electric hand mixer: Stirring by hand can get the job done for most recipes, but investing in a mixer, whether it is a stand mixer or a handheld model, will save you tons of time and effort. Plus, you simply can't whip egg whites well without one. I use my KitchenAid almost daily. I can whip cream in a matter of minutes; prepare mousse-like desserts with a wonderfully smooth texture; and mix cookie batter, cake batter, and bread dough with this fantastic appliance. If you don't have the counter space or budget for a stand mixer, the next best thing is a electric hand mixer.

Waffle maker: If you have kids and want to prep breakfast ahead, making waffles is an amazing option. Make a big batch on the weekend and store them in the fridge or freezer. I prefer using a waffle maker that makes four waffles at a time. Chef's Choice has a good one that is perfect for thick keto batters.

Tools and Gadgets

Cookie scoops: Useful for more than just dishing out cookie batter, these scoops are available in many sizes. I use them all the time for scooping cookie dough and ice cream, making perfectly sized meatballs, and portioning muffin and cupcake batter. They give a perfect shape and help you work more efficiently. I have a set of three sizes, each with an easy trigger release. If you're dealing with a sticky batter, it's helpful to grease the cookie scoop for an even smoother release. You can find a huge selection on Amazon.

Dessert decorating tool: I use the Wilton brand and find this tool easier to use than a pastry bag with tips. It's perfect for decorating any cake, especially my Triple-Layer Chocolate Cake (page 250), and can also pipe filling for Cannoli (page 228).

Digital kitchen scale: I use my scale every day. Weighing low-carb flours like coconut, sesame, and almond really does help the outcome of a recipe, as it gives you a more accurate measurement. Plus, it helps with portion sizes for finished foods. I don't know about you, but my eyes deceive me every time. I always think I have less food than I do. Once I weigh it, I'm accountable. I don't think I could stick to my macros without a scale.

Microplane grater: From grating cheeses to zesting lemons and limes and even grating ginger, garlic, and onion, this tool is a must-have in any kitchen.

Parchment paper: A silicone baking mat works just as well as parchment paper, but if you don't feel like having to clean the mat after it's used, parchment paper is the way to go. I love the convenience and easy cleanup when I need to line a cake pan or cookie sheet, wrap fish to bake, or roll out fathead dough to make my Cinnamon Rolls (page 86). Don't confuse waxed paper with parchment, as waxed paper is not heat resistant and cannot be used in the oven.

Serrated peeler: You don't need a spiral slicer if you have limited space. A serrated peeler is great for removing skin from fruits and vegetables, but it can also carve cucumbers and zucchini into neat ribbons. So while you may not get those long spaghetti-like strands that a spiral slicer would produce, you can still get a similar effect with a shorter veggie noodle.

Spiral vegetable slicer: A spiral slicer cuts vegetables and fruits into curly ribbons resembling spaghetti. It's wonderful for making zucchini noodles, cucumber noodles, beet noodles, and many more. I use a Paderno three-blade spiral slicer.

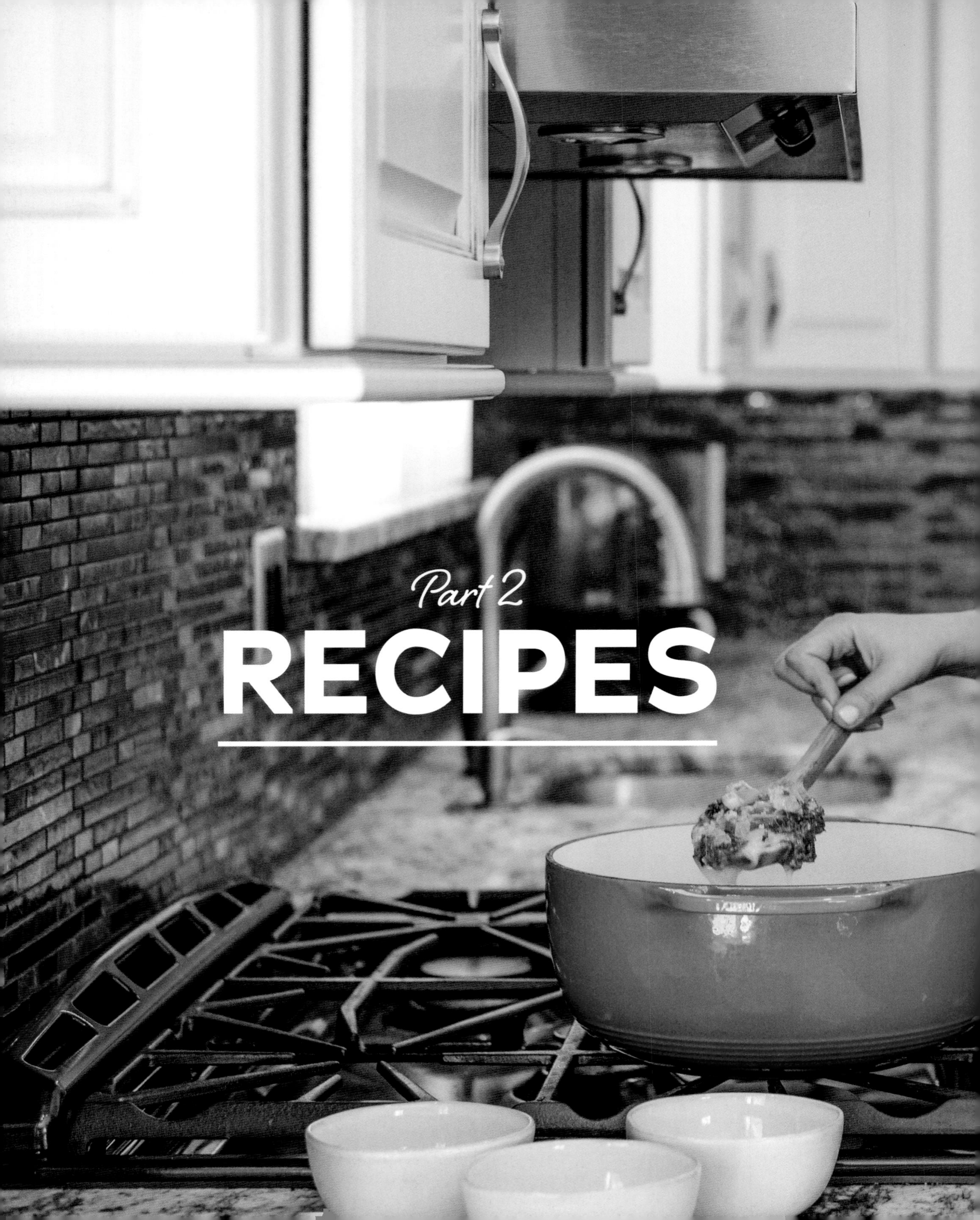

Part 2

RECIPES

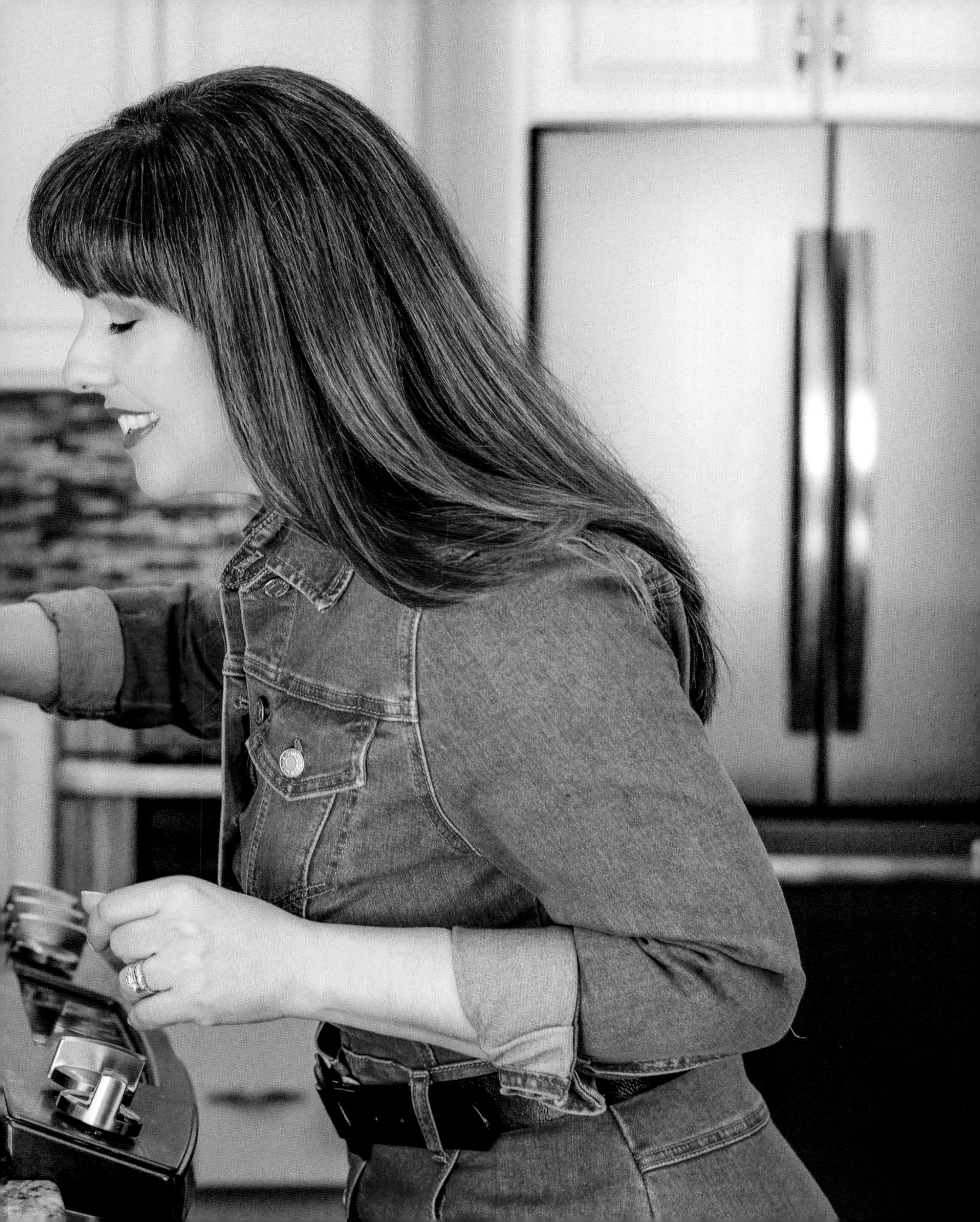

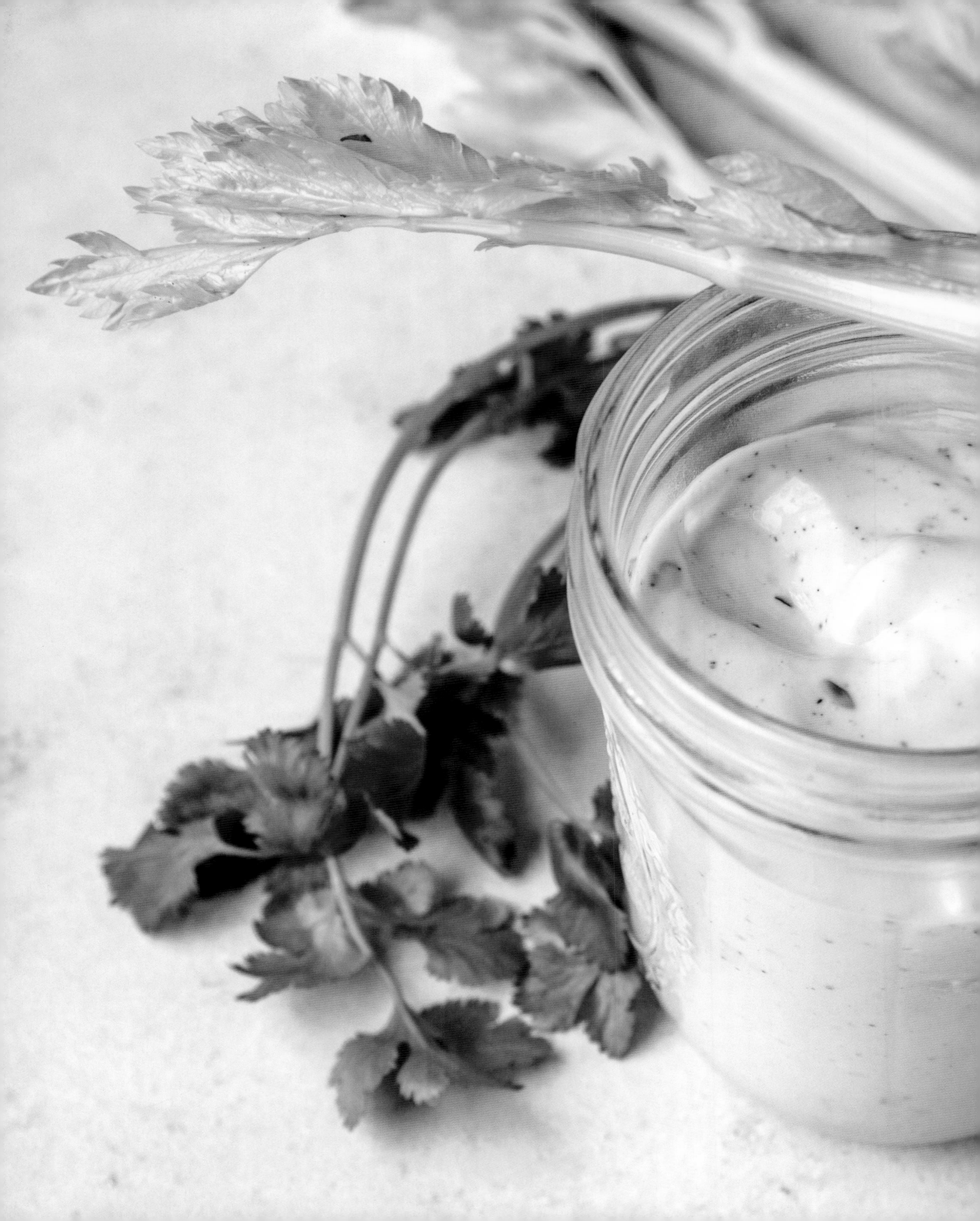

Basics

ALFREDO SAUCE

YIELD: 1½ cups (2 tablespoons per serving)

PREP TIME: 5 minutes

COOK TIME: 20 minutes

If you're a lover of cheese, Alfredo sauce is a must. Those shirataki or zucchini noodles (page 217) will taste even better topped with this sauce! You can also use it for my Chicken Crust Pizza (page 176).

¼ cup (½ stick) plus 1 tablespoon salted butter, divided

2 cups heavy whipping cream

1 teaspoon minced garlic

1 large egg yolk

½ teaspoon onion powder

¼ teaspoon fine sea salt

¼ teaspoon ground white pepper

¼ cup grated Parmesan cheese

OPTIONAL INGREDIENTS

1 teaspoon grated lemon zest

¼ teaspoon ground nutmeg

Chopped fresh flat-leaf parsley

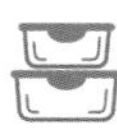

Store in an airtight container in the refrigerator for up to 1 week. Reheat before serving.

1. Bring ¼ cup of the butter, the cream, and garlic to a boil in a large saucepan over medium heat. Reduce the heat to a simmer and stir in the egg yolk until well incorporated.
2. Stir in the onion powder, salt, and pepper. Continue to simmer, stirring, until the sauce thickens, about 15 minutes.
3. Remove from the heat and stir in the Parmesan cheese, the remaining 1 tablespoon of butter, and any optional ingredients, if desired.
4. Serve warm.

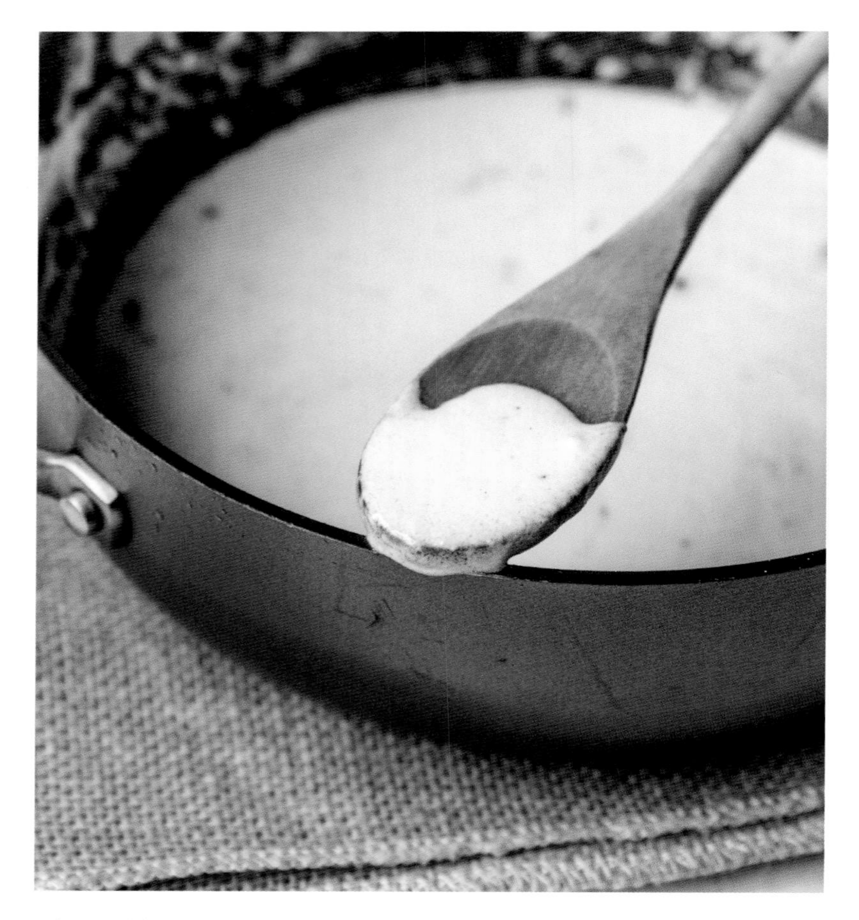

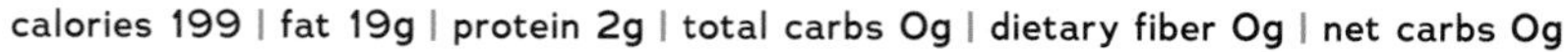

calories 199 | fat 19g | protein 2g | total carbs 0g | dietary fiber 0g | net carbs 0g

BBQ SAUCE

YIELD: 2 cups (2 tablespoons per serving)

PREP TIME: 3 minutes

Make your own sugar-free ketchup to use in this recipe or purchase a store-bought version, and you'll have one tasty keto BBQ sauce for ribs or chicken.

1½ cups sugar-free ketchup, store-bought or homemade (page 50)

¼ cup apple cider vinegar

1 tablespoon yacón syrup or sugar-free maple syrup, store-bought or homemade (page 70)

1 teaspoon maple extract

¼ cup packed Swerve brown sugar sweetener

2 tablespoons smoked paprika

Pinch of fine sea salt

Store in an airtight container in the refrigerator for up to 1 month.

Place all of the ingredients in a blender and blend until smooth. Taste and add more sweetener and/or salt, if desired.

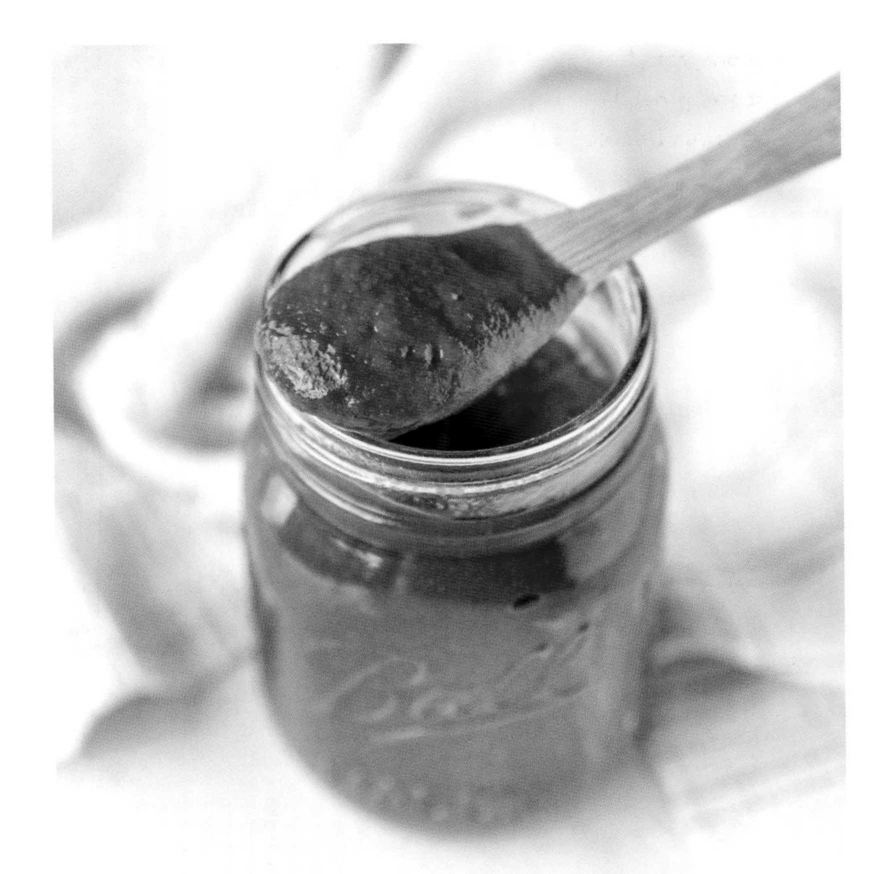

calories 14 | fat 0g | protein 0g | total carbs 3g | dietary fiber 0g | net carbs 3g

BEEF SPICE RUB

YIELD: 1 cup (1 tablespoon per serving)

PREP TIME: 5 minutes

This spice rub makes the most succulent ribs, but you can use it on any cut of beef or even pork if you like! Use 2 tablespoons per pound of meat.

- ¼ cup smoked paprika
- 2 tablespoons fine sea salt
- 2 tablespoons freshly ground black pepper
- 2 tablespoons garlic powder
- 2 tablespoons granulated onion
- 2 tablespoons ground cumin
- 1 tablespoon chili powder
- 1 tablespoon mustard powder

Store in an airtight container in the pantry for up to 1 year.

Place all of the ingredients in a medium bowl and whisk to combine.

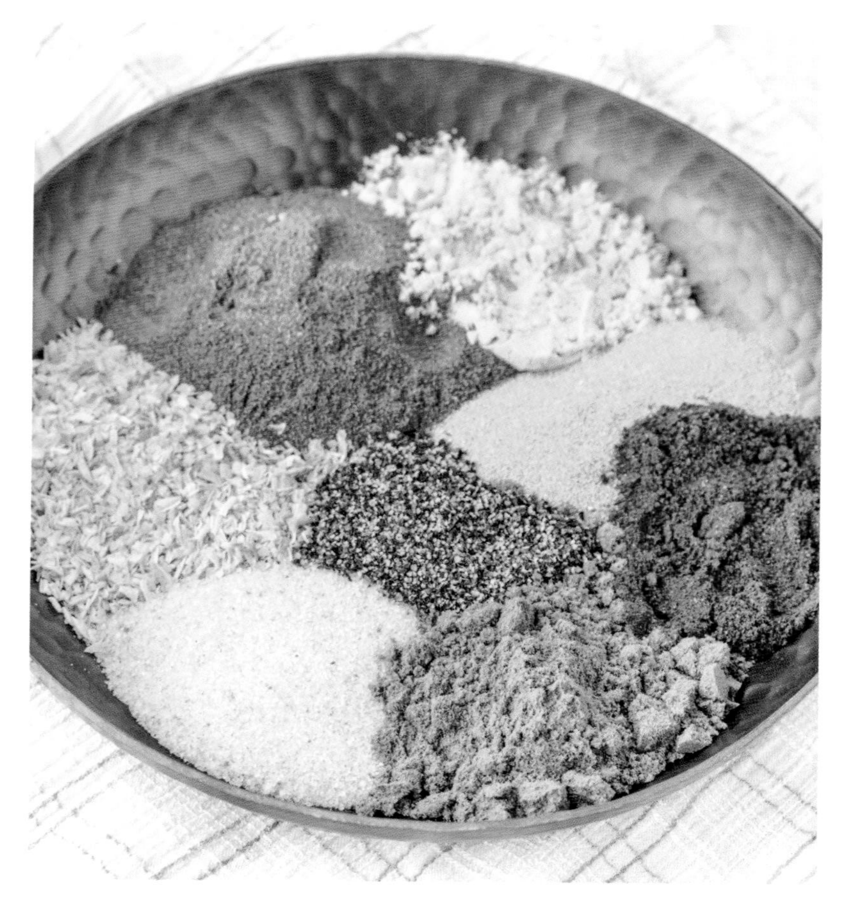

calories 16 | fat 0g | protein 0g | total carbs 3g | dietary fiber 1g | net carbs 2g

CHICKEN SPICE RUB

YIELD: ¾ cup (1 tablespoon per serving)

PREP TIME: 5 minutes

Whenever you want to spice up plain chicken, try this rub! Use 2 tablespoons per pound of meat.

¼ cup smoked paprika

2 tablespoons coarse sea salt

2 tablespoons ground cumin

1 tablespoon dried onion flakes

1 tablespoon dried oregano leaves

1 tablespoon freshly ground black pepper

1 tablespoon garlic powder

½ to 1 tablespoon cayenne pepper, depending on heat preference (optional)

Store in an airtight container in the pantry for up to 1 year.

Place all of the ingredients in a medium bowl and whisk to combine.

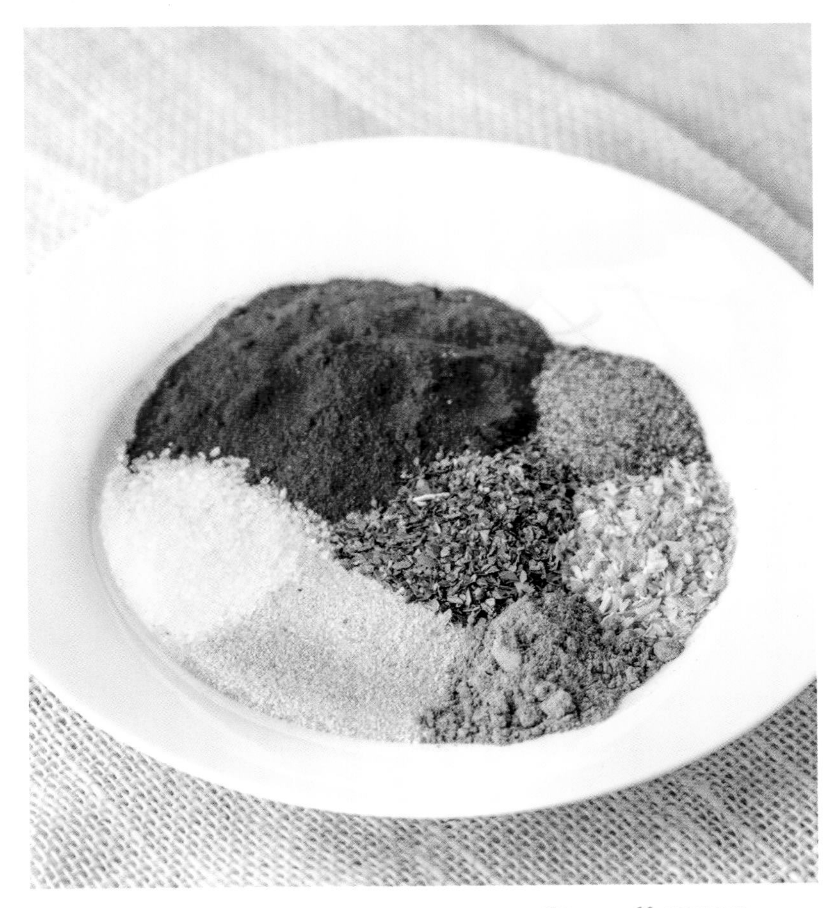

calories 16 | fat 0g | protein 0g | total carbs 3g | dietary fiber 1g | net carbs 3g

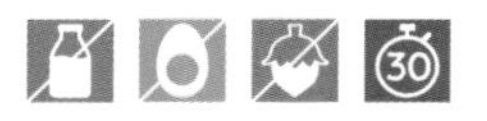

EGG-FREE MAYO

YIELD: 2½ cups (2 tablespoons per serving)

PREP TIME: 5 minutes

COOK TIME: 2 minutes

Maybe you're like me and have always been wary of making homemade mayonnaise because of the use of raw eggs. I can tell you that this version tastes just like traditional egg-based mayo, but because of the gelatin, it will continue to thicken up in the fridge. A simple reheating will bring it back to the right texture, or you can just halve the recipe if you'd rather not have much mayo left over. Please note: Collagen peptides will not work as a substitute for the gelatin here; collagen will not cause the mayo to thicken up as it should.

1 tablespoon unflavored gelatin

3 tablespoons water, divided

1 cup avocado oil

1 tablespoon distilled vinegar

1 tablespoon freshly squeezed lemon juice

1 tablespoon Dijon mustard

½ teaspoon fine sea salt

SPECIAL EQUIPMENT:

Immersion blender

1. Place the gelatin in a small bowl and stir in 1 tablespoon of the water. Mix until a thick paste forms.

2. Pour the remaining 2 tablespoons of water into a small ramekin and microwave until boiling, then pour the boiling water into the gelatin mixture. Stir until dissolved. Set aside.

3. Whisk the remaining ingredients in a small bowl, then add the gelatin mixture. Using an immersion blender, blend on high until the mixture is smooth and has the texture of traditional mayonnaise.

4. Taste and add more salt, if desired.

5. Best if used immediately. If you're going to be using all of the mayo the same day it's made, you don't need to refrigerate it. To keep it longer, cover and refrigerate. When ready to use again, you will need to heat the mayo in the microwave for 30 seconds or in a saucepan over low heat since it gels when refrigerated.

calories 105 | fat 11g | protein 0g | total carbs 0g | dietary fiber 0g | net carbs 0g

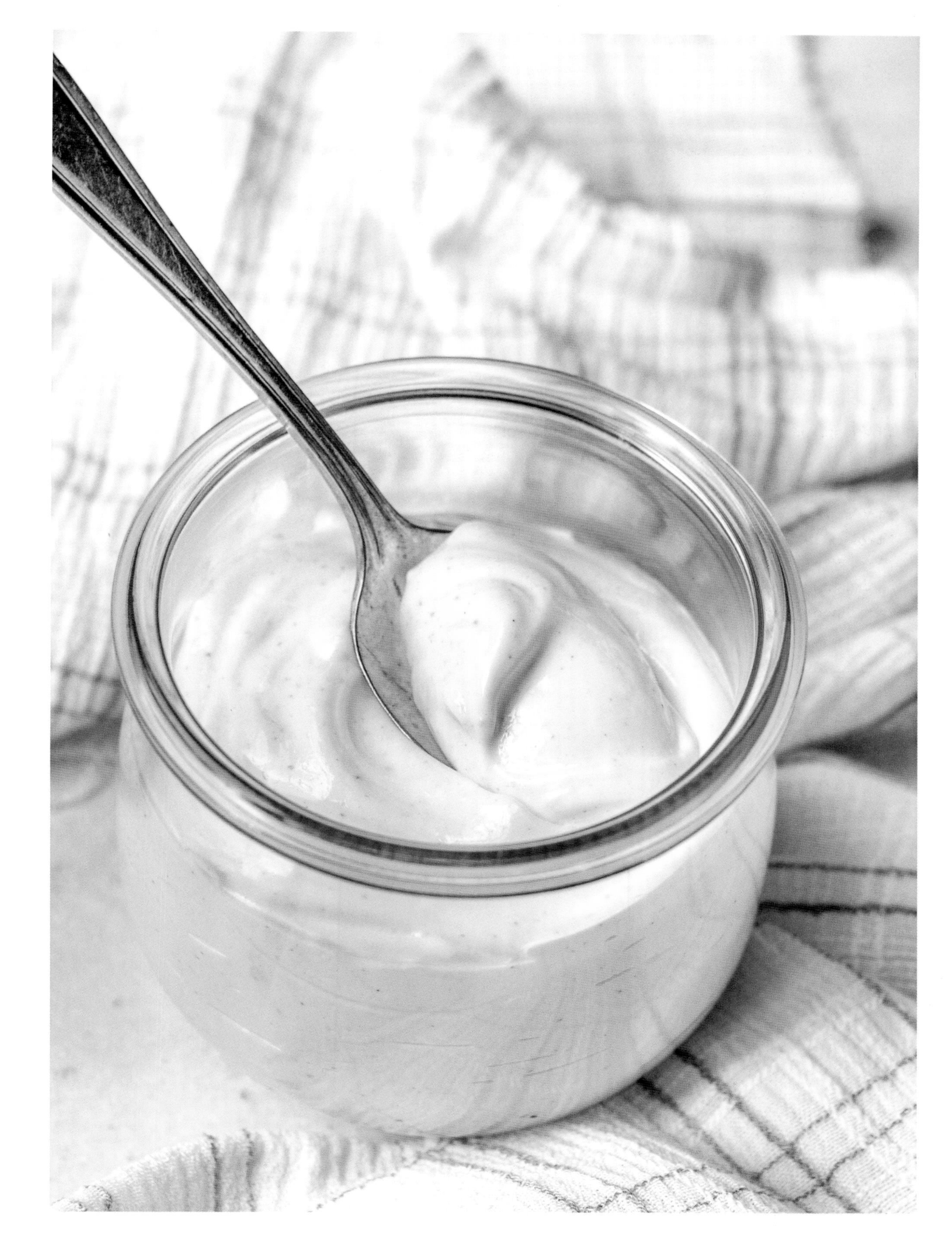

EASY BLENDER KETCHUP

YIELD: 4¾ cups (¼ cup per serving)

PREP TIME: 5 minutes

This recipe makes a whole lot of ketchup. Feel free to cut the ingredients in half if your family just doesn't use this much. You can always use extra ketchup for Fry Sauce (page 52) and/or BBQ Sauce (page 45). I often use the blender method because it's quicker, but the stovetop method really marries all of the flavors, giving the ketchup an unbeatable depth of flavor.

- 1 (28-ounce) can tomato puree
- 1 (6-ounce) can tomato paste
- ¼ cup apple cider vinegar
- ¼ cup red wine vinegar
- 2 tablespoons yacón syrup, or ¼ cup Swerve confectioners'-style sweetener
- 2 cloves garlic, minced
- 1 tablespoon extra-virgin olive oil
- 1 tablespoon dried minced onions
- 1 teaspoon fine sea salt
- ½ teaspoon dried oregano leaves
- ¼ teaspoon ground cloves

Store in a glass jar in the refrigerator for up to 6 months.

STOVETOP OPTION: *Place all of the ingredients in an enameled Dutch oven or other heavy nonreactive pot and stir to combine. Bring to a boil, then lower the heat and simmer until the ketchup is reduced and thickened, 15 to 20 minutes. Use an immersion blender to blend the ketchup for a smoother texture. Taste and adjust the spices and sweetener, if desired. Makes 3¾ cups.*

Place all of the ingredients in a blender and pulse until the ketchup has the desired consistency. Taste and adjust the spices and sweetener, if desired.

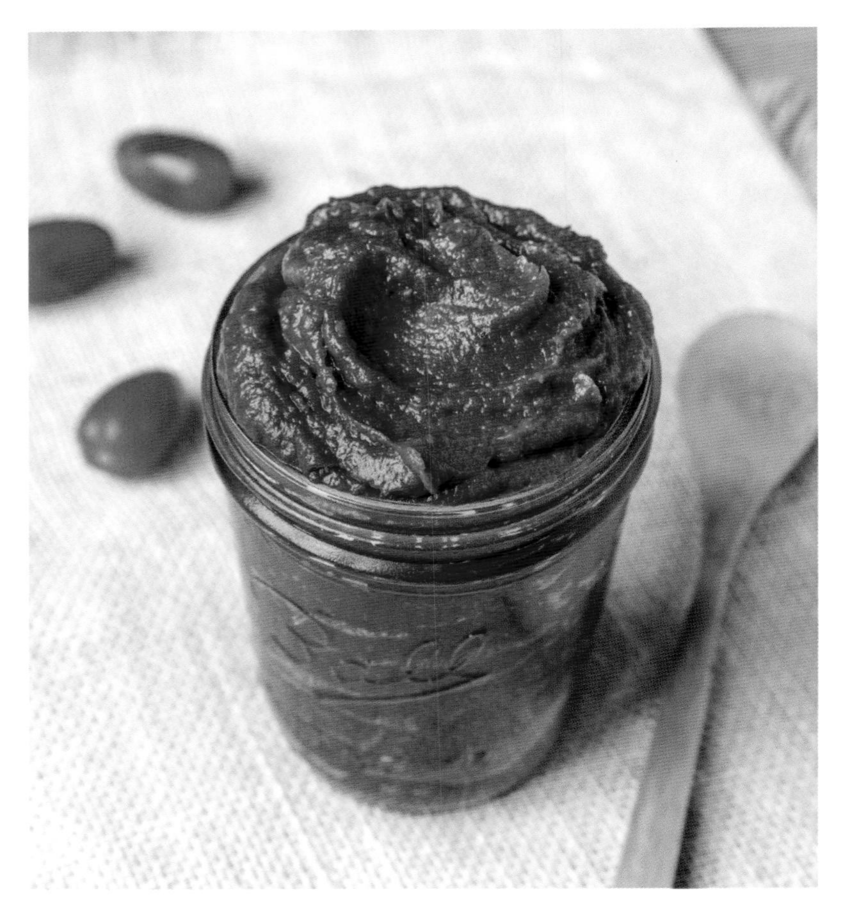

calories 15 | fat 0g | protein 0g | total carbs 2g | dietary fiber 0g | net carbs 2g

LEMON AIOLI

YIELD: 1½ cups (2 tablespoons per serving)

PREP TIME: 5 minutes

Aioli is a sauce made with garlic and olive oil and sometimes emulsified with an egg. Often, at least in the Italian home I grew up in, it is served with fish and pasta. My dad will cringe when he sees that I make this version with mayonnaise, because that isn't typical. Since I opted to leave out the egg yolk, I use mayonnaise to get that creamy texture. Use this sauce for dipping Focaccia (page 118) or Crispy Brussels Sprouts (page 214).

- 1 cup avocado oil mayonnaise (for egg-free, use Egg-Free Mayo, page 48)
- ⅓ cup extra-virgin olive oil
- 2 cloves garlic, minced
- 2 tablespoons freshly squeezed lemon juice
- ½ teaspoon fine sea salt
- Freshly ground black pepper, to taste

Store in an airtight container in the refrigerator for up to 3 months.

Note: You can use homemade egg-free mayo (page 48) in this recipe if you will be using the aioli immediately. If you need to refrigerate leftover aioli, it will need to be warmed slightly, as the mayo will gel in the fridge.

Place all of the ingredients in a blender and blend, or whisk together in a medium bowl, until smooth. Taste and add more salt and pepper, if desired.

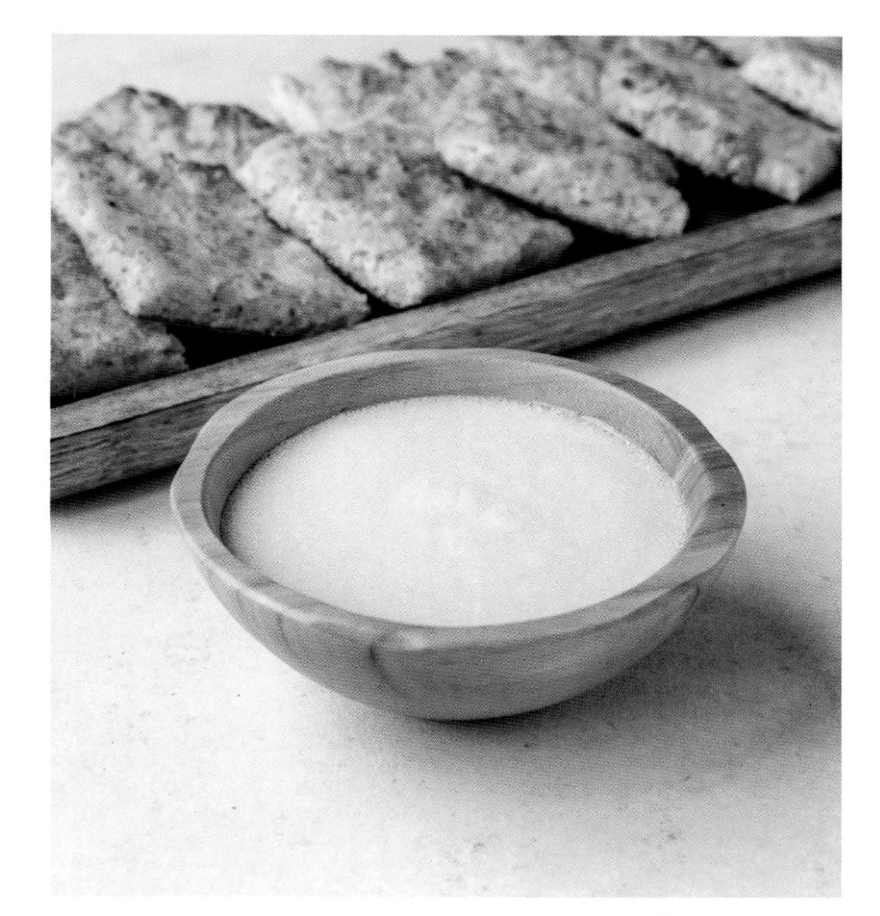

calories 187 | fat 22g | protein 0g | total carbs 0g | dietary fiber 0g | net carbs 0g

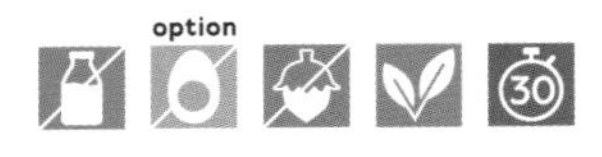

FRY SAUCE

YIELD: 1½ cups (2 tablespoons per serving)

PREP TIME: 2 minutes

This super simple, quick sauce is delicious with Zucchini Fries (page 206), Jicama Fries (page 216), and burgers too!

1 cup avocado oil mayonnaise (for egg-free, use Egg-Free Mayo, page 48)

½ cup sugar-free ketchup, store-bought or homemade (page 50)

Store in an airtight container in the refrigerator for up to 6 months.

Note: You can use homemade egg-free mayo in this recipe if you will be using the sauce immediately. If you need to refrigerate leftover sauce, it will need to be warmed slightly, as the mayo will gel in the fridge.

Place the ingredients in a blender and blend, or whisk together in a small bowl, until thoroughly combined.

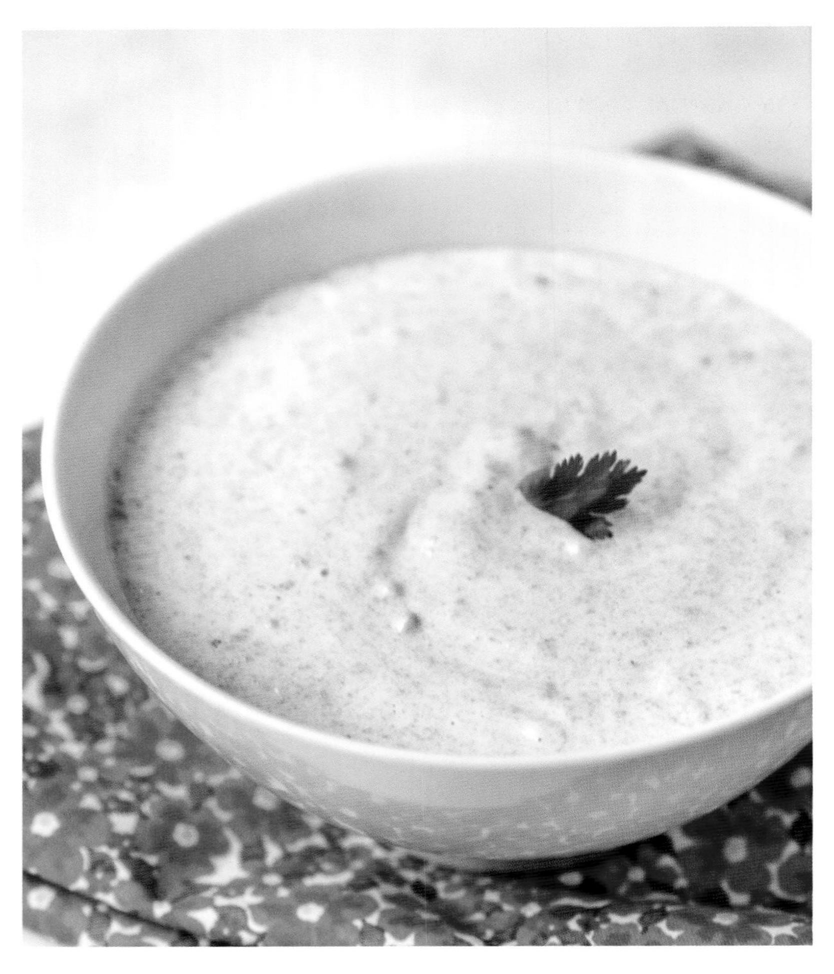

calories 137 | fat 16g | protein 0g | total carbs 0g | dietary fiber 0g | net carbs 0g

QUICK MARINARA SAUCE

YIELD: 8 cups (1/2 cup per serving)

PREP TIME: 5 minutes

COOK TIME: 35 minutes

This is an authentic Italian marinara sauce, but it comes together in just over 30 minutes. You'll never go back to jarred sauce again!

2 (28-ounce) cans tomato puree

1 cup water

2 tablespoons extra-virgin olive oil

2 cloves garlic, minced

2 teaspoons dried basil

2 teaspoons dried parsley

2 teaspoons fine sea salt

1 teaspoon freshly ground black pepper

1 teaspoon dried fennel seeds

FOR GARNISH (OPTIONAL)

Red pepper flakes

Chopped fresh basil

Chopped fresh flat-leaf parsley

Store in an airtight container in the refrigerator for up to 5 days or in the freezer for up to 3 months.

1. Place all of the ingredients in an enameled Dutch oven or other large nonreactive pot with a lid over medium-high heat. Stir to combine well and bring to a boil.

2. Reduce the heat to medium-low, cover, and simmer for 30 minutes. Taste and add more salt and pepper, if desired. Serve.

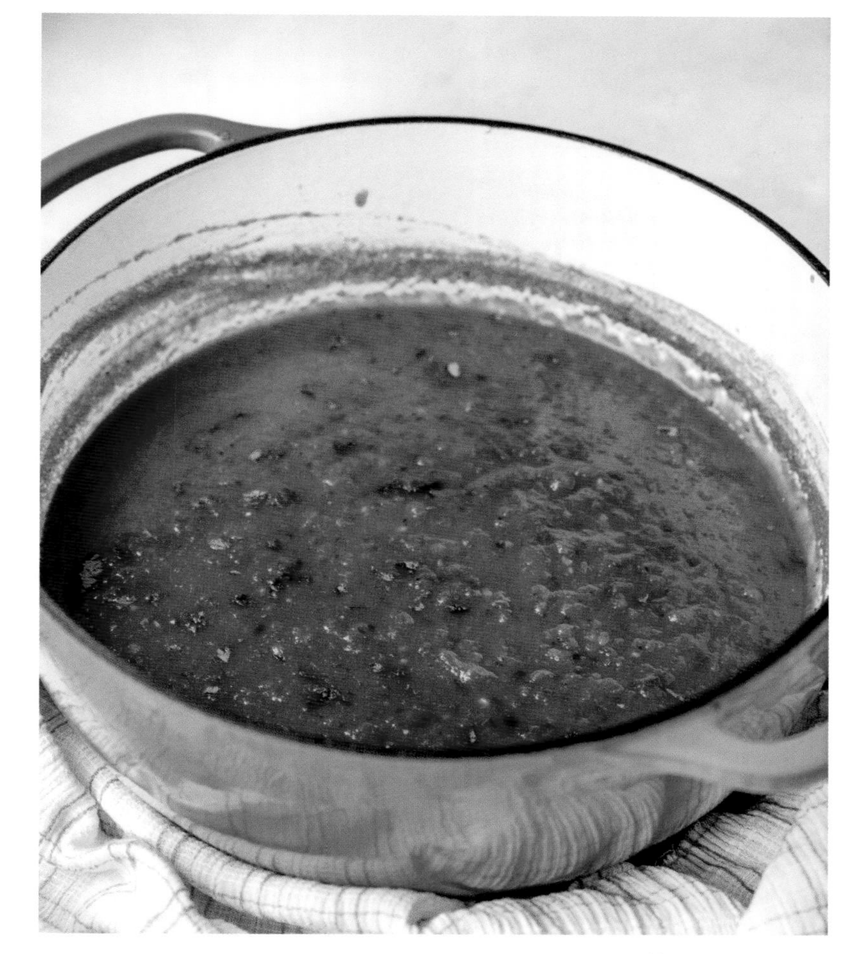

calories 33 | fat 1g | protein 0g | total carbs 4g | dietary fiber 1g | net carbs 3g

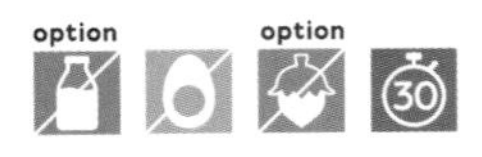

PESTO

YIELD: 1 cup (2 tablespoons per serving)

PREP TIME: 10 minutes

Traditional pesto contains pine nuts, but because my youngest child has a tree nut allergy, I make it without the pine nuts, and it really doesn't taste any less delicious. You can certainly include the pine nuts if you like; just keep in mind that doing so will alter the nutritional information.

1 bunch fresh basil, stems removed (about 1 cup)

1 cup packed fresh flat-leaf parsley leaves

2 cloves garlic

½ cup extra-virgin olive oil

½ cup grated Parmesan cheese (or nutritional yeast for dairy-free)

¼ cup pine nuts (optional)

¼ teaspoon fine sea salt

Pinch of freshly ground black pepper

Store in an airtight container in the refrigerator for up to 1 week or in the freezer for up to 6 months.

1. Place the basil, parsley, and garlic in a food processor and process until chopped.

2. Add the remaining ingredients and process to combine. Taste and add more salt and pepper, if desired.

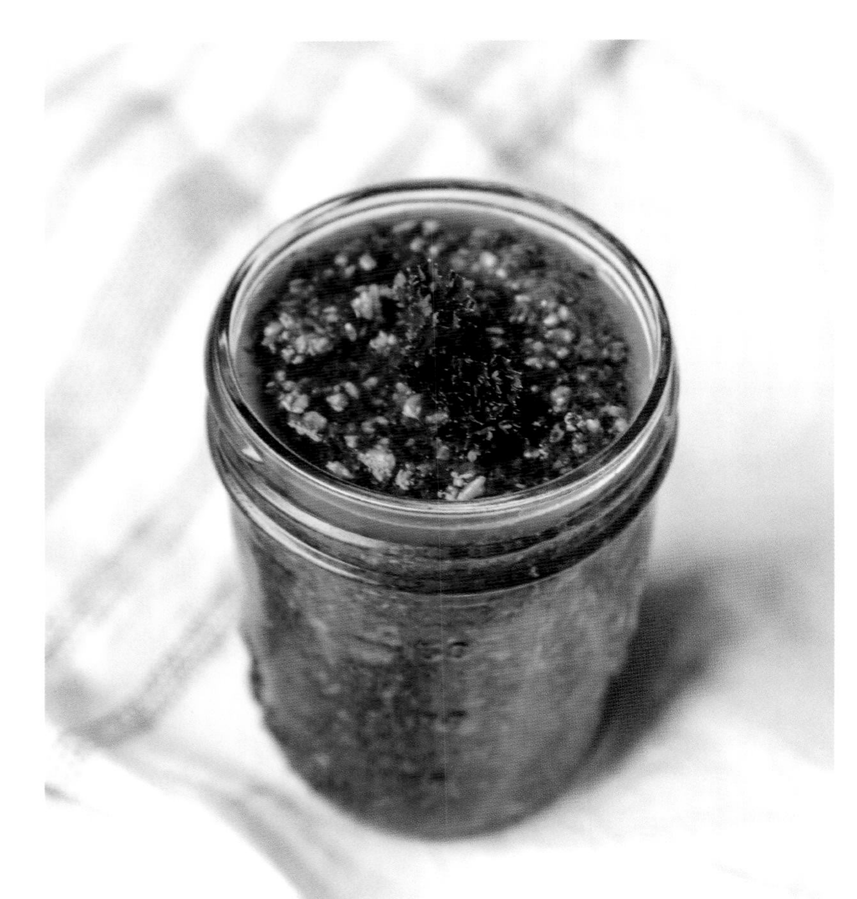

calories 152 | fat 15g | protein 2g | total carbs 1g | dietary fiber 0g | net carbs 1g

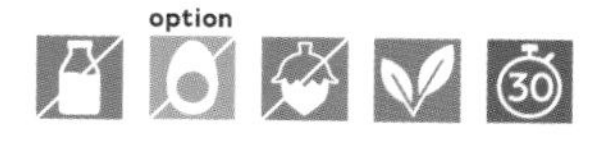

SECRET BURGER SAUCE

YIELD: 1½ cups (2 tablespoons per serving)

PREP TIME: 5 minutes

I made this special sauce for my daughter, who has been having issues with dairy, so she doesn't feel deprived when having a burger without cheese. This sauce really makes the burger delicious, and she doesn't feel like she's missing out on anything! Enjoy it on my Cheeseburger Salad Bowls (page 140) or just on top of a burger.

1 cup avocado oil mayonnaise (for egg-free, use Egg-Free Mayo, page 48)

⅓ cup sugar-free ketchup, store-bought or homemade (page 50)

3 tablespoons dill pickle relish

1 tablespoon onion powder

1 teaspoon smoked paprika

½ teaspoon apple cider vinegar

½ teaspoon garlic powder

½ teaspoon fine sea salt

1. Place all of the ingredients in a blender and blend, or whisk together in a medium bowl, until smooth.
2. Taste and adjust the spices, if desired.

Store in an airtight container in the refrigerator for up to 3 weeks.

Note: You can use homemade egg-free mayo in this recipe if using the sauce immediately. Leftover sauce will need to be warmed slightly after being refrigerated, as the mayo will gel in the fridge.

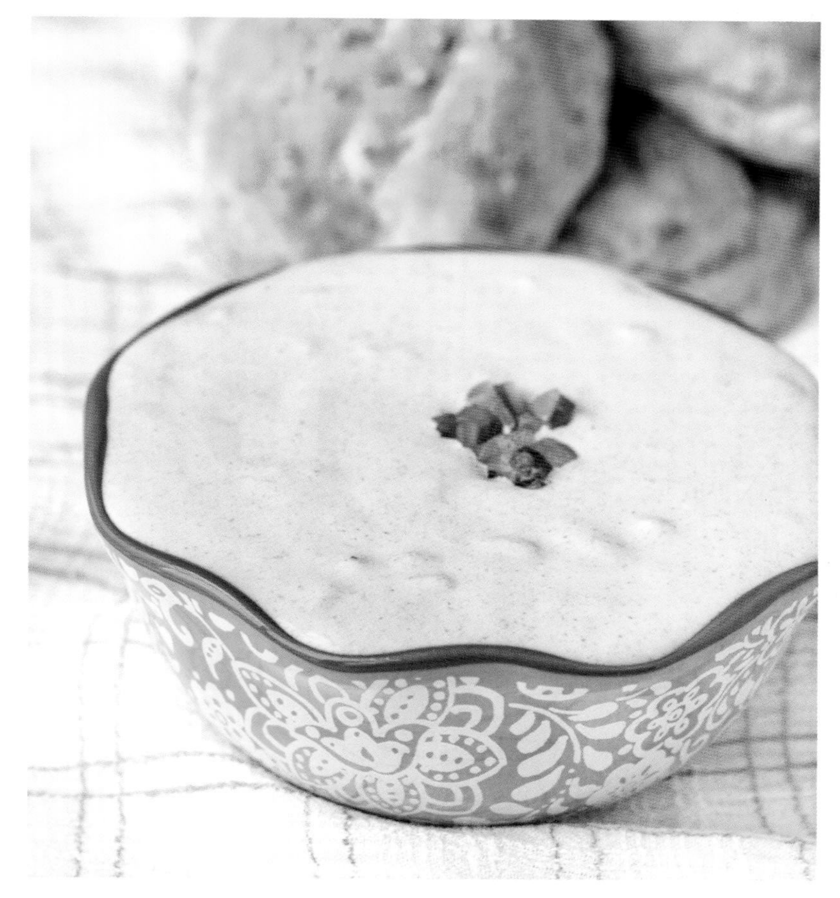

calories 133 | fat 14g | protein 0g | total carbs 1g | dietary fiber 0g | net carbs 1g

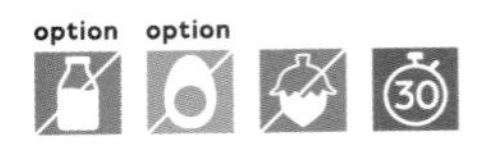

KETO BREADING

YIELD: 2 cups (2 tablespoons per serving)

PREP TIME: 5 minutes

This is the ultimate breading for just about everything. Use it to coat the chicken for my Skillet Chicken Parmesan (page 196) or for frying fish or even veggies.

- 1 cup crushed pork rinds
- 1 cup unflavored whey protein powder or egg white protein powder
- 1 tablespoon baking powder
- 1 teaspoon Italian seasoning
- 1 teaspoon fine sea salt
- ½ teaspoon freshly ground black pepper
- ½ teaspoon garlic powder
- ½ teaspoon onion powder

Store in an airtight container in the pantry for up to 1 month.

Sift all of the ingredients together into a medium bowl.

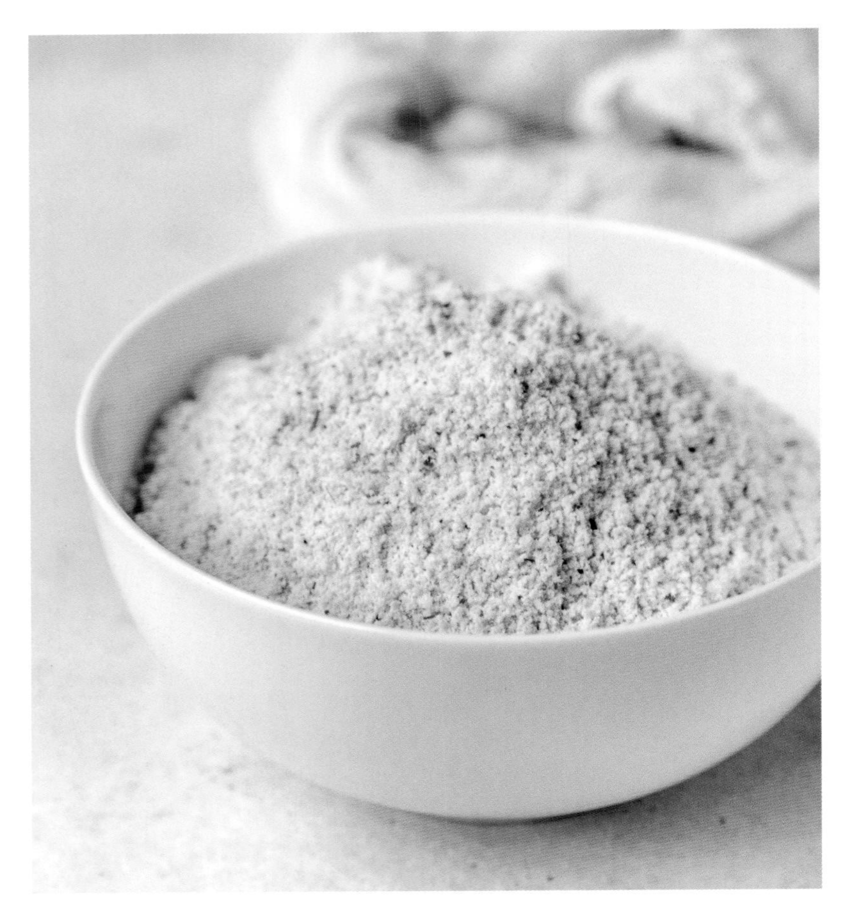

calories 39 | fat 1g | protein 8g | total carbs 1g | dietary fiber 1g | net carbs 0g

OLIVE SAUCE

YIELD: ½ cup (1 tablespoon per serving)

PREP TIME: 10 minutes

COOK TIME: 15 minutes

Enjoy this chunky olive sauce, a play on tapenade, over chicken or fish or with Focaccia (page 118) or Sesame Crackers (page 126).

- ⅓ cup balsamic vinegar
- ¼ cup sliced green olives
- ¼ cup pitted and sliced Kalamata olives
- 1 clove garlic, minced
- 3 tablespoons chopped fresh basil
- 2 tablespoons chopped fresh flat-leaf parsley
- 2 tablespoons extra-virgin olive oil
- 1 tablespoon freshly squeezed lemon juice
- 2 teaspoons drained capers
- 1 teaspoon anchovy paste
- 1 tablespoon water (optional)

Store in an airtight container in the refrigerator for up to 3 days.

1. Pour the balsamic vinegar into a small saucepan over medium-low heat and simmer for 10 to 15 minutes, or until it has thickened and reduced to about ¼ cup. Set aside to cool.

2. Place the remaining ingredients, except the water, in a small bowl and stir to combine.

3. Stir the thickened balsamic vinegar into the olive mixture. If the vinegar is too thick to pour into the olive mixture, simply stir in the water to make it pourable.

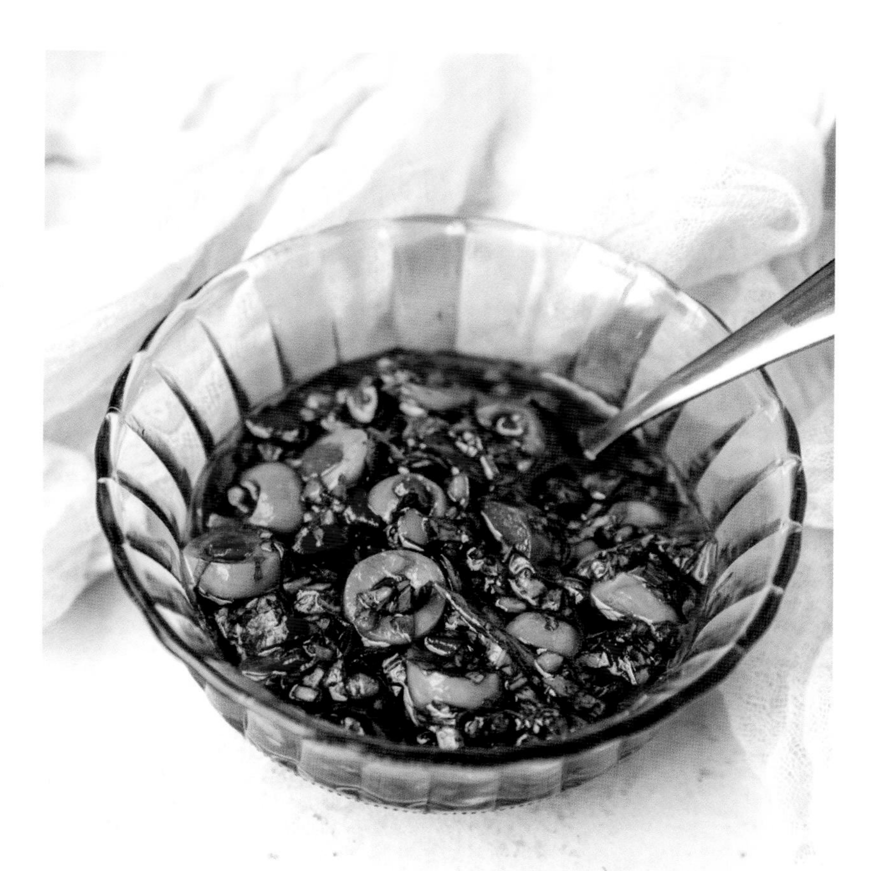

calories 55 | fat 4g | protein 0g | total carbs 2g | dietary fiber 0g | net carbs 2g

MIRACLE DOUGH PIZZA CRUST

YIELD: one 12 by 16-inch pizza crust or two 12-inch round crusts

PREP TIME: 15 minutes

Although I call this a pizza crust, there are so many options for using miracle dough—think bagels, cinnamon rolls, and so on. This recipe is perfect for making one large or two small pizzas. Plan to use it immediately; the dough doesn't store well.

4 cups (450g) shredded part-skim mozzarella cheese

4 ounces cream cheese (½ cup), softened

4 large eggs, beaten

1 cup (120g) coconut flour

1 teaspoon baking powder

1 teaspoon baking soda

½ teaspoon xanthan gum

½ teaspoon dried oregano leaves

½ teaspoon dried basil

½ teaspoon garlic powder

½ teaspoon fine sea salt

¼ teaspoon dried parsley

¼ teaspoon onion powder

TO MAKE THE DOUGH:

1. Place all of the ingredients in a food processor and process until combined.

2. Transfer the dough to a microwave-safe bowl and microwave for 2 minutes, or until melted. (If you prefer not to use a microwave, you can melt the ingredients in a saucepan over low heat.) Wet your hands with water, then knead the dough until everything is well combined.

TO USE FOR PIZZA:

1. Preheat the oven to 425°F. Line a sheet pan with parchment paper.

2. Wet your hands with water and divide the dough in half for two small pizzas, if desired. Spread the dough on the lined sheet pan as evenly as you can into one 12 by 16-inch rectangle or two 12-inch circles. Continue to wet your hands as needed to prevent the dough from sticking. Using a fork, poke holes in the crust(s).

3. Par-bake for 12 to 15 minutes, or until slightly browned. Add your desired toppings, such as tomato sauce (or marinara sauce, page 53), shredded mozzarella cheese, and sliced pepperoni and bake for 5 more minutes to melt the cheese.

calories 200 | fat 13.3g | protein 13.4g | total carbs 8.7g | dietary fiber 4g | net carbs 4.7g

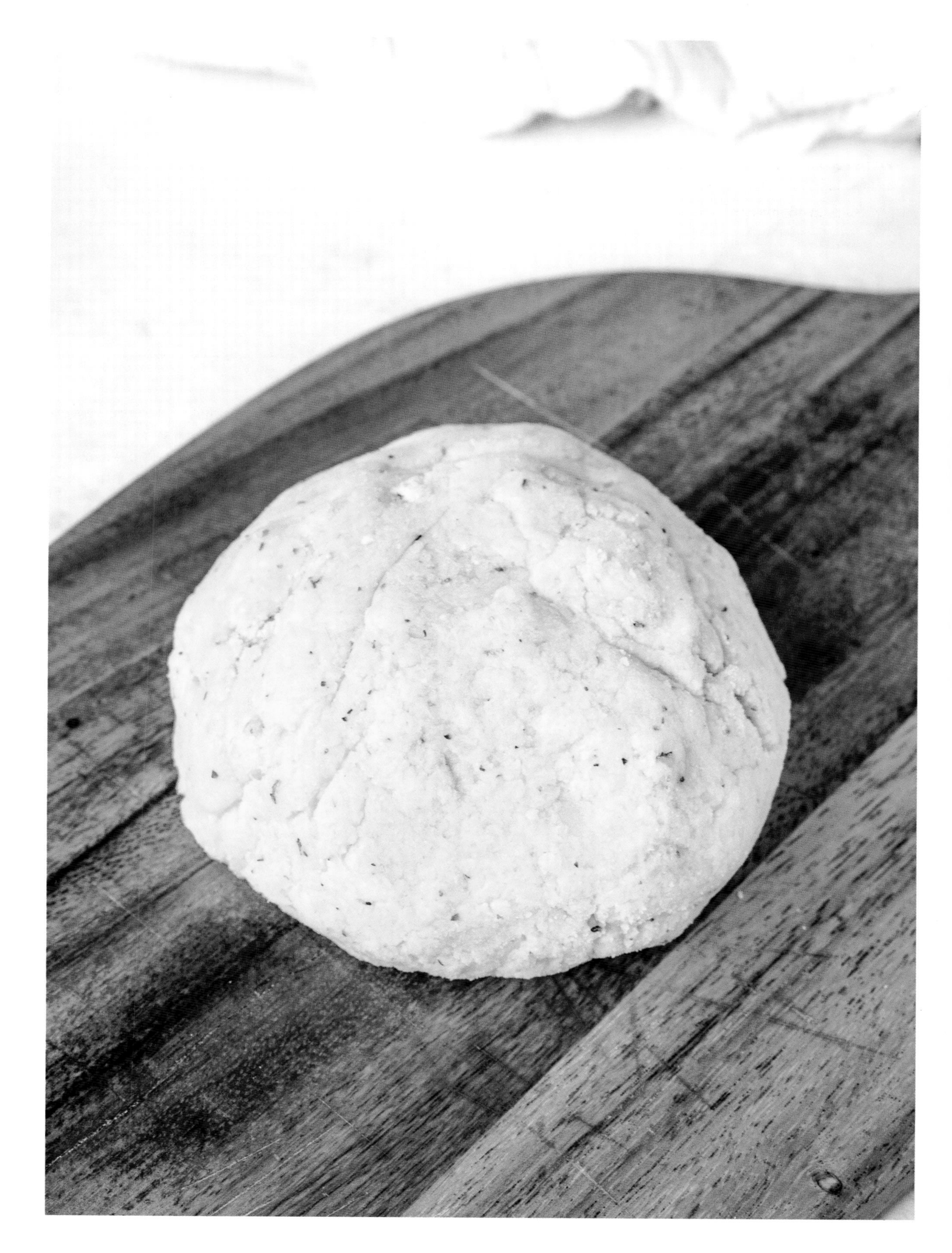

option

CAESAR DRESSING

YIELD: 2 cups (1 tablespoon per serving)

PREP TIME: 5 minutes

Creamy Caesar dressing is easy to make at home. You can leave out the anchovy paste, but if you've never tried it, I suggest keeping it in this recipe. You won't even realize it's there, but it really makes this dressing over-the-top delicious and authentic in taste, even without the traditional raw egg.

- 1 cup avocado oil mayonnaise (for egg-free, use Egg-Free Mayo, page 48)
- 1/3 cup extra-virgin olive oil
- 1/3 cup grated Parmesan cheese
- 2 1/2 tablespoons freshly squeezed lemon juice
- 2 teaspoons prepared yellow mustard
- 2 teaspoons anchovy paste (optional)
- 2 cloves garlic, minced
- 1/2 teaspoon fine sea salt
- 1/4 teaspoon freshly ground black pepper

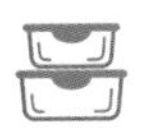
Store in an airtight container in the refrigerator for up to 1 week.

Place all of the ingredients in a blender and blend until smooth and combined. Taste and add more salt and pepper, if desired.

Note: You can use homemade egg-free mayo in this recipe if using the dressing immediately. If you need to refrigerate leftover dressing, it will need to be warmed slightly before use, as the mayo will gel in the fridge.

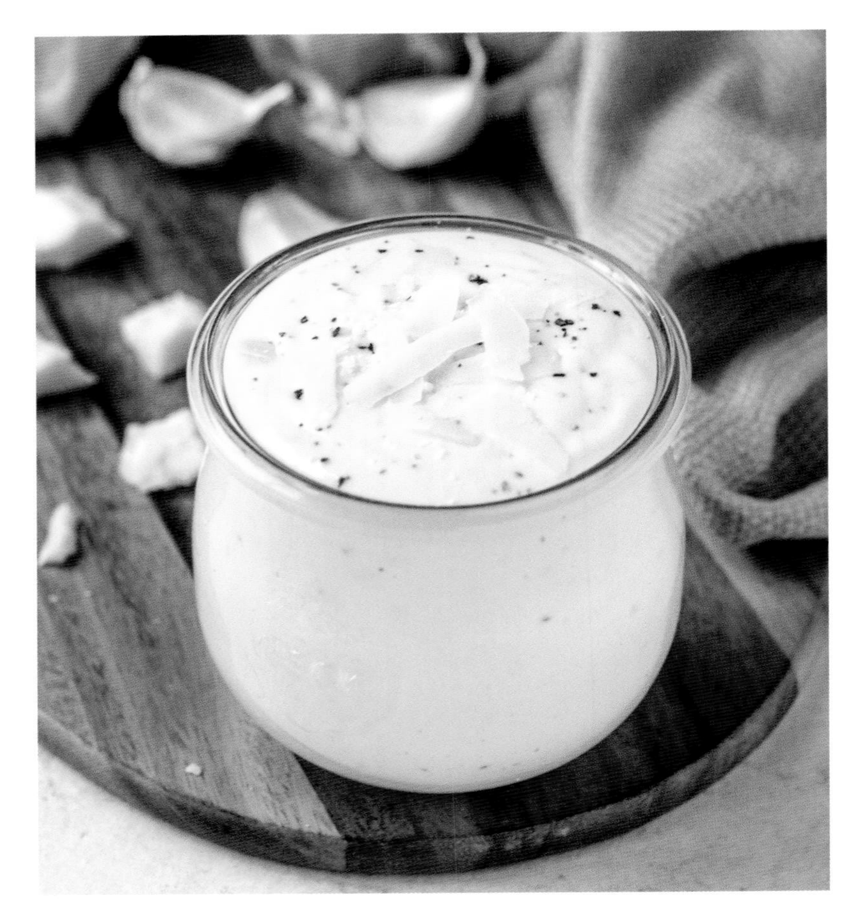

calories 152 | fat 17g | protein 1g | total carbs 0g | dietary fiber 0g | net carbs 0g

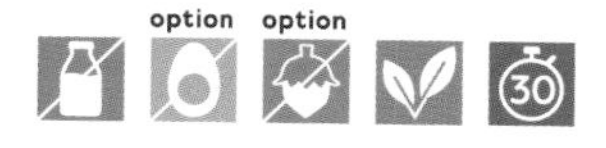

RANCH DRESSING

YIELD: 1½ cups (2 tablespoons per serving)

PREP TIME: 5 minutes

I don't know about your kids, but mine want to dip everything in ranch dressing. I'm happy to oblige and offer them this keto-friendly version with an amazing flavor!

- 1 cup avocado oil mayonnaise (for egg-free, use Egg-Free Mayo, page 48)
- ½ cup unsweetened coconut milk or nut milk of choice
- ¼ cup chopped fresh flat-leaf parsley
- 1 tablespoon freshly squeezed lemon juice
- ½ teaspoon garlic powder
- ½ teaspoon onion powder
- ½ teaspoon fine sea salt
- ¼ teaspoon freshly ground black pepper

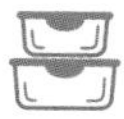

Store in an airtight container in the refrigerator for up to 10 days.

Place all of the ingredients in a blender and blend, or whisk in a medium bowl, until smooth. Taste and add more salt and pepper, if desired.

Note: You can use homemade egg-free mayo (page 48) in this recipe if using the dressing immediately. If you need to refrigerate leftover dressing, it will need to be warmed slightly, as the mayo will gel in the fridge.

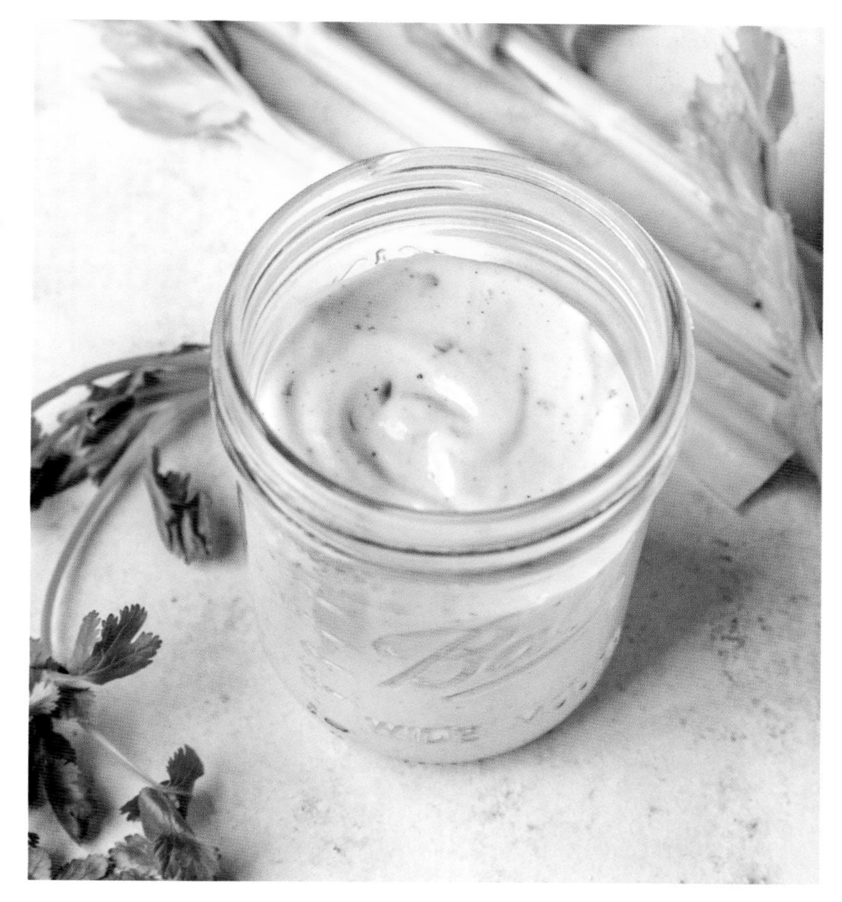

calories 157 | fat 18g | protein 0g | total carbs 0g | dietary fiber 0g | net carbs 0g

TACO SEASONING

YIELD: about 1½ cups (1 tablespoon per serving)

PREP TIME: 2 minutes

Homemade taco seasoning is perfect for simple tacos, or you can use it anytime you cook some ground beef. It's even great on chicken! Use ¼ cup per pound of meat, or more to your taste.

- ¼ cup plus 2 tablespoons chili powder
- ¼ cup plus 1 tablespoon ground cumin
- 3 tablespoons smoked paprika
- 3 tablespoons dried oregano leaves
- 3 tablespoons onion powder
- 3 tablespoons fine sea salt
- 2 tablespoons garlic powder

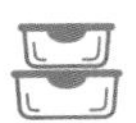 *Store in an airtight container in the pantry for up to 1 year.*

Place all of the ingredients in a small bowl and whisk to combine.

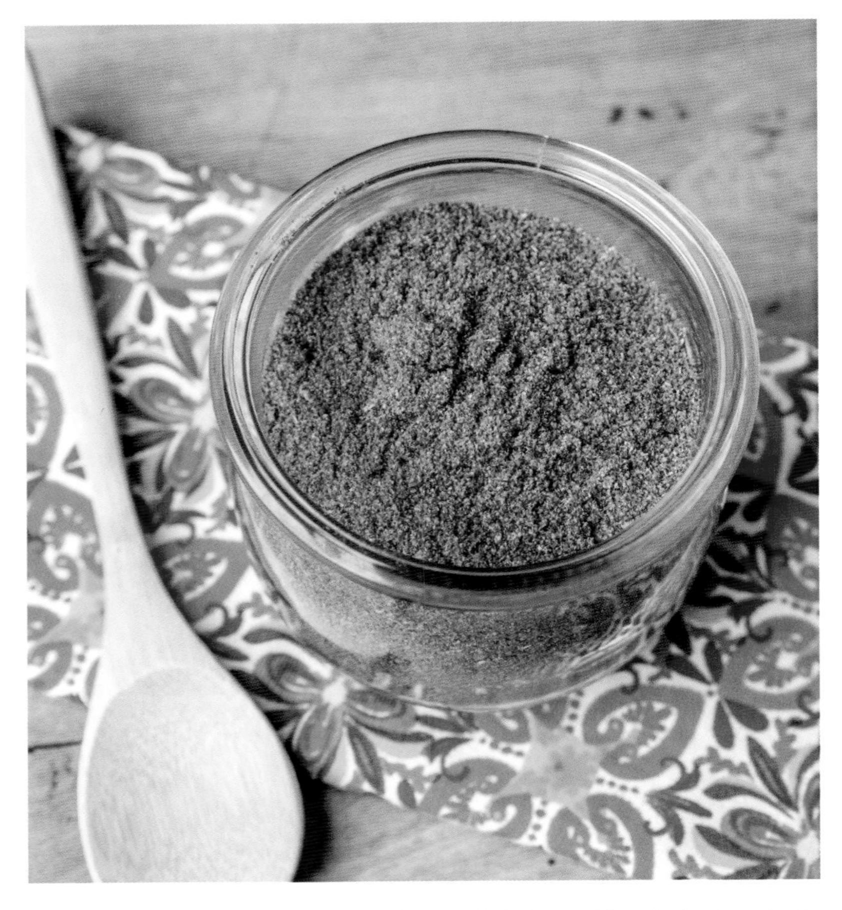

calories 9 | fat 0g | protein 0g | total carbs 2g | dietary fiber 0g | net carbs 2g

CARAMEL SAUCE

YIELD: 1¼ cups (2 tablespoons per serving)

PREP TIME: 5 minutes

COOK TIME: 20 minutes

Having a homemade caramel sauce that is keto-friendly is important in my house. My kids never feel deprived (and neither do I) when they can enjoy this sauce over Vanilla Gelato (page 254) or Apple Crisp (page 222)!

- 6 tablespoons (¾ stick) unsalted butter
- 1 cup heavy whipping cream
- ½ cup packed Swerve brown sugar sweetener
- 2 tablespoons yacón syrup or sugar-free maple syrup, store-bought or homemade (page 70)
- 2 teaspoons caramel extract
- 1 teaspoon vanilla extract
- ½ teaspoon ground cinnamon
- ¼ teaspoon fine sea salt
- ¼ teaspoon xanthan gum

Store in an airtight container in the refrigerator for up to 1 month. It will continue to thicken as it cools. Rewarm before serving.

1. Brown the butter in a large saucepan over medium heat. Once it's dark in color, add the cream and reduce the heat to low.
2. Whisk in the remaining ingredients and bring to a boil over medium heat. Continue to stir for 3 to 5 minutes, or until the sauce thickens. If using an electric stove, to help manage the temperature, lift the pan on and off the heat as needed so the sauce doesn't boil over.
3. Allow to cool slightly before serving.

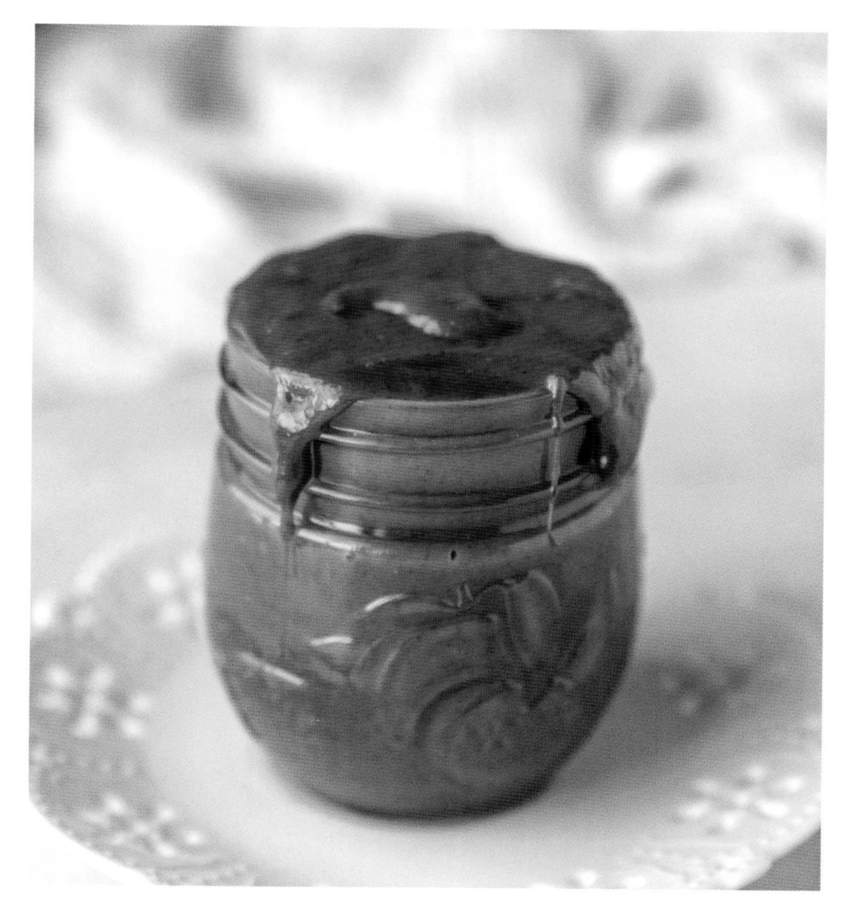

calories 144 | fat 14g | protein 0g | total carbs 1g | dietary fiber 0g | net carbs 1g

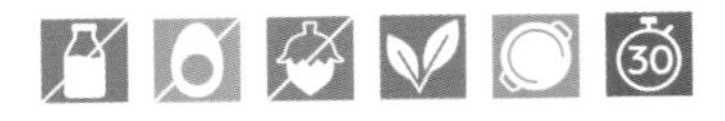

BLUEBERRY SYRUP

YIELD: 1 cup (2 tablespoons per serving)

PREP TIME: 5 minutes

COOK TIME: 15 minutes

This berry syrup is delicious served warm over Fluffy Keto Pancakes (page 96) or Coconut Flour Waffles (page 95), or served chilled in my Mini Crustless Blueberry Lemon Cheesecakes (page 242) or over keto ice cream.

8 ounces fresh blueberries

1/2 cup water

2 tablespoons freshly squeezed lemon juice

1/3 cup Swerve confectioners'-style sweetener

Pinch of fine sea salt

1. Place all of the ingredients in a small saucepan and bring to a boil.

2. Simmer the berries, smashing and stirring them constantly, until thickened, 10 to 12 minutes. Let cool slightly, then serve warm, or refrigerate and serve chilled.

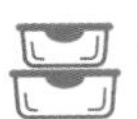

Store in an airtight container in the refrigerator for up to 1 week.

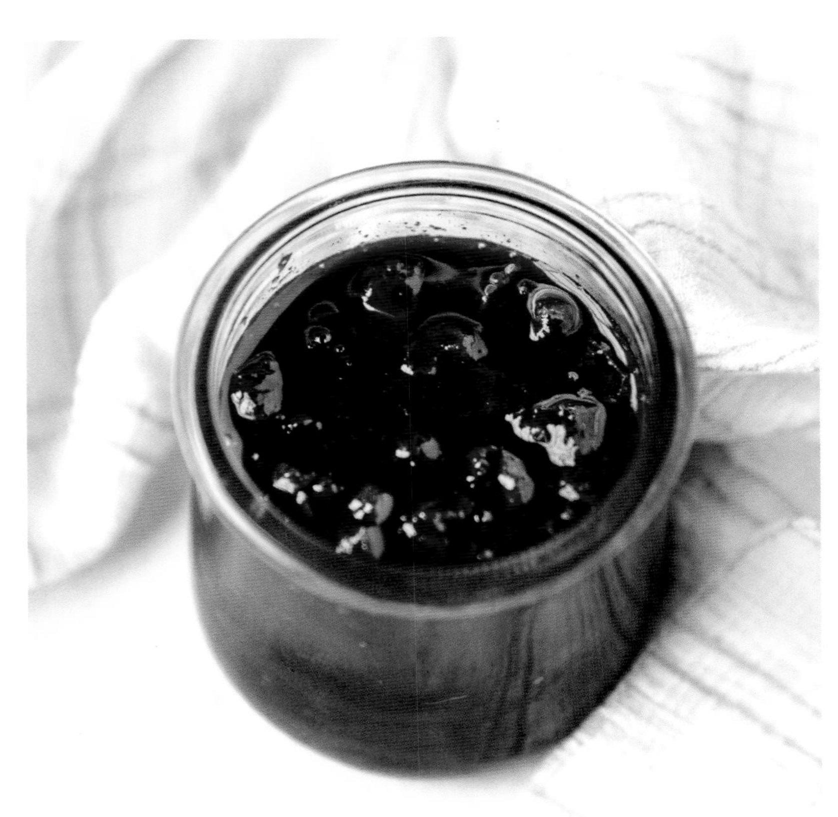

calories 16 | fat 0g | protein 0g | total carbs 4g | dietary fiber 0g | net carbs 4g

HOT FUDGE SAUCE

YIELD: 2¾ cups (2 tablespoons per serving)

PREP TIME: 5 minutes

COOK TIME: 15 minutes

This hot fudge sauce is the perfect accompaniment for ice cream or simply for topping whipped cream. After it thickens in the refrigerator, you can spoon it out and roll it up like a truffle if you want.

4 ounces dark chocolate (85% cacao), chopped

½ cup (1 stick) unsalted butter

1½ cups heavy whipping cream

⅓ cup Swerve confectioners'-style sweetener

½ teaspoon instant espresso powder or instant coffee granules

⅛ teaspoon fine sea salt

2 teaspoons vanilla extract

¼ teaspoon chocolate- or vanilla-flavored liquid stevia

Store in an airtight container in the refrigerator for up to 2 weeks. Place a piece of plastic wrap directly on top of the sauce to prevent a skin from forming. This sauce will thicken in the refrigerator and will need a quick reheating on the stovetop over low heat, or microwave for 1 minute to warm it through.

1. Melt the chocolate and butter in a heavy saucepan over low heat. Stir until smooth.

2. Whisk in the cream, confectioners'-style sweetener, espresso powder, and salt. Bring to a boil, stirring continuously. If using an electric stove, you may need to move your pan on and off the heat to manage the temperature. Cook for about 5 minutes, or until the sauce is bubbling and thickened.

3. Remove from the heat and stir in the vanilla extract and stevia. Serve warm.

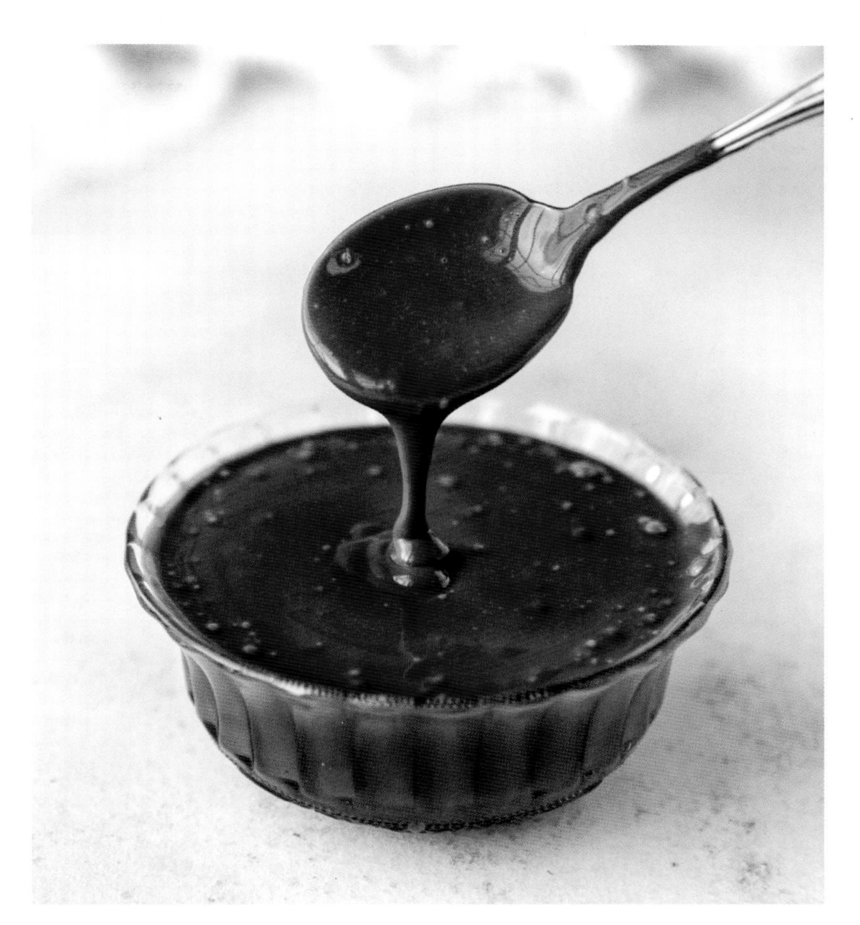

calories 153 | fat 14g | protein 0g | total carbs 2g | dietary fiber 1g | net carbs 1g

COCONUT WHIPPED CREAM

YIELD: ¾ cup (2 tablespoons per serving)

PREP TIME: 10 minutes, plus time to chill coconut milk

Dairy-free, sugar-free whipped cream made with canned coconut milk is a fantastic alternative to dairy whipped cream! The key to making this coconut whipped cream is letting the can sit overnight in the refrigerator. This will produce a thick cream that rises to the top, which you will scoop out for this recipe; leave the coconut water at the bottom of the can for use in a smoothie or another recipe. Whipped coconut cream will continue to thicken in the fridge. Enjoy on top of my Quick Strawberry Shortcakes (page 248).

1 (13½-ounce) can full-fat coconut milk (see Notes)

1 tablespoon Swerve confectioners'-style sweetener

¼ teaspoon vanilla-flavored liquid stevia

½ teaspoon vanilla extract

1. Without shaking the can, place the can of coconut milk in the refrigerator overnight. This will allow the cream to rise to the top of the can.

2. Remove the can from the refrigerator and flip it upside down. This will allow the watery coconut milk to easily be removed from the can. Open the can and discard the watery liquid. Scoop the chilled coconut cream into the bowl of a stand mixer (or a medium bowl if using an electric hand mixer).

3. Add the sweeteners and vanilla extract and, using the whisk attachment, beat on high speed until the mixture becomes thick; it may take up to 10 minutes.

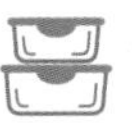

Store in an airtight container in the refrigerator for up to 5 days.

Notes: This recipe will not work with anything other than canned full-fat coconut milk that contains guar gum. The brands that work best for me are Thai Kitchen, Native Forest, and 365 Whole Foods.

If you would like your whipped cream to have a lighter, airier texture, you can include some of the separated coconut water from the can of coconut milk rather than discard all of the liquid. Some brands yield more liquid than others, so measure the amount of coconut water in the can. Use no more than ⅓ cup of the coconut water—any more than that and your coconut milk will not whip to the right consistency.

calories 52 | fat 5g | protein 0g | total carbs 1g | dietary fiber 0g | net carbs 1g

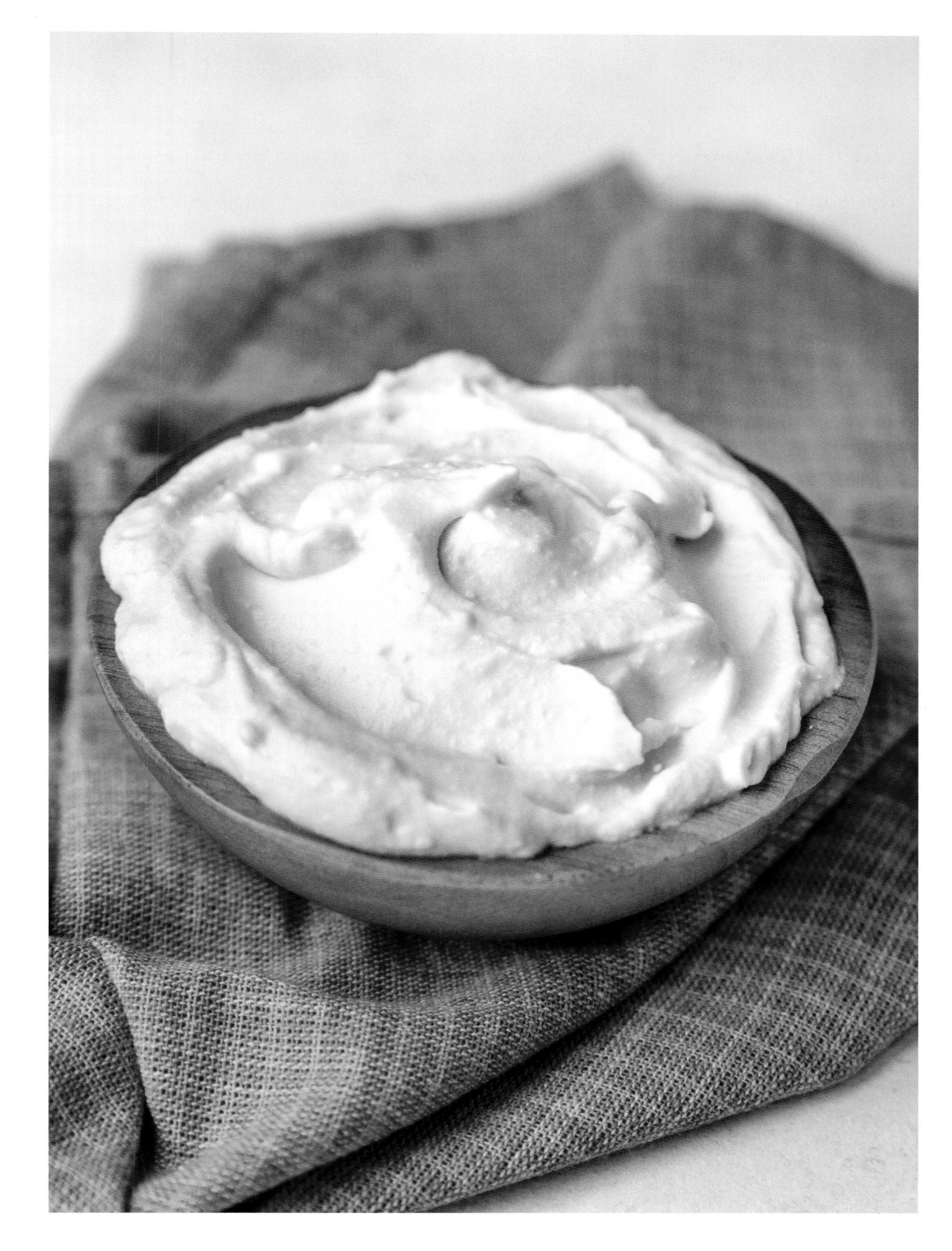

option

COCONUT FLOUR PIE CRUST

YIELD: one 9-inch pie crust (12 servings)

PREP TIME: 10 minutes

COOK TIME: 10 minutes

Every keto cook needs a recipe for a perfectly flaky pie crust that can easily work for both sweet and savory pies. I perfected this one years ago. Even my Italian mother couldn't believe how flaky this crust is. I use it for quiche and for sweet pies, and everyone, including non-keto family members and friends, loves it!

2 large eggs

1 tablespoon extra-virgin olive oil

1 teaspoon vanilla extract

1 cup (120g) coconut flour

1/4 cup (56g) Swerve granular sweetener

1/4 teaspoon fine sea salt

1/2 cup (1 stick) cold salted butter (or softened coconut oil for dairy-free), cut into cubes

1. Preheat the oven to 400°F. Grease a 9-inch pie pan or line it with parchment paper.

2. Place the eggs, oil, and vanilla extract in a food processor and pulse until combined.

3. Add the flour, sweetener, and salt and process until combined.

4. Add the cubed butter and pulse until fine crumbles form.

5. Remove the dough from the processor and place in the prepared pie pan. Wet your hands with water. Using your fingers, press the dough out, as evenly as possible, across the bottom and up the sides of the pan. Use a fork to randomly poke holes in the bottom of the crust.

6. If using this crust for a pie that will be baked further, cover the edges with aluminum foil. (If you will be adding a no-bake filling, there is no need to cover the edges.) Bake the crust for 10 minutes, or until golden. Remove from the oven and let cool.

7. Once cool, add your filling.

VARIATION: SAVORY PIE CRUST. If using this crust for a savory pie, omit the vanilla extract and Swerve granular sweetener.

calories 129 | fat 10g | protein 2g | total carbs 5g | dietary fiber 3g | net carbs 2g

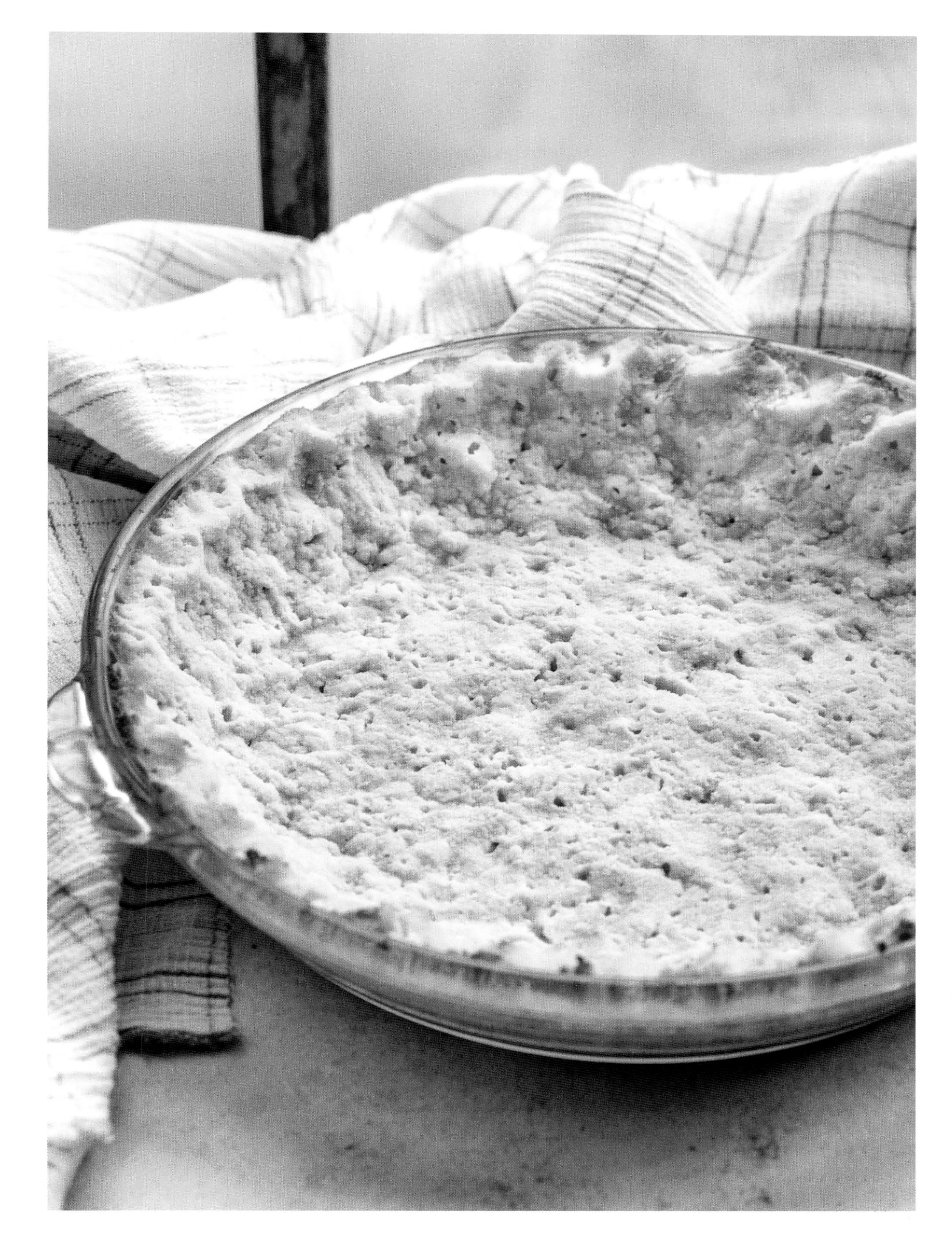

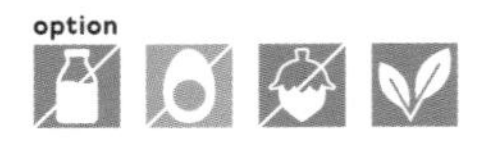

SUGAR-FREE MAPLE SYRUP

YIELD: 1¼ cups (2 tablespoons per serving)

PREP TIME: 5 minutes, plus 30 minutes to cool

COOK TIME: 20 minutes

You can certainly buy sugar-free maple syrup, but it can be costly. Making it at home ensures that you can choose your sweetener as well as how sweet you like the syrup to be. It's best to use a brown sugar substitute if you want that authentic maple syrup flavor. If you don't have yacón syrup, you can use molasses in its place; it will not change the carb count.

1 tablespoon unsalted butter, ghee, or coconut oil

1½ cups water

1 tablespoon yacón syrup or molasses

½ cup packed Swerve brown sugar sweetener

½ teaspoon ground cinnamon

¼ teaspoon fine sea salt

½ teaspoon xanthan gum

2 teaspoons maple extract

1 teaspoon vanilla extract

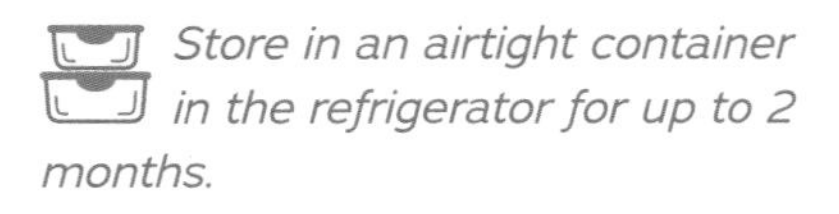

Store in an airtight container in the refrigerator for up to 2 months.

1. Brown the butter in a saucepan over medium-high heat.
2. Pour in the water, yacón syrup, brown sugar sweetener, cinnamon, and salt. Whisk together and bring to a boil, then reduce the heat to a simmer.
3. Sprinkle in the xanthan gum a little at a time while whisking. Continue simmering for about 10 minutes, or until the syrup thickens.
4. Remove from the heat and stir in the extracts. Allow the syrup to cool for 30 minutes; it will thicken as it cools. Serve warm.

calories 15 | fat 1g | protein 0g | total carbs 1g | dietary fiber 0g | net carbs 1g

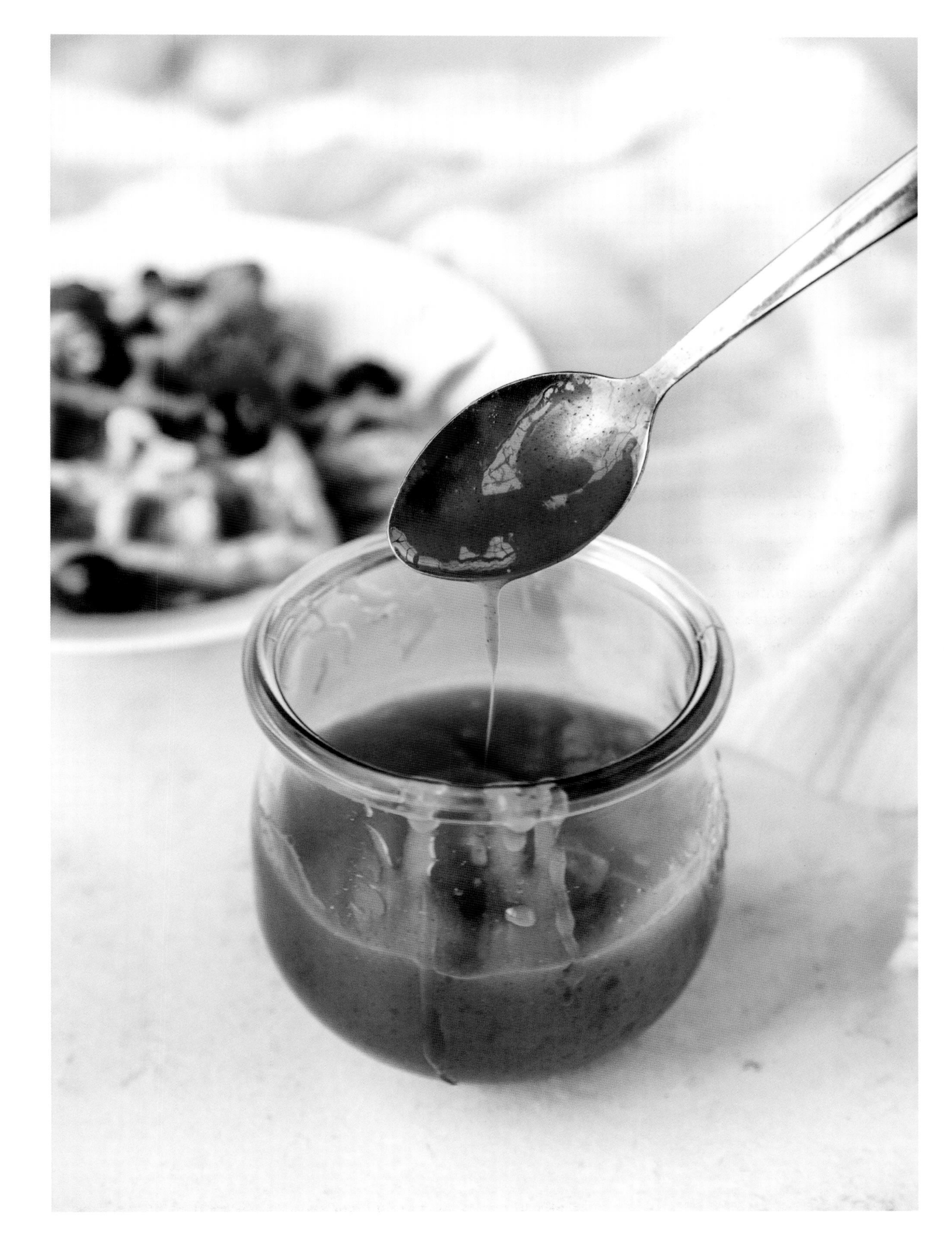

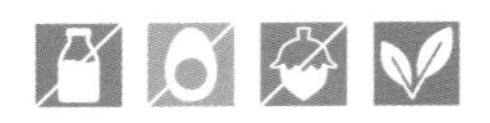

RASPBERRY CHIA JAM

YIELD: ¾ cup (2 tablespoons per serving)

PREP TIME: 2 minutes, plus 1 hour to chill

This simple but delicious jam is terrific on my 2-Minute English Muffins (page 88)!

- 2 cups fresh raspberries
- 2 tablespoons Swerve confectioners'-style sweetener
- 1 tablespoon freshly squeezed lemon juice
- 1 tablespoon water
- ½ teaspoon lemon-flavored liquid stevia
- Pinch of fine sea salt
- 3 tablespoons chia seeds

Store in an airtight container in the refrigerator for up to 2 weeks.

1. Place all of the ingredients except the chia seeds in a high-powered blender or food processor and blend on high until smooth or to the desired texture. Taste and add more sweetener and/or salt, if desired.
2. Add the chia seeds and pulse two or three times to combine. Allow to cool.
3. Pour the jam into a mason jar, cover, and refrigerate for 1 hour before using.

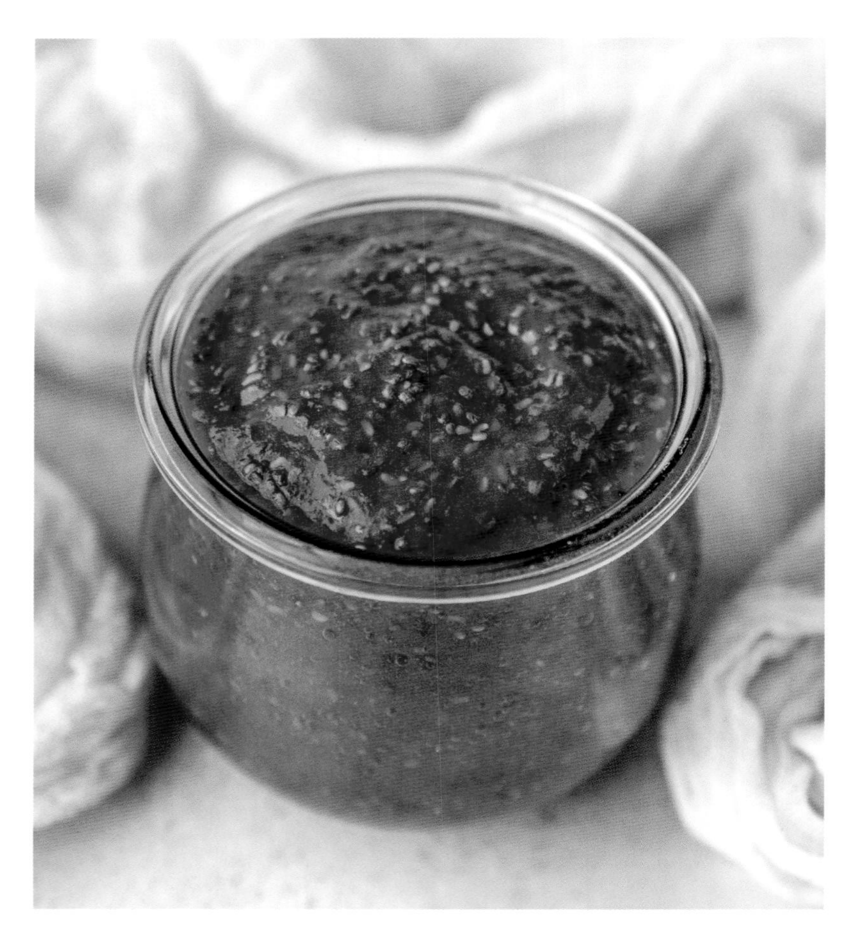

calories 50 | fat 2g | protein 1g | total carbs 7g | dietary fiber 4g | net carbs 3g

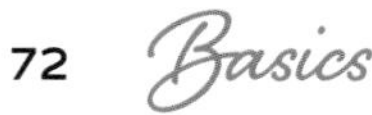

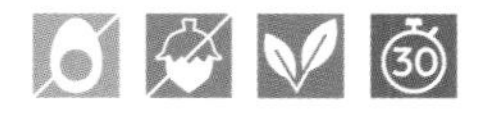

WHIPPED CREAM

YIELD: 2 cups (1/4 cup per serving)

PREP TIME: 5 minutes

I enjoy whipped cream on just about everything. In fact, I even enjoy it on top of a couple tablespoons of peanut butter! For you, I suggest trying it on iced coffee or any dessert.

1 cup heavy whipping cream

1/4 cup Swerve confectioners'-style sweetener

1/2 teaspoon vanilla extract

1/4 teaspoon vanilla-flavored liquid stevia (optional)

Place all of the ingredients in the bowl of a stand mixer fitted with the whisk attachment (or a medium bowl if using an electric hand mixer). Whisk on high until soft peaks form, 3 to 4 minutes.

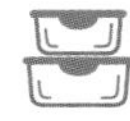

Store in an airtight container in the refrigerator for up to 2 days.

Tip: Place the whisk attachment and mixing bowl in the freezer for 10 minutes to make beating the cream even quicker!

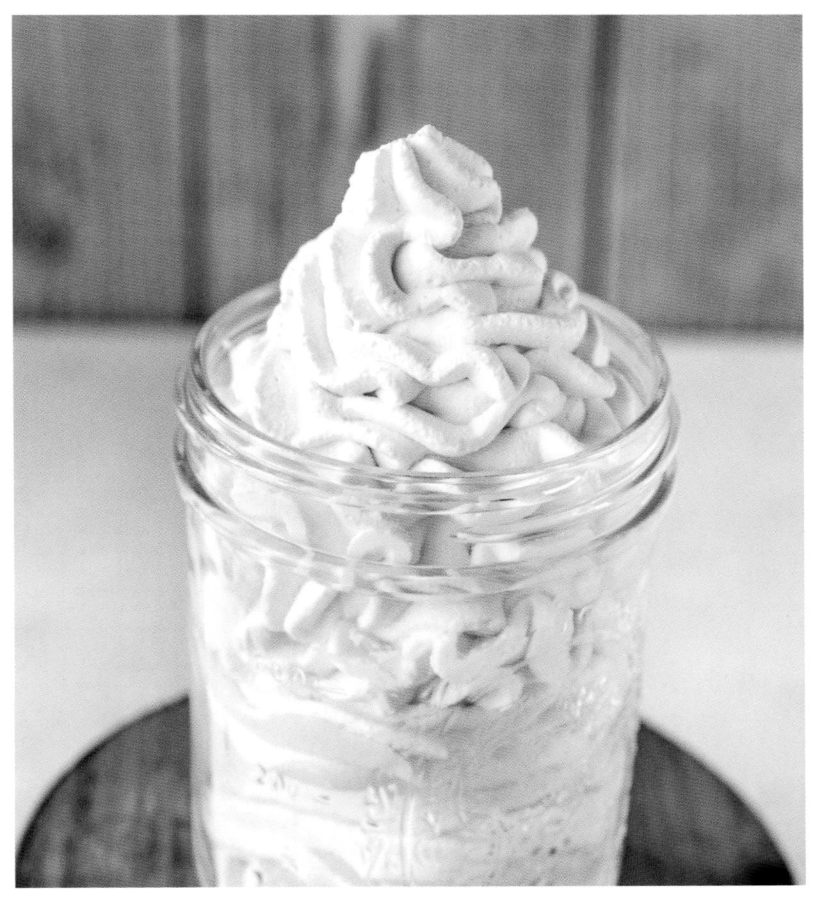

calories 100 | fat 10g | protein 0g | total carbs 0g | dietary fiber 0g | net carbs 0g

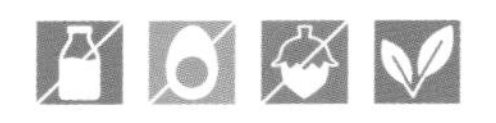

SALTED CARAMEL SUNFLOWER SEED BUTTER

YIELD: 2 cups (2 tablespoons per serving)

PREP TIME: 20 minutes

COOK TIME: 12 minutes

If you have a nut allergy and have bought sunflower seed butter, you know how hard it is to find one that does not contain sugar. And when you do find it, it's expensive. You won't need to buy it anymore. In fact, I can say that this homemade version tastes even better than store-bought.

2 cups raw sunflower seeds

1/3 cup packed Swerve brown sugar sweetener

3 tablespoons coconut oil, plus more if needed

1/2 teaspoon ground cinnamon

1/2 teaspoon fine sea salt

1/2 teaspoon cinnamon-flavored liquid stevia (optional)

Store in an airtight container in the refrigerator for up to 3 months.

1. Preheat the oven to 325°F.

2. Spread the sunflower seeds in an even layer on a sheet pan and bake for 10 to 12 minutes, or until golden. Let cool.

3. Put the cooled seeds in a food processor along with the brown sugar sweetener and coconut oil. Blend for a few minutes, then stop and scrape down the sides of the processor. Continue to process until the butter is smooth or has the texture you prefer. You can add more coconut oil and process more to make the butter even smoother.

4. Add the cinnamon, salt, and stevia, if desired, and pulse until combined. Taste and add more salt, if needed.

calories 120 | fat 24g | protein 3g | total carbs 3g | dietary fiber 1g | net carbs 2g

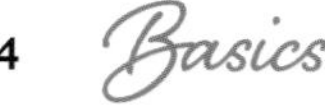

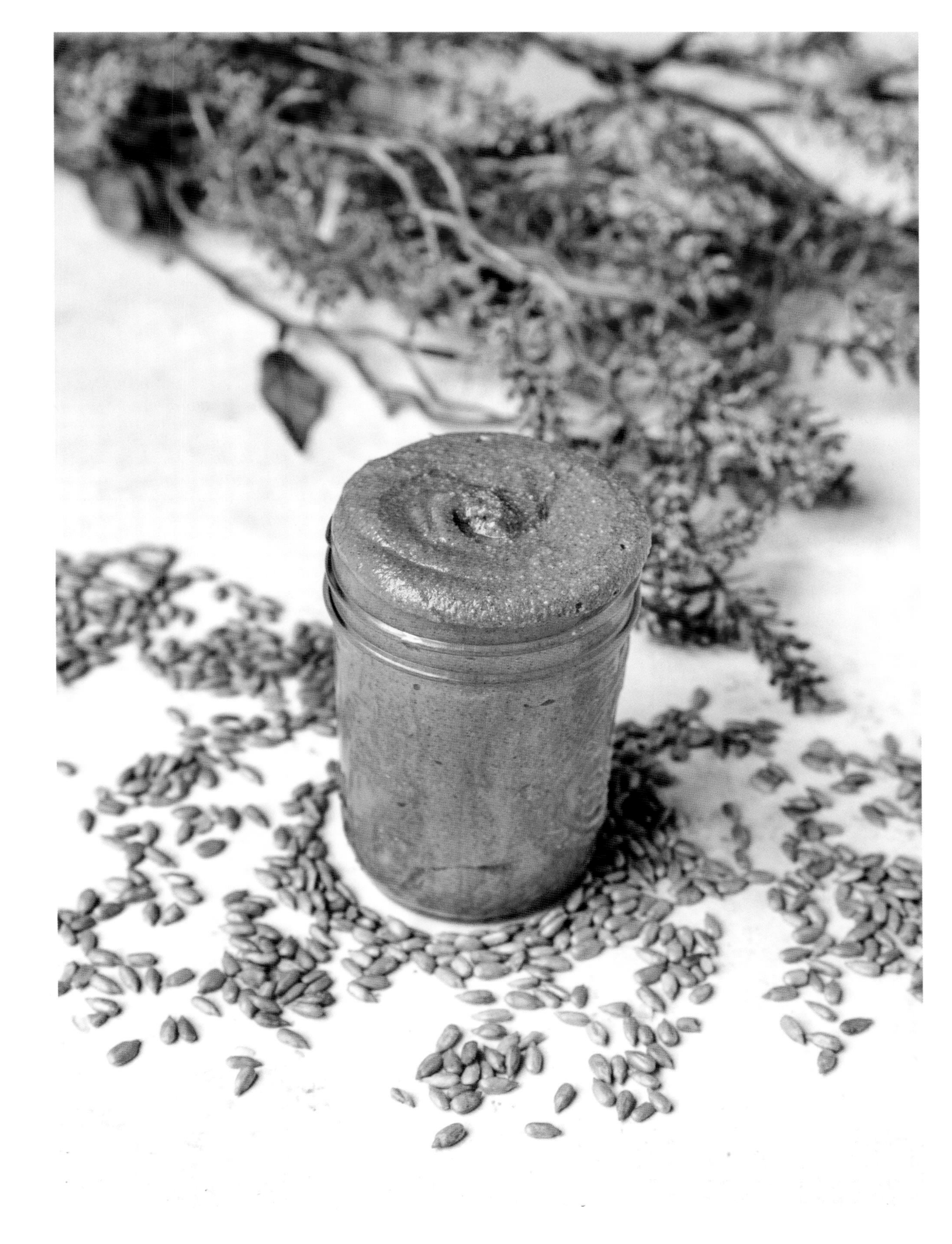

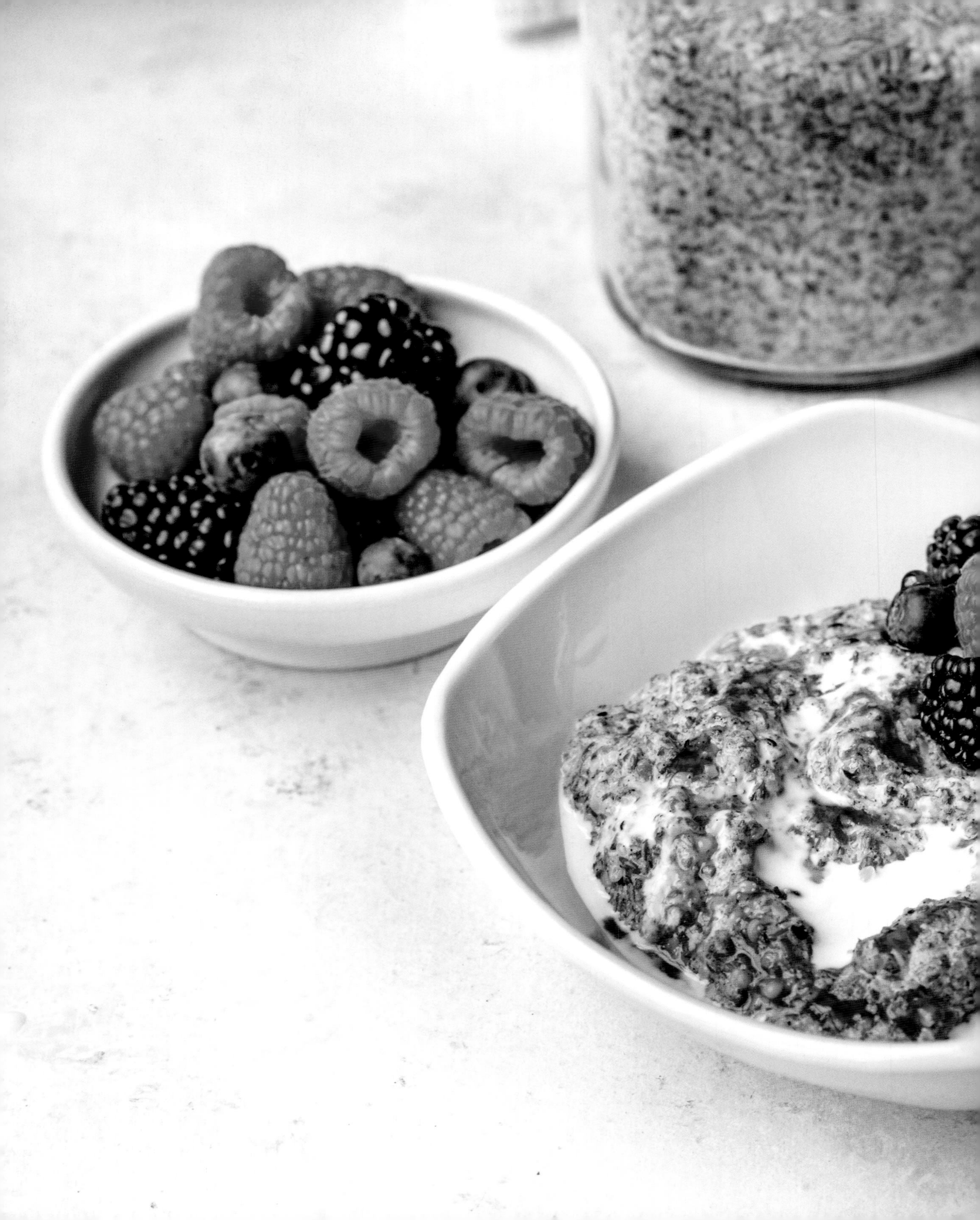

Breakfast

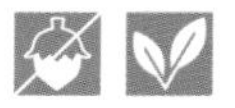

BAKED FRENCH TOAST

YIELD: 12 servings

PREP TIME: 5 minutes, plus 1 hour to chill (not including time to make bread)

COOK TIME: 40 minutes

I'm always looking to get the biggest bang for my buck in the kitchen, so to speak. I honestly hate standing at the stove to cook large amounts of food. That's why I opted to bake this French toast instead of cooking it the traditional way. Stovetop directions are also provided if you prefer.

- 1 batch Cloud Bread Loaf (made without garlic and onion powder) (page 112)
- 4 large eggs
- 3/4 cup heavy whipping cream
- 1 tablespoon vanilla extract
- 1 teaspoon vanilla-flavored liquid stevia, or 1/3 cup Swerve granular sweetener
- 1 teaspoon ground cinnamon
- 1/4 teaspoon fine sea salt
- 1/4 cup (1/2 stick) salted butter
- 1/2 cup packed Swerve brown sugar sweetener
- Swerve confectioners'-style sweetener, for sprinkling (optional)

1. Cut the bread into 12 slices and set aside.
2. In a large bowl, whisk together the eggs, cream, vanilla extract, stevia, cinnamon, and salt, then pour the mixture into a 13 by 9-inch baking dish. Lay the slices of bread in the dish and flip them over to coat the other side. Cover and refrigerate for at least 1 hour, preferably overnight.
3. When ready to bake, preheat the oven to 350°F. Remove the dish from the refrigerator and place the soaked bread slices on a sheet pan.
4. Melt the butter, then mix in the brown sugar sweetener until thoroughly combined. Pour the brown sugar mixture over the bread slices and cover with aluminum foil.
5. Bake for 30 minutes, remove the foil, and bake for an additional 5 to 10 minutes, or until the outer edges look crisp. Sprinkle with confectioners'-style sweetener before serving, if desired.

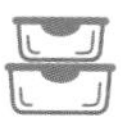

Store in an airtight container in the refrigerator for up to 3 days.

STOVETOP OPTION: *Follow instructions through Step 2. Heat half of the butter in a large skillet over medium-high heat. Place half of the slices into the hot pan and cook for a couple of minutes until the bottom of each slice of bread is nicely browned. While it's cooking, sprinkle half of the brown sugar sweetener over the slices. Once cooked on the bottom, flip the slices over and cook for a few more minutes until nicely browned. Repeat with the remaining slices, butter, and brown sugar sweetener. Top with confectioners'-style sweetener before serving, if desired, and enjoy!*

calories 192 | fat 14g | protein 9g | total carbs 1g | dietary fiber 0g | net carbs 1g

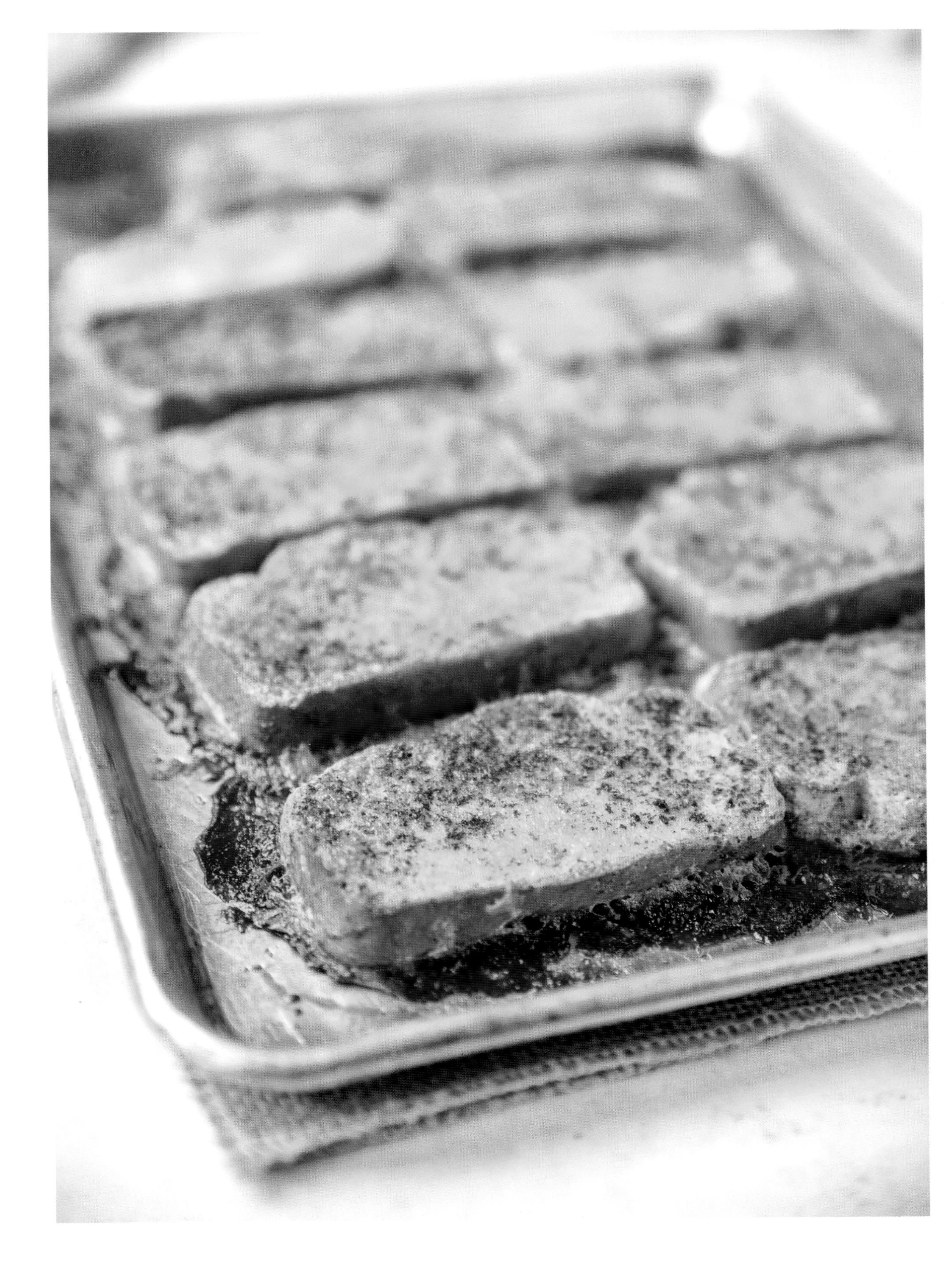

BISCUITS AND GRAVY

YIELD: 6 servings

PREP TIME: 2 minutes (not including time to make rolls)

COOK TIME: 20 minutes

If it weren't for my husband, I probably never would have tried biscuits and gravy. I'm Italian, and we like our sausage in tomato sauce, not a white sauce. But I married a man who, although he wasn't born in the South, has traveled extensively, and he loves a good biscuits and gravy for breakfast. I have become a fan, and I hope you will, too.

1 pound bulk breakfast sausage

¼ cup (½ stick) salted butter

1 cup beef bone broth

1 cup heavy whipping cream

1 teaspoon freshly ground black pepper

½ teaspoon xanthan gum

6 Hamburger Rolls (page 122)

Chopped fresh flat-leaf parsley, for garnish

Store the gravy in an airtight container in the refrigerator for up to 3 days.

1. Cook the sausage in a large skillet over medium-high heat, stirring often to crumble the meat, until browned and no longer pink, about 10 minutes.

2. Reduce the heat to low and remove the sausage with a slotted spoon, leaving the drippings in the skillet. Add the butter and heat until melted.

3. Stir in the broth and cream, increase the heat to medium-high, and bring to a boil, scraping the browned bits on the bottom of the pan.

4. Once boiling, reduce the heat to a simmer. Add the pepper and sprinkle the gravy with the xanthan gum, then continue to stir until thickened, about 5 minutes.

5. Return the sausage to the skillet and stir to coat with the gravy. Serve the gravy over the rolls and garnish with parsley, if desired.

calories 637 | fat 56g | protein 13g | total carbs 10g | dietary fiber 5g | net carbs 5g

| GRAVY ONLY | calories 438 | fat 41g | protein 12g | total carbs 0g | dietary fiber 0g | net carbs 0g

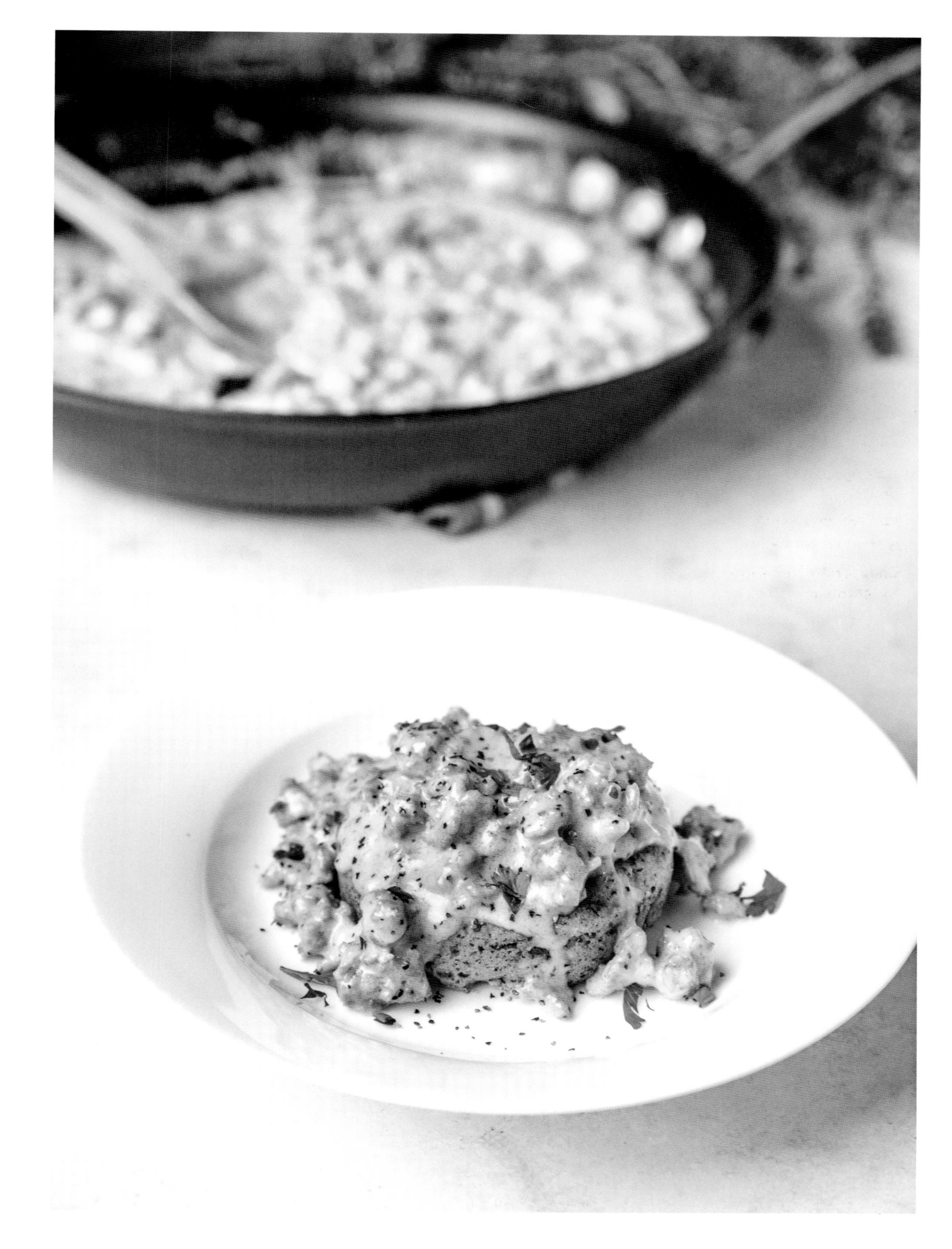

CINNAMON CRUMB MUFFINS

YIELD: 12 muffins (1 per serving)

PREP TIME: 20 minutes

COOK TIME: 35 minutes

These muffins were adapted from my popular chocolate chip muffin recipe on my website. The crumb topping makes them extra special!

- 1/2 cup (1 stick) unsalted butter, softened
- 1/2 cup sour cream
- 1 cup (120g) coconut flour
- 1/2 cup (95g) packed Swerve brown sugar sweetener
- 2 teaspoons ground cinnamon
- 1 teaspoon baking powder
- 1 teaspoon baking soda
- 1 teaspoon xanthan gum
- 1/2 teaspoon fine sea salt
- 6 large eggs (see Tip)
- 1/2 cup heavy whipping cream
- 1 teaspoon maple extract
- 1/2 teaspoon vanilla-flavored liquid stevia

FOR THE CINNAMON CRUMB TOPPING

- 1/4 cup (1/2 stick) salted butter, softened
- 1/2 cup coconut flour
- 1/2 cup packed Swerve brown sugar sweetener
- 1 teaspoon ground cinnamon

1. Preheat the oven to 350°F. Grease a standard-size 12-well muffin pan or use 12 silicone cupcake liners.

2. Place the butter, sour cream, coconut flour, brown sugar sweetener, cinnamon, baking powder, baking soda, xanthan gum, and salt in the bowl of a stand mixer (or a medium bowl if using an electric hand mixer) and mix on high until well combined.

3. Turn the mixer to low speed and add the eggs one at a time, mixing until incorporated before each addition. Add the cream, maple extract, and stevia and mix until combined.

4. Spoon the batter evenly into the prepared muffin pan.

5. Make the cinnamon crumb topping: Place all of the topping ingredients in a small bowl. Mix well until crumbs form. Sprinkle the topping over the muffins.

6. Bake for 20 minutes, then remove from the oven and cover the muffins loosely with aluminum foil to prevent the crumb topping from burning. Bake for another 10 to 15 minutes, or until a toothpick inserted in the center of a muffin comes out clean.

7. Let cool in the pan for 10 minutes before removing. Enjoy!

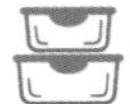

Store in an airtight container in the refrigerator for up to 5 days.

Tip: Some eggs are larger than others—especially if you use farm-fresh eggs. To achieve the perfect result, remember that one large egg in the shell weighs about 2 ounces, and the yolk and white measure about 1/4 cup.

calories 249 | fat 20g | protein 5g | total carbs 9g | dietary fiber 5g | net carbs 4g

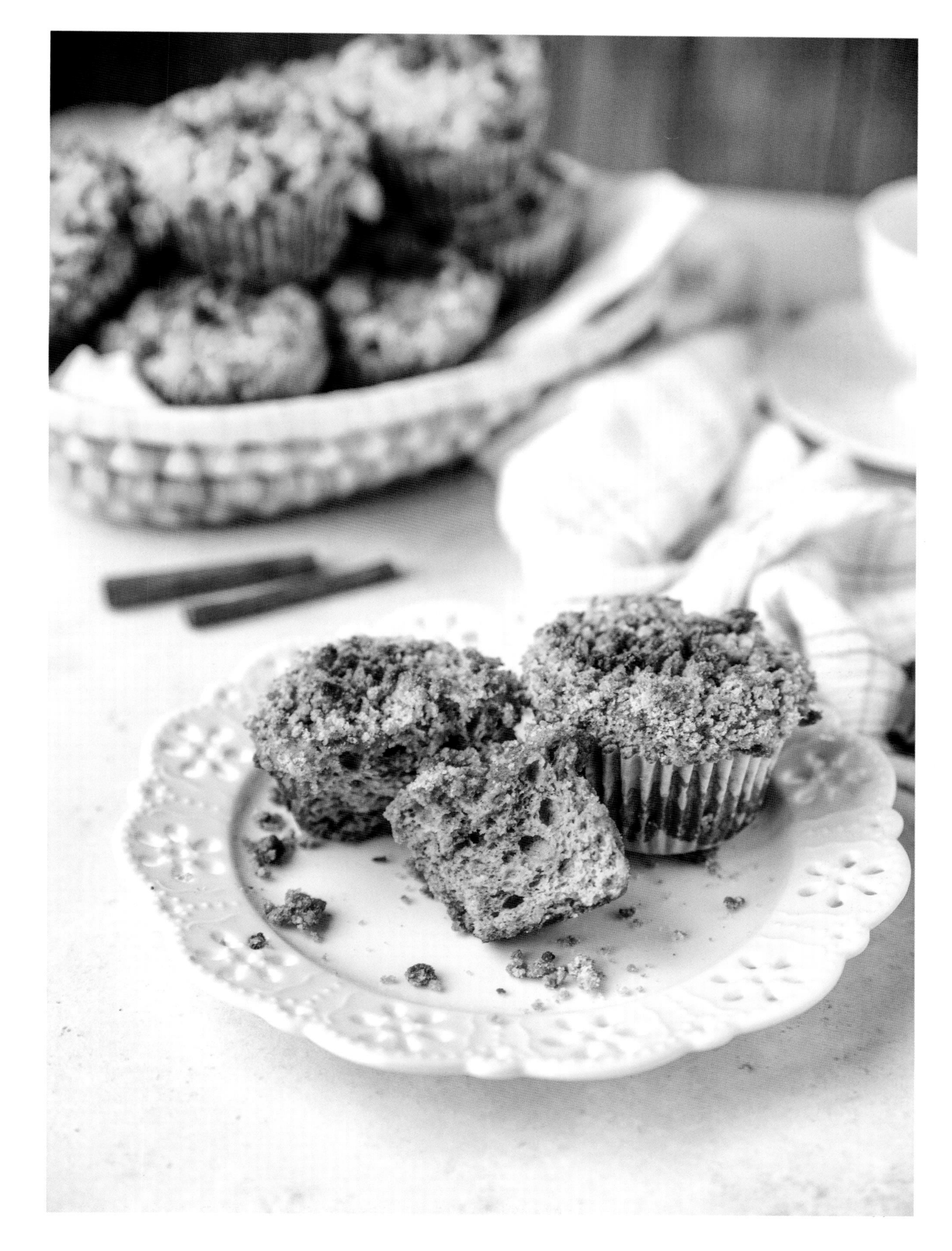

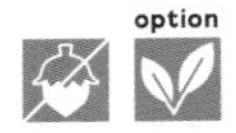

MIRACLE DOUGH BAGELS

YIELD: 6 bagels (1 per serving)

PREP TIME: 20 minutes

COOK TIME: 15 minutes

You can double this recipe to make 12 bagels—have half of them over the weekend and freeze the rest for later use during the work/school week! Adding whey protein powder to my basic Miracle Dough recipe gives these bagels that chewiness we love!

FOR THE DOUGH

2 cups (225g) shredded part-skim mozzarella cheese

1/2 cup (60g) coconut flour

2 large eggs

2 ounces cream cheese (1/4 cup), softened

2 tablespoons unflavored whey protein powder

1 tablespoon baking powder

1 teaspoon baking soda

1/2 teaspoon xanthan gum or unflavored gelatin

1/4 teaspoon fine sea salt

1/8 teaspoon garlic powder

1/8 teaspoon onion powder

TOPPINGS

1 large egg, beaten, for egg wash (optional)

1/4 cup sesame seeds, for topping (optional)

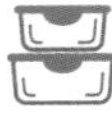

Store in an airtight container in the refrigerator for up to 1 week.

1. Preheat the oven to 425°F. Line a sheet pan with parchment paper.

2. Make the dough: Place all of the ingredients in a food processor or the bowl of a stand mixer (or a large bowl if using an electric hand mixer) and mix until a sticky dough forms.

3. Transfer the dough to a microwave-safe bowl and microwave for 2 minutes, or until melted. (If you prefer not to use a microwave, you can warm the ingredients in a saucepan over medium heat until the cheese is melted.) Turn out the dough onto a clean work surface and knead it back into a mass.

4. Separate the dough into 6 equal-sized portions, roll each portion into a ball, and place on the prepared sheet pan. Make a hole in the center of each ball using your index finger or thumb.

5. If you'd like the bagels to have a golden color, use the additional beaten egg as an egg wash and brush it over the top of each bagel. Sprinkle on the sesame seeds, if desired.

6. Bake for 13 to 15 minutes, or until browned. If the holes disappeared while baking, insert the end of a wooden spoon handle into the center of each still-warm bagel and twist to enlarge the hole. Let cool slightly before eating.

calories 199 | fat 12g | protein 14g | total carbs 8g | dietary fiber 3g | net carbs 5g

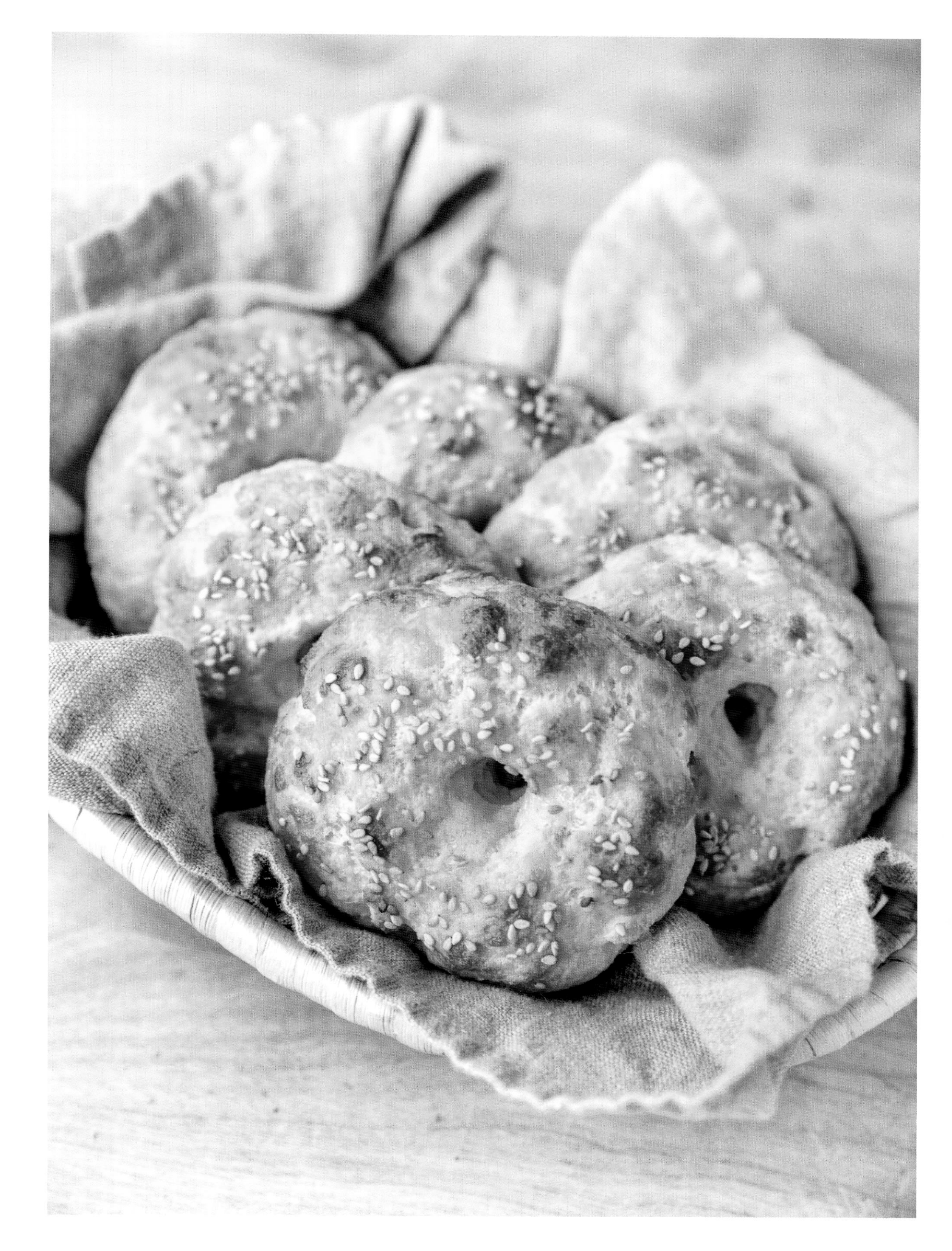

CINNAMON ROLLS

YIELD: 12 rolls (1 per serving)

PREP TIME: 15 minutes

COOK TIME: 20 minutes

Who doesn't love a yummy cinnamon roll, especially around the holidays? It doesn't need to be Christmastime to enjoy these luscious just-like-traditional-but-keto cinnamon rolls! It's truly shocking how close these are in texture to conventional sugar-filled cinnamon rolls. You might be skeptical of the famous keto miracle dough, but don't knock it until you've tried it. Read the rave reviews on my website, Sugar-Free Mom!

FOR THE DOUGH

2 cups (225g) shredded part-skim mozzarella cheese

3 ounces cream cheese (¼ cup plus 2 tablespoons), softened

½ cup (60g) coconut flour

¼ cup (32g) Swerve confectioners'-style sweetener

1 tablespoon baking powder

1 teaspoon baking soda

½ teaspoon xanthan gum

¼ teaspoon fine sea salt

2 large eggs

1 teaspoon vanilla extract

½ teaspoon vanilla-flavored liquid stevia

FOR THE CINNAMON "SUGAR"

½ cup (1 stick) unsalted butter, melted

⅓ cup packed Swerve brown sugar sweetener

2 teaspoons ground cinnamon

FOR THE CREAM CHEESE ICING

3 ounces cream cheese (¼ cup plus 2 tablespoons), softened

3 tablespoons heavy whipping cream

1 tablespoon Swerve confectioners'-style sweetener

½ teaspoon vanilla extract

1. Preheat the oven to 400°F. Grease a 9-inch pie pan or line it with parchment paper.

2. Make the dough: Place all of the dough ingredients in a food processor and process until a sticky dough forms. Remove the dough from the food processor and place it in a microwave-safe bowl. Microwave for 2 minutes, or until melted, then knead the dough to combine the melted cheese back into a mass. (If you prefer not to use the microwave, you can warm the dough in a saucepan over medium heat until the cheese is melted.)

3. Set an 18-inch length of parchment paper on the counter. Place the dough on the parchment paper, then top it with another sheet of parchment. Using your hands, press the dough to flatten it into a rough rectangle, then use a rolling pin to roll the dough out to a 16 by 8-inch rectangle.

4. Remove the top sheet of parchment paper. If necessary, turn the dough so that the long side is facing you. Set aside.

5. Make the cinnamon "sugar": Put the melted butter, sweetener, and cinnamon in a small bowl and mix together. Sprinkle half of the cinnamon sugar over the dough. Using the parchment paper to guide you, roll the long side of the dough over onto itself until it is all rolled up.

6. Make sure the rolled dough is seam side down on the parchment paper and cut into 12 slices. Place the slices, cut sides down, in the prepared pie pan. Sprinkle the remaining cinnamon sugar over the tops of the cinnamon rolls.

7. Bake for 15 to 20 minutes, or until the rolls have doubled in size, are fluffy looking, and are nicely browned.

8. Meanwhile, make the icing: Put all of the icing ingredients in a blender and blend until smooth.

9. As soon as the rolls come out of the oven, spread the icing over the tops. Allow to cool in the pan for about 5 minutes, then enjoy!

calories 219 | fat 19g | protein 6g | total carbs 4g | dietary fiber 2g | net carbs 2g

Store in an airtight container in the refrigerator for up to 3 days.

Make-ahead tip: You can prepare the rolls one day ahead, then bake and ice them the next day. Use your preferred method of preparing the pie pan in Step 1 and complete Steps 2 through 6 above, then cover and refrigerate. When you are ready to bake the rolls, allow them to come to room temperature on the counter for 1 hour, then bake as instructed. You may need to bake rolls that have been refrigerated overnight for 10 to 15 minutes longer. If they are looking too browned but haven't yet doubled in size, cover the dish loosely with aluminum foil and check every 5 minutes until they have doubled in size. While the rolls are in the oven, make the icing (Step 8), then spread the icing over the hot rolls (Step 9).

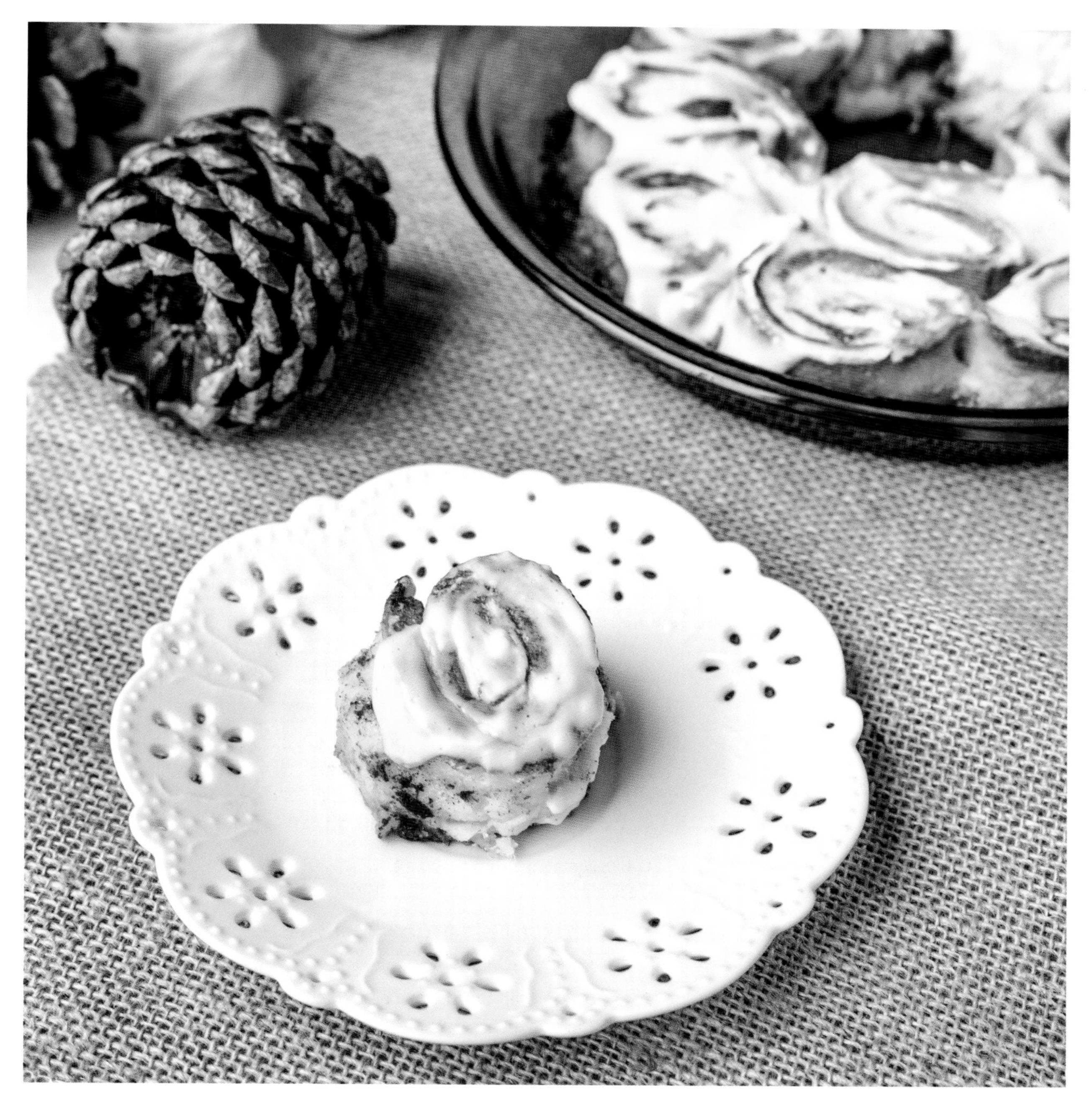

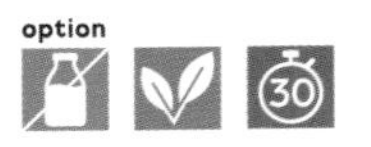

2-MINUTE ENGLISH MUFFINS

YIELD: 2 muffins (1 per serving)

PREP TIME: 5 minutes

COOK TIME: 2 minutes

I created this incredible English muffin recipe quite a few years ago for my website, and it became popular for good reason. These English muffins have real nooks and crannies, just like the traditional ones made with wheat flour.

You can swap out the almond butter for any nut butter you prefer, though I suggest you steer clear of peanut butter—its flavor is too strong for this recipe. You can also swap out the almond milk for another nondairy milk of your choice, such as coconut milk, or for heavy whipping cream or even water. If you want lots of nooks and crannies, don't overmix the batter—the less you work it, the more "holes" in the muffins you will get. You want to just combine the wet and dry ingredients.

For flatter English muffins that are about the size of traditional ones, I use shallow quiche dishes, about 4¼ inches in diameter and 1 inch tall. But 7-ounce ramekins will work just fine, too—the muffins just won't be as wide.

---

2 tablespoons unsweetened almond butter

1 tablespoon salted butter or coconut oil

2 tablespoons blanched almond flour

½ teaspoon baking powder

⅛ teaspoon fine sea salt

1 tablespoon unsweetened almond milk

1 large egg, beaten

Butter, for serving (omit for dairy-free)

SPECIAL EQUIPMENT:

2 (4-ounce) quiche dishes or 7-ounce ramekins

Store the untoasted muffins in an airtight container in the refrigerator for up to 5 days. Toast when ready to enjoy.

1. Grease two 4-ounce quiche dishes or 7-ounce ramekins with olive oil or coconut oil spray.

2. Put the almond butter and butter in a small microwave-safe bowl. Microwave for 30 seconds, or until melted, then mix until smooth. Set aside to cool.

3. In another small bowl, whisk the almond flour, baking powder, and salt together.

4. Pour the almond milk and egg into the dry ingredients and stir until just combined. Stir in the almond butter mixture until combined. Remember not to overmix the batter.

5. Pour the batter evenly into the prepared quiche dishes or ramekins. Microwave one at a time for 1 minute. Check the center with a toothpick; if it comes out clean, the muffin is done. If not, continue to microwave in 30-second intervals until the center is done. (If you used a shallow quiche dish, the muffin will likely be done in 1 minute.)

6. Allow to cool for a few minutes, then remove the muffins from the dishes and slice in half.

7. Toast, if desired, and enjoy with some butter!

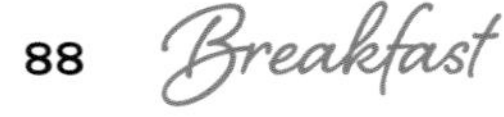

calories 222 | fat 19.4g | protein 8.3g | total carbs 4.8g | dietary fiber 2.8g | net carbs 2g

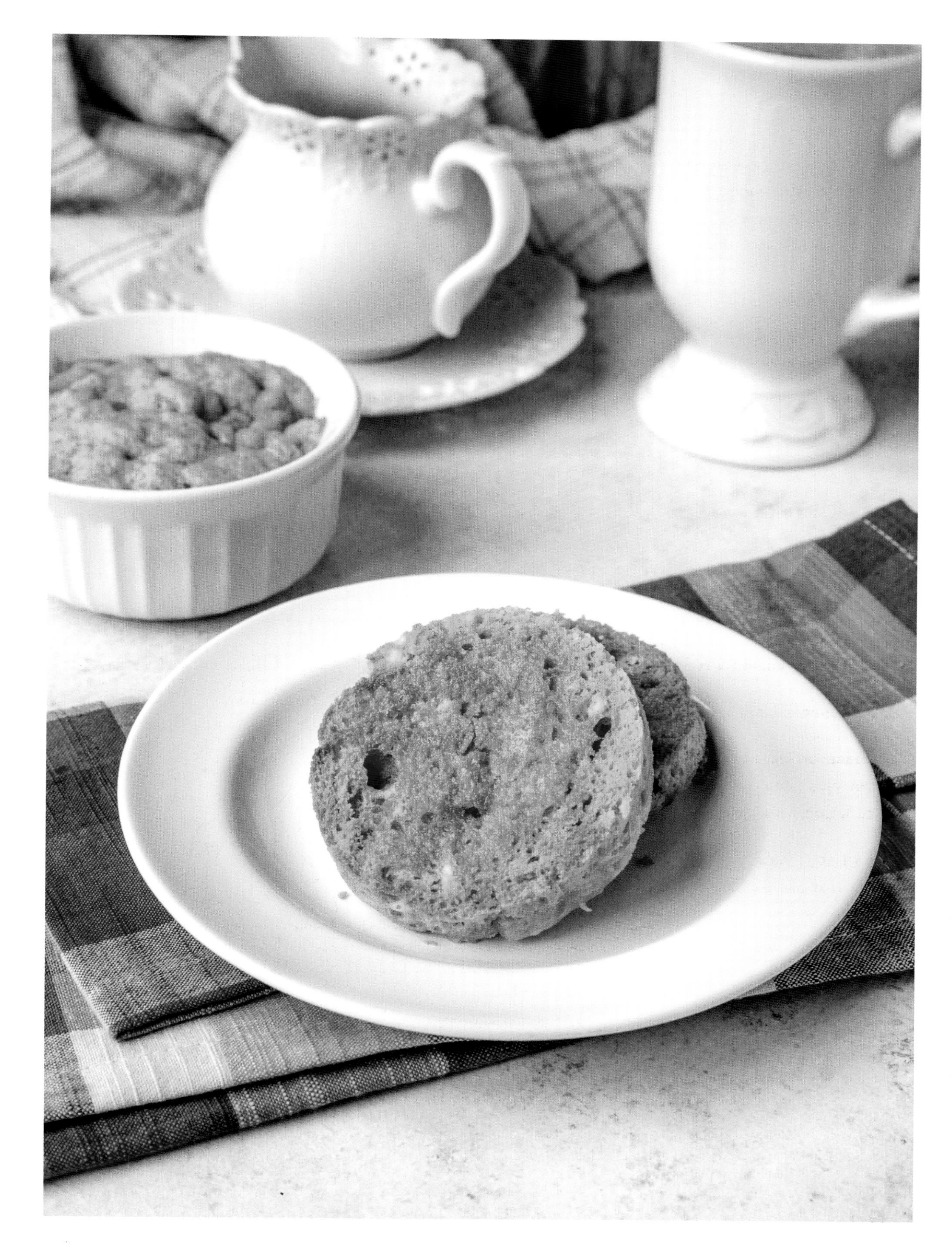

PANCETTA AND GRUYÈRE EGG BITES

YIELD: 12 bites (1 per serving)

PREP TIME: 20 minutes

COOK TIME: 35 minutes

These are my take on the famous Starbucks egg bites. I don't want to toot my own horn, but I think mine are even better, and so does my family!

4 ounces pancetta or bacon, chopped

10 large eggs (see Tip, page 82)

⅓ cup heavy whipping cream

¼ teaspoon fine sea salt

¼ teaspoon freshly ground black pepper

4 ounces Gruyère cheese, shredded (about 1 cup)

Store in an airtight container in the refrigerator for up to 5 days or in the freezer for up to 2 months. Reheat in the microwave for 1 to 2 minutes or in a preheated 325°F oven for 15 minutes.

1. Preheat the oven to 325°F. Insert a silicone or paper cupcake liner into each well of a standard-size 12-well muffin pan, or grease the pan well.

2. Cook the pancetta in a small skillet until crisp, about 5 minutes. Set aside to cool.

3. In a large bowl, whisk the eggs with the cream, salt, and pepper. Stir in the cheese.

4. Distribute half of the pancetta evenly among the muffin cups, then fill the cups evenly with the egg and cheese mixture. Add the remaining pancetta to the muffin cups.

5. Place the muffin pan inside a larger roasting pan and fill the roasting pan with enough hot water to come three-quarters of the way up the sides of the muffin pan (approximately 6 cups).

6. Bake for 25 to 30 minutes, or until the egg bites are puffed up and the centers are set. Enjoy immediately.

calories 153 | fat 12g | protein 8g | total carbs 0g | dietary fiber 0g | net carbs 0g

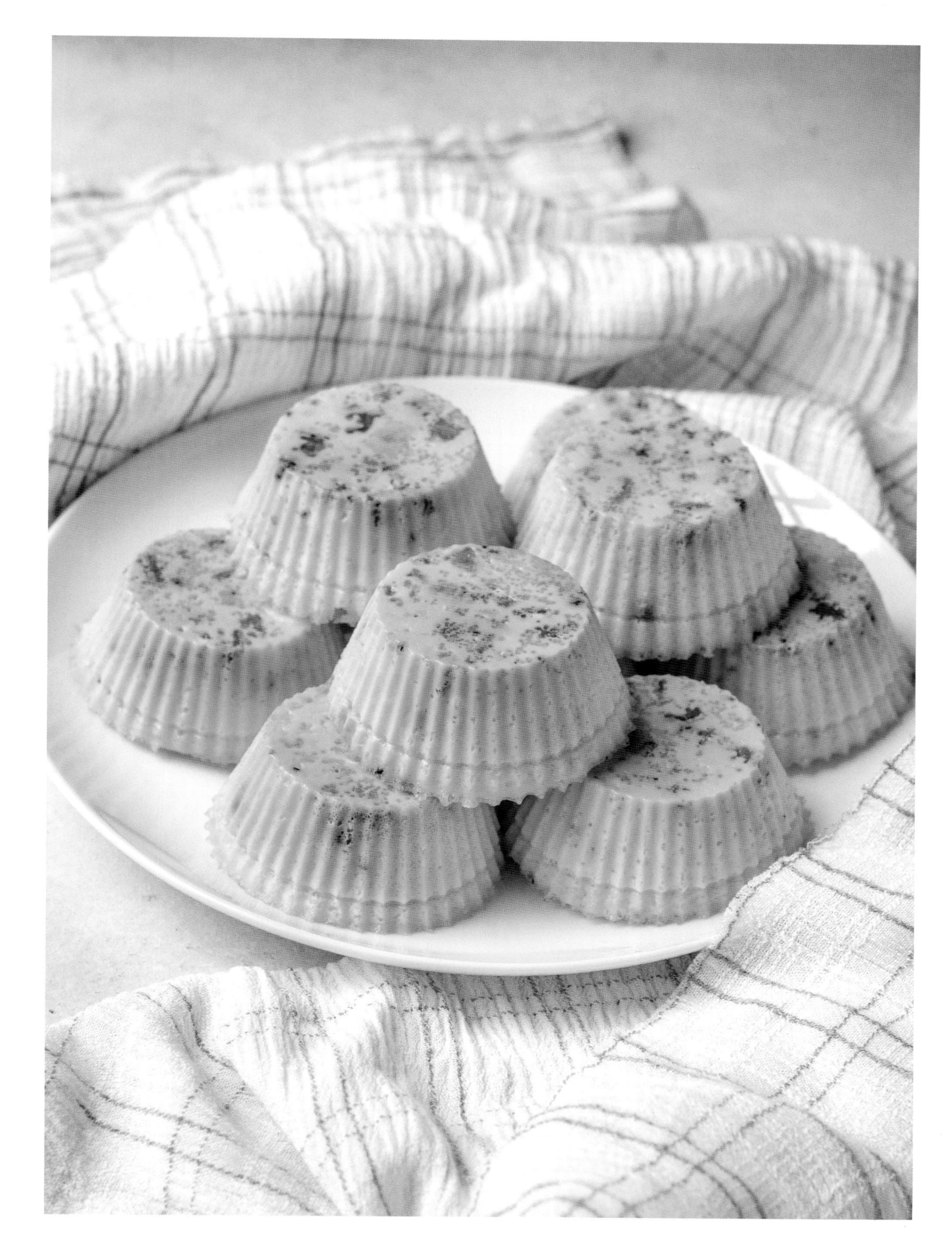

SLOW COOKER GRANOLA

YIELD: 6 cups (1/2 cup per serving)

PREP TIME: 10 minutes

COOK TIME: 2 hours

Super simple to make, this is a fantastic granola to prep for the week ahead for breakfast with a little coconut or almond milk or as a snack. Using a slow cooker frees you up: no need to watch the granola constantly to avoid burning it. But you can certainly bake it in the oven if you prefer (see the oven option below).

- 1/3 cup coconut oil
- 1 teaspoon vanilla extract
- 1 teaspoon vanilla-flavored liquid stevia
- 1/2 cup sliced raw almonds
- 1/2 cup raw hazelnuts, chopped
- 1/2 cup raw pecans, chopped
- 1/2 cup raw walnuts, chopped
- 1 cup raw pumpkin seeds
- 1 cup raw sunflower seeds
- 1 cup unsweetened shredded coconut
- 1/2 cup Swerve granular sweetener or other keto sweetener of choice
- 1 teaspoon ground cinnamon
- 1 teaspoon fine sea salt

1. Put the coconut oil in a 6-quart slow cooker and turn it to low.
2. Once the oil is melted, add the vanilla extract and stevia and stir to combine. Add the nuts, seeds, and shredded coconut to the slow cooker and stir until the granola mixture is well coated in the oil.
3. Whisk the granular sweetener, cinnamon, and salt together in a small bowl, then sprinkle over the granola mixture in the slow cooker.
4. Cover and cook on low, stirring every 30 minutes, until the granola is aromatic and toasted, about 2 hours.
5. Pour the granola onto a sheet pan, spread it out, and allow to cool to room temperature. The granola will form nice big chunks as it cools.

Store the cooled granola in a large glass jar or a gallon-sized zip-top plastic bag and store in the refrigerator for up to 2 weeks. It can also be stored in the pantry for up to 1 week, but my family finds that it stays nice and crisp when stored in the fridge.

OVEN OPTION: *Preheat the oven to 325°F. Place the nuts, seeds, and shredded coconut in a large mixing bowl. Melt the oil in a small saucepan over low heat, then stir in the vanilla extract and stevia. Pour the coconut oil mixture over the nut and seed mixture and toss to coat. Pour the granola mixture onto a sheet pan. Whisk the granular sweetener, cinnamon, and salt together in a small bowl, then sprinkle over the granola mixture. Bake for 30 minutes, then stir well. If the nuts aren't as roasted as you prefer, continue baking until the granola is done to your preference, stirring every 15 minutes and watching it carefully to avoid burning. Remove from the oven and allow to cool to room temperature.*

calories 327 | fat 31g | protein 7g | total carbs 8g | dietary fiber 4g | net carbs 4g

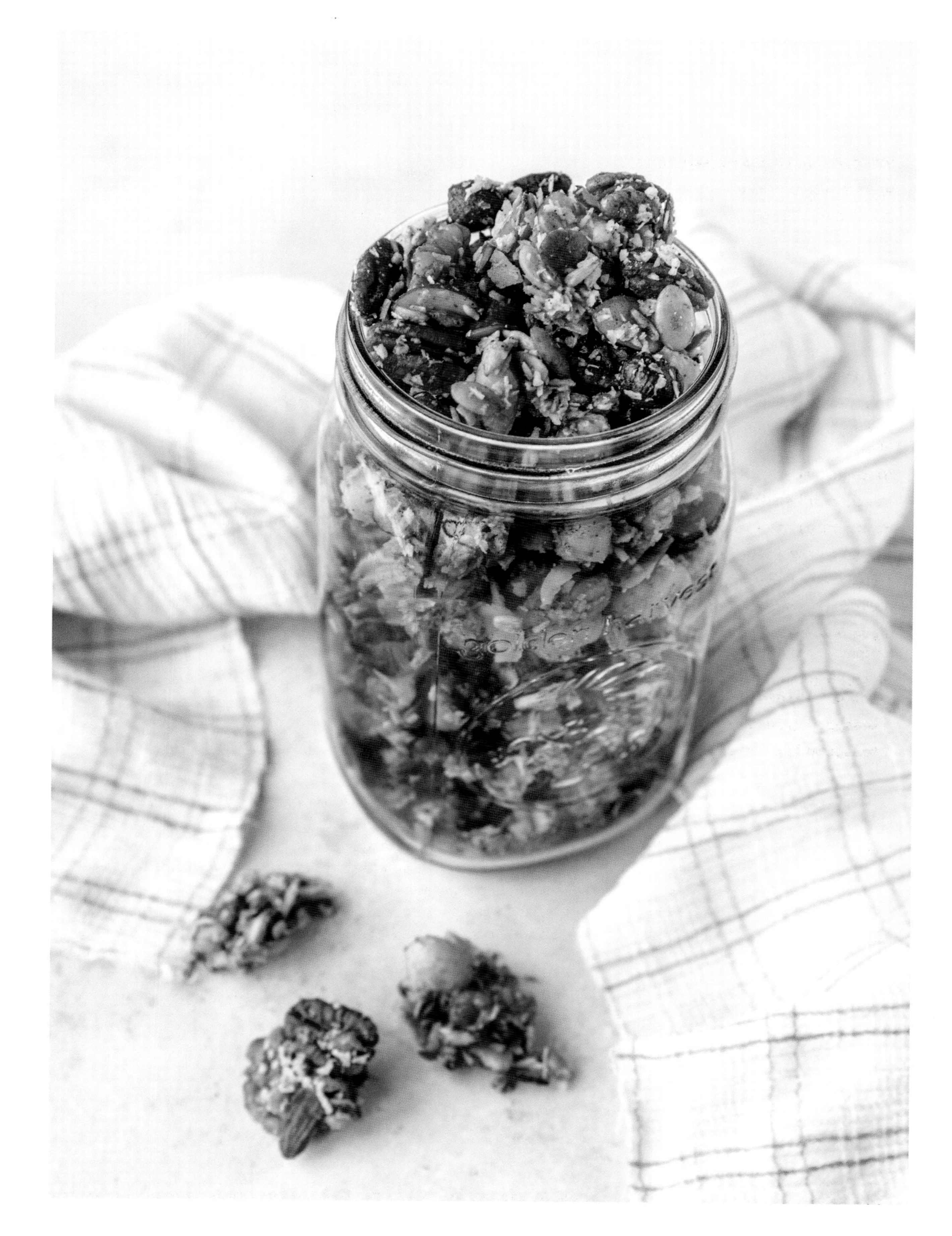

PREP-AHEAD HOT CINNAMON CEREAL

YIELD: 3 cups (1/3 cup per serving)

PREP TIME: 5 minutes

COOK TIME: 2 minutes

I don't know about you, but I prefer to get the most out of my time in the kitchen. I love making recipes once that can be enjoyed multiple times, and prepping ahead is key for me. My hubby and I love this hot cereal topped with fresh berries and sugar-free maple syrup.

1 cup hemp hearts
1 cup blanched almond flour
1 cup ground flaxseed
3 tablespoons chia seeds
1 teaspoon ground cinnamon
1/2 teaspoon fine sea salt

FOR SERVING

1/3 cup unsweetened almond milk, other nut milk of choice, or water

TOPPINGS (OPTIONAL)

Heavy whipping cream (omit for dairy-free)
Sugar-free maple syrup, store-bought or homemade (page 70)
Chopped nuts
Fresh berries

Store the dry cereal in an airtight container in the refrigerator for up to 6 months.

1. In a medium bowl, whisk together all of the dry ingredients. Place in a covered mason jar in the refrigerator until ready to serve.

2. To serve: Pour 1/3 cup of cereal into a microwave-safe bowl. Stir in the almond milk.

3. Microwave for 1 to 2 minutes, or until the cereal has the desired consistency. If you'd like it a bit thinner, add more almond milk. (If you prefer not to use a microwave, you can heat the cereal in a saucepan over medium-low heat until it thickens.)

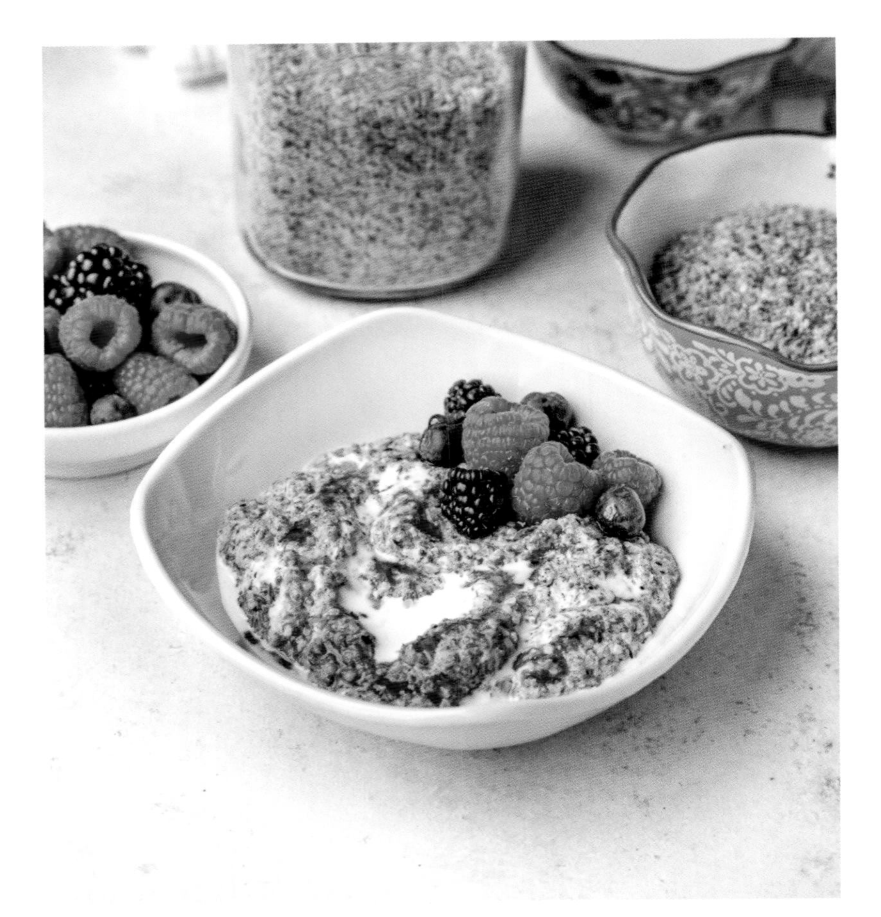

calories 291 | fat 23g | protein 11g | total carbs 10g | dietary fiber 8g | net carbs 2g

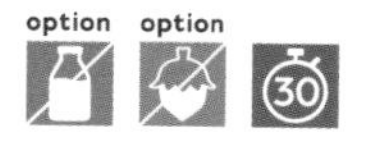

COCONUT FLOUR WAFFLES

YIELD: 14 Belgian-style waffle pieces or 16 regular waffles (1 piece per serving)

PREP TIME: 5 minutes

COOK TIME: about 25 minutes

These waffles can be made in either a Belgian-style waffle maker or a traditional one. A Belgian waffle maker requires more batter and will provide only fourteen waffle pieces, whereas a traditional waffle maker uses less batter per waffle and will yield sixteen waffles.

1½ cups water, unsweetened almond milk, or coconut milk

6 large eggs (see Tip, page 82)

¾ cup (90g) coconut flour

½ cup (1 stick) salted butter or coconut oil, softened

¼ cup (28g) ground flaxseed

3 tablespoons Swerve granular sweetener

2 tablespoons unflavored gelatin

1 tablespoon baking powder

1 teaspoon maple extract

½ teaspoon xanthan gum

½ teaspoon fine sea salt

FOR SERVING (OPTIONAL)

Butter

Sugar-free maple syrup, store-bought or homemade (page 70)

Fresh berries

Store in an airtight container in the refrigerator for up to 1 week or in the freezer for up to 2 months.

1. Place all of the ingredients in a high-powered blender or food processor and blend until incorporated. The batter will be thick.

2. Preheat and prepare a waffle maker according to the manufacturer's directions. Place 1 cup of the batter in the center of a Belgian-style waffle iron or ¼ cup of the batter in the center of a traditional waffle maker and cook the waffle according to the manufacturer's directions. Repeat with the remaining batter; if making Belgian waffles, your last batch will be ½ waffle.

3. Serve immediately with butter, maple syrup, and/or fresh berries, if desired.

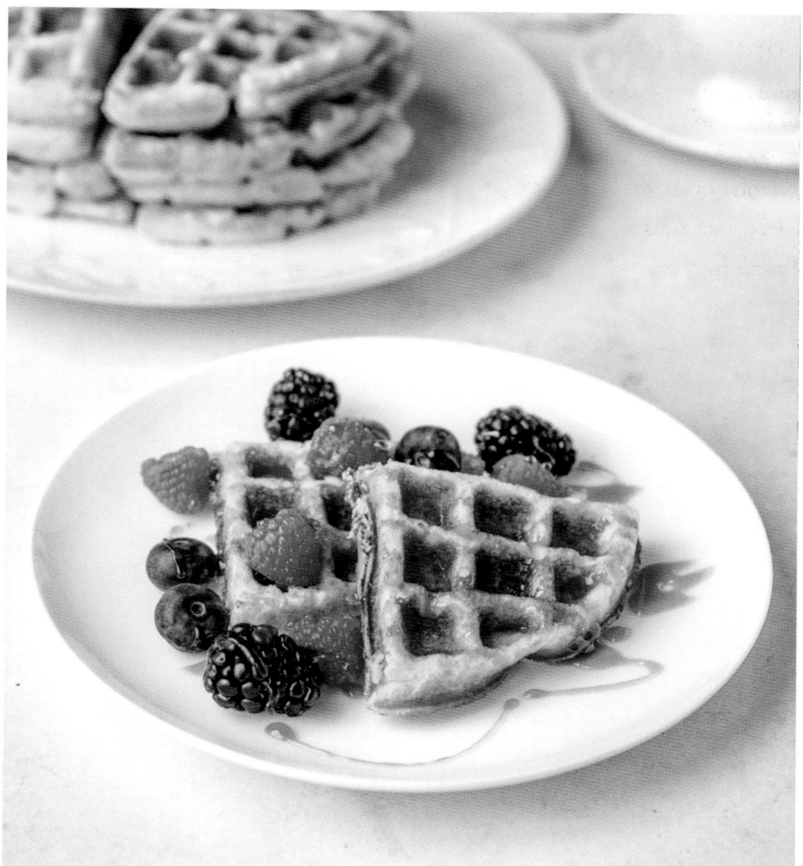

|FOR BELGIAN-STYLE WAFFLES|

calories 131 | fat 10g | protein 4g | total carbs 4g | dietary fiber 3g | net carbs 1g

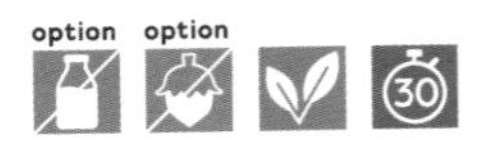

FLUFFY KETO PANCAKES

YIELD: 8 pancakes (1 per serving)

PREP TIME: 5 minutes

COOK TIME: 25 minutes

These pancakes are a family favorite, and they're great for meal prepping. I often double the recipe so the kids can reheat them for breakfast during the week.

½ cup (60g) coconut flour
¼ cup Swerve granular sweetener
1 teaspoon baking powder
½ teaspoon xanthan gum
½ teaspoon ground cinnamon
¼ teaspoon fine sea salt
4 large eggs
1 cup heavy whipping cream (or water, unsweetened almond milk, or coconut milk for dairy-free)
2 teaspoons vanilla extract
¼ teaspoon vanilla-flavored or unflavored liquid stevia
Coconut oil or butter, for the pan

FOR SERVING (OPTIONAL)
Butter
Sugar-free maple syrup, store-bought or homemade (page 70)
Fresh berries

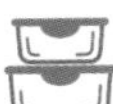

Store in an airtight container in the refrigerator for up to 1 week or in the freezer for up to 2 months.

1. In a large bowl, whisk together the coconut flour, granular sweetener, baking powder, xanthan gum, cinnamon, and salt. (You can also combine the dry ingredients and store in the refrigerator for up to 1 week.)
2. Stir in the eggs, cream, vanilla extract, and stevia and mix well.
3. Preheat a large nonstick skillet over medium-high heat. Put the coconut oil in the hot skillet.
4. Once the coconut oil is melted, spread ¼ cup of the batter in the skillet, making a pancake about 4 inches in diameter. Repeat to make a second pancake. Cover the pan and cook until the edges of the pancakes look set and bubbles have formed in the center, 2 to 3 minutes. Flip and cook for another 2 to 3 minutes. Remove to a plate or serving platter and repeat with the remaining batter. You can keep the pancakes warm by stacking them in a covered casserole dish.
5. Serve immediately with the toppings of your choice.

calories 111 | fat 8g | protein 2g | total carbs 3g | dietary fiber 1g | net carbs 2g

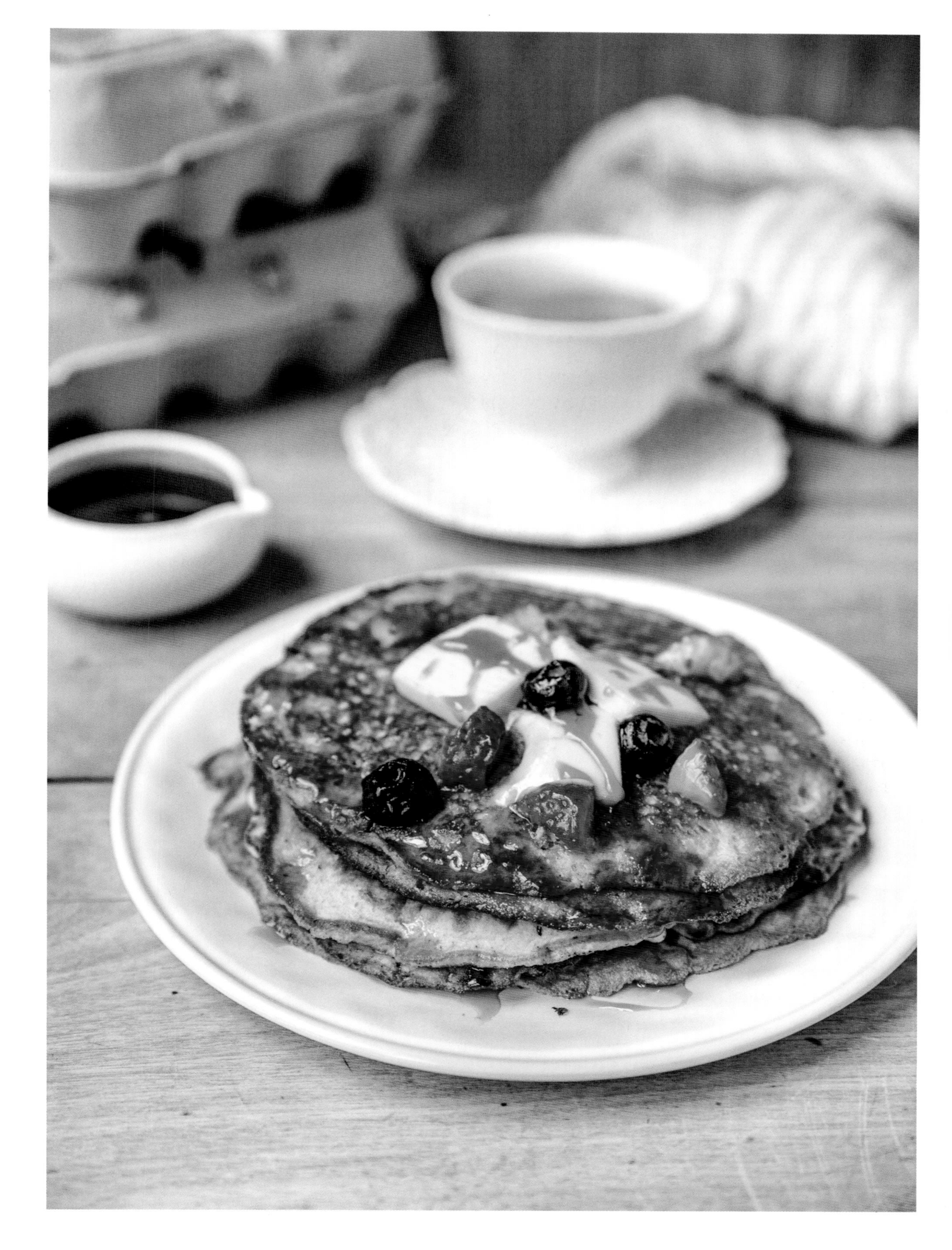

PUMPKIN DONUTS

YIELD: 9 donuts (1 per serving)

PREP TIME: 10 minutes

COOK TIME: 17 minutes

Call it a donut for breakfast and everyone comes running. The chocolate glaze is totally optional, but it makes the first bite just heavenly!

½ cup pumpkin puree (not pie filling)

¼ cup heavy whipping cream or coconut cream

4 large eggs

2 tablespoons avocado oil

1 teaspoon vanilla extract

1 teaspoon vanilla-flavored liquid stevia

½ cup (60g) coconut flour

2 teaspoons pumpkin pie spice

1 teaspoon baking powder

¼ teaspoon baking soda

½ cup (95g) packed Swerve brown sugar sweetener

⅛ teaspoon fine sea salt

FOR THE CHOCOLATE GLAZE (OPTIONAL)

½ cup sugar-free chocolate chips, store-bought or homemade (page 230)

2 tablespoons salted butter

SPECIAL EQUIPMENT:

2 (6-well) donut pans

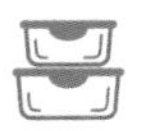

Store in an airtight container in the refrigerator for up to 3 days.

1. Preheat the oven to 350°F. Grease 9 wells of two 6-well donut pans.
2. Place the pumpkin puree, cream, eggs, oil, vanilla extract, and stevia in the bowl of a stand mixer (or a large bowl if using an electric hand mixer) and mix on medium-high until smooth.
3. In a medium bowl, whisk together the remaining ingredients for the donuts.
4. Turn the mixer to low and slowly add the dry ingredients to the wet ingredients until thoroughly combined.
5. Evenly pour the batter into the greased wells of the donut pans.
6. Bake for 15 minutes, or until the donuts bounce back when you touch them. Remove from the oven and loosen the edges of the donuts with a knife. Let cool for about 15 minutes before removing from the pans.
7. Make the glaze, if using: Put the ingredients in a microwave-safe bowl and microwave for 1 to 2 minutes, or until melted, then stir until smooth. Spoon the glaze over the cooled donuts and allow to set for about 5 minutes before serving.

| WITHOUT GLAZE |

calories 100 | fat 6g | protein 3g | total carbs 5g | dietary fiber 2g | net carbs 3g

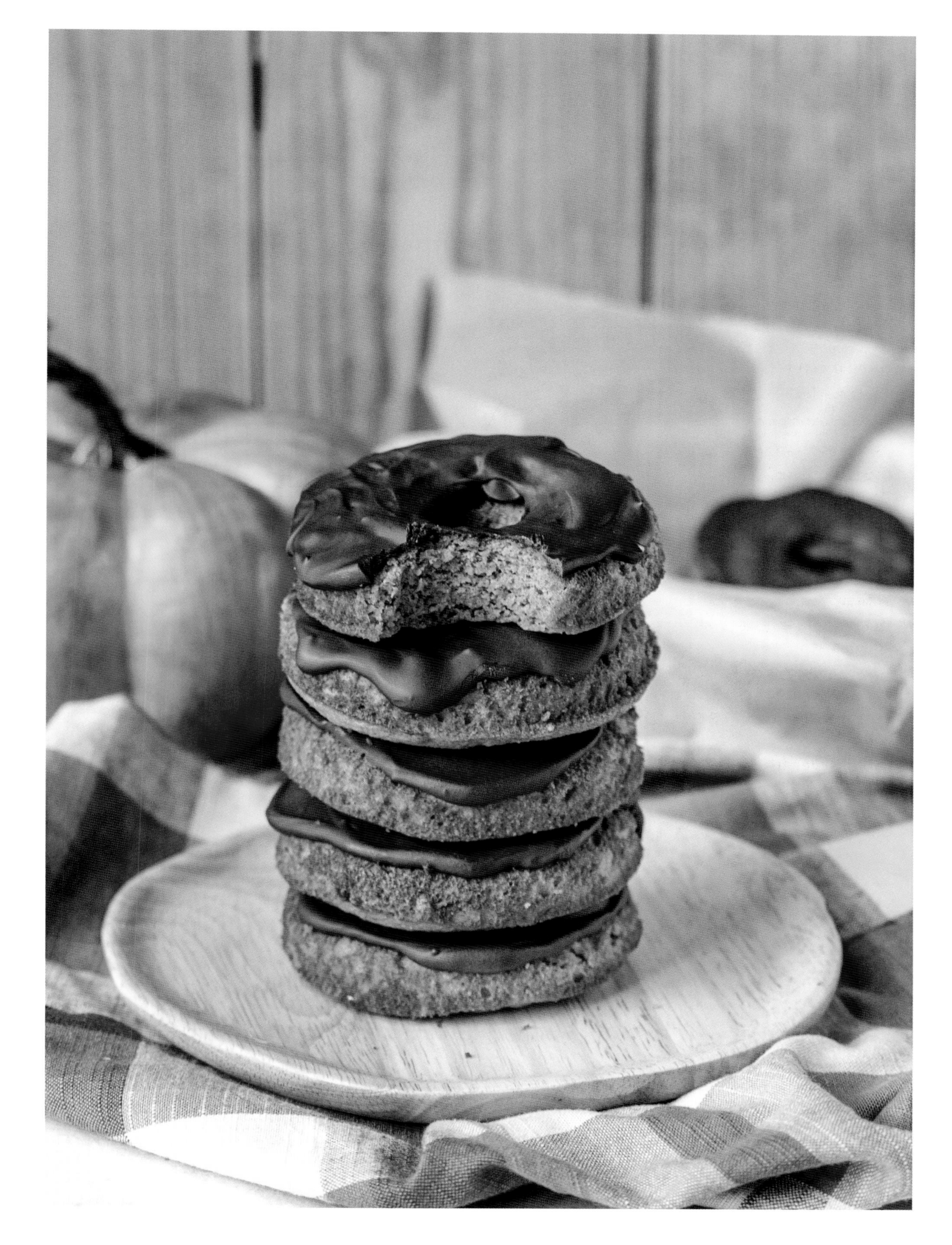

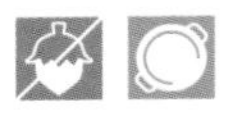

SAUSAGE AND BACON QUICHE

YIELD: 8 servings

PREP TIME: 10 minutes

COOK TIME: 1 hour 15 minutes

Whether you eat this quiche for breakfast or dinner, it's a family-friendly recipe. It starts on the stovetop and finishes in the oven, so getting this dish on the table is not going to take you a whole lot of effort. If you don't have a cast-iron skillet, simply place the cooked sausage, bacon, and cream cheese mixture in a 9-inch pie pan with the remaining ingredients and bake the quiche.

12 ounces bulk breakfast sausage

8 ounces bacon, chopped

1 (8-ounce) package cream cheese

4 large eggs

1½ cups heavy whipping cream

Pinch of fine sea salt

¼ teaspoon freshly ground black pepper

1½ cups shredded cheddar cheese (about 6 ounces)

Chopped fresh flat-leaf parsley, for garnish

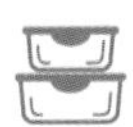

Store in an airtight container in the refrigerator for up to 4 days.

1. Preheat the oven to 350°F.

2. Cook the sausage and bacon in a large cast-iron skillet over medium-high heat, stirring often to crumble the sausage, until the sausage is browned and the bacon is crisp, about 10 minutes. Drain some of the fat, leaving about a tablespoon in the skillet.

3. Reduce the heat to medium-low and stir in the cream cheese until melted, about 5 minutes. Scrape the bottom of the skillet while stirring the cream cheese to get all of the browned bits off the bottom.

4. In a medium bowl, whisk the eggs and cream. Stir in the salt, pepper, and shredded cheese. Pour the egg mixture over the sausage and bacon in the skillet.

5. Place the skillet in the oven and bake for 50 to 60 minutes, until the quiche is slightly browned and set in the center. Allow to cool for about 10 minutes before slicing. Garnish with parsley and serve.

calories 611 | fat 56g | protein 19g | total carbs 2g | dietary fiber 0g | net carbs 2g

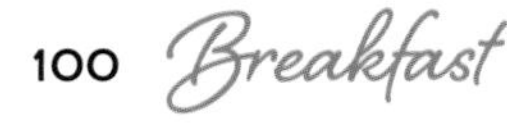

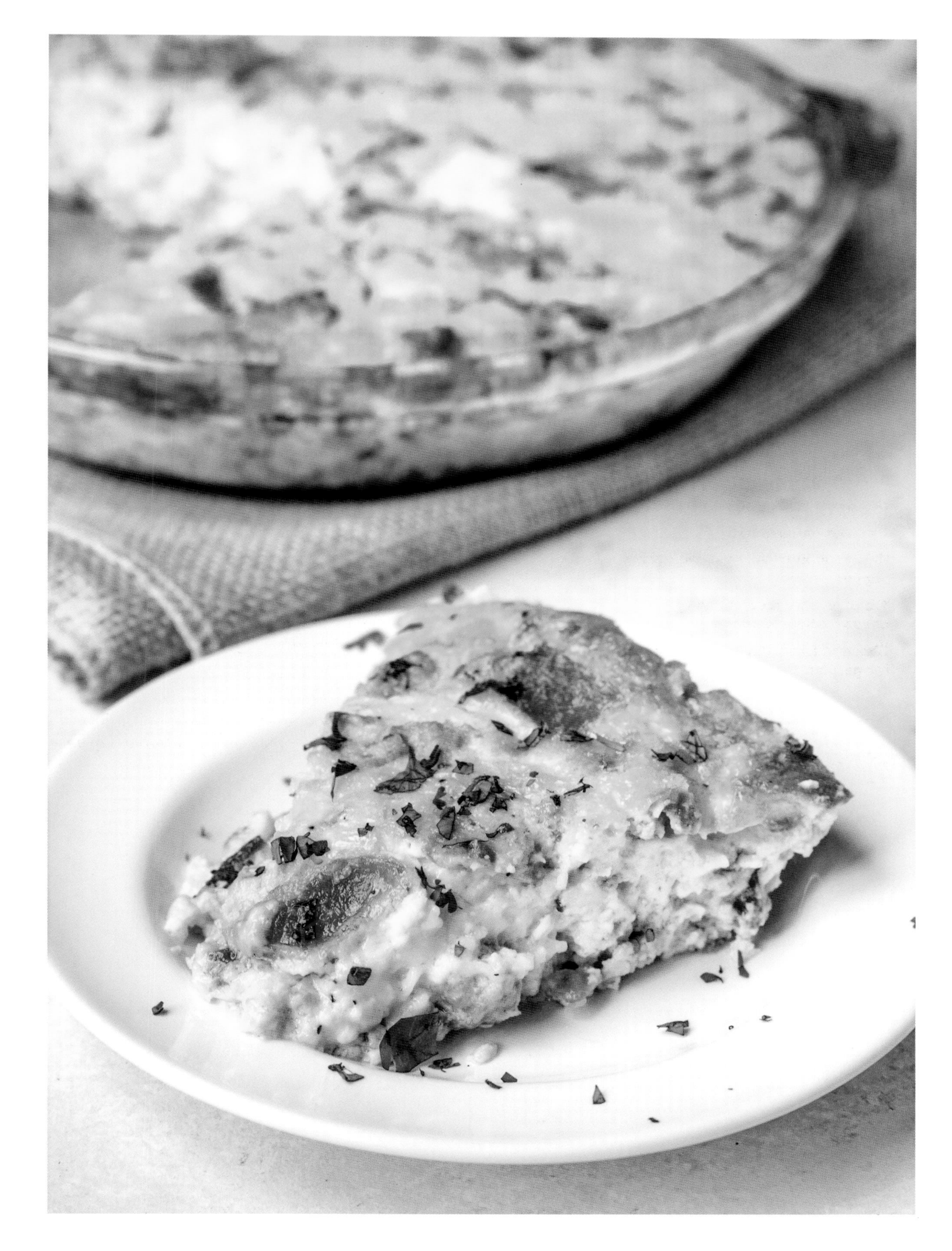

VANILLA BEAN SCONES

YIELD: 8 scones (1 per serving)

PREP TIME: 25 minutes

COOK TIME: 17 minutes

I don't make scones often, but when I do, I want them to taste like I remember scones tasting prior to my low-carb days. I tested this recipe using coconut flour, almond flour, and sesame flour and found that both coconut and almond flour gave the scones a lighter texture while sesame flour created a denser texture, which is more like a traditional scone.

1 cup (120g) sesame flour

1/3 cup (75g) Swerve granular sweetener

2 tablespoons ground flaxseed

2 tablespoons unflavored gelatin

1 tablespoon baking powder

1 teaspoon baking soda

1/2 teaspoon xanthan gum

1/2 teaspoon ground cinnamon

1/4 teaspoon fine sea salt

1/4 cup (1/2 stick) unsalted butter, cold, cubed

1/4 cup heavy whipping cream

2 large eggs

2 tablespoons sugar-free maple syrup, store-bought or homemade (page 70)

Seeds scraped from 1 vanilla bean, or 2 teaspoons vanilla extract

1/2 teaspoon vanilla-flavored liquid stevia

FOR THE VANILLA BEAN GLAZE

1/2 cup Swerve confectioners'-style sweetener

2 tablespoons water

1/2 teaspoon vanilla bean paste or vanilla extract

Store in an airtight container in the refrigerator for up to 3 days.

1. Preheat the oven to 375°F and line a sheet pan with parchment paper.
2. Place the sesame flour, granular sweetener, ground flaxseed, gelatin, baking powder, baking soda, xanthan gum, cinnamon, and salt in a food processor and process until combined.
3. Add the butter to the processor and pulse until the mixture looks like crumbs.
4. Add the cream, eggs, maple syrup, vanilla bean seeds, and stevia and process until a dough forms. Remove from the processor and place on the lined sheet pan.
5. Wet your hands with water and form the dough into a circle about an inch thick. Lightly grease a pizza cutter or knife and cut the circle into 8 triangles. Grease a spatula and use it to separate the triangles so they are not touching.
6. Bake for 15 to 17 minutes, or until slightly golden. Let cool for 10 minutes before topping with the glaze.
7. Make the glaze: Place all of the ingredients in a small bowl and stir until smooth. Spoon over the tops of the cooled scones and allow to set about 5 minutes, then serve.

calories 156 | fat 11g | protein 10g | total carbs 5g | dietary fiber 2g | net carbs 3g

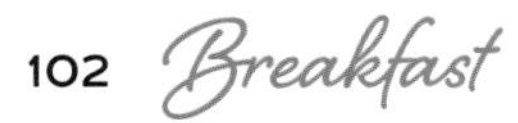

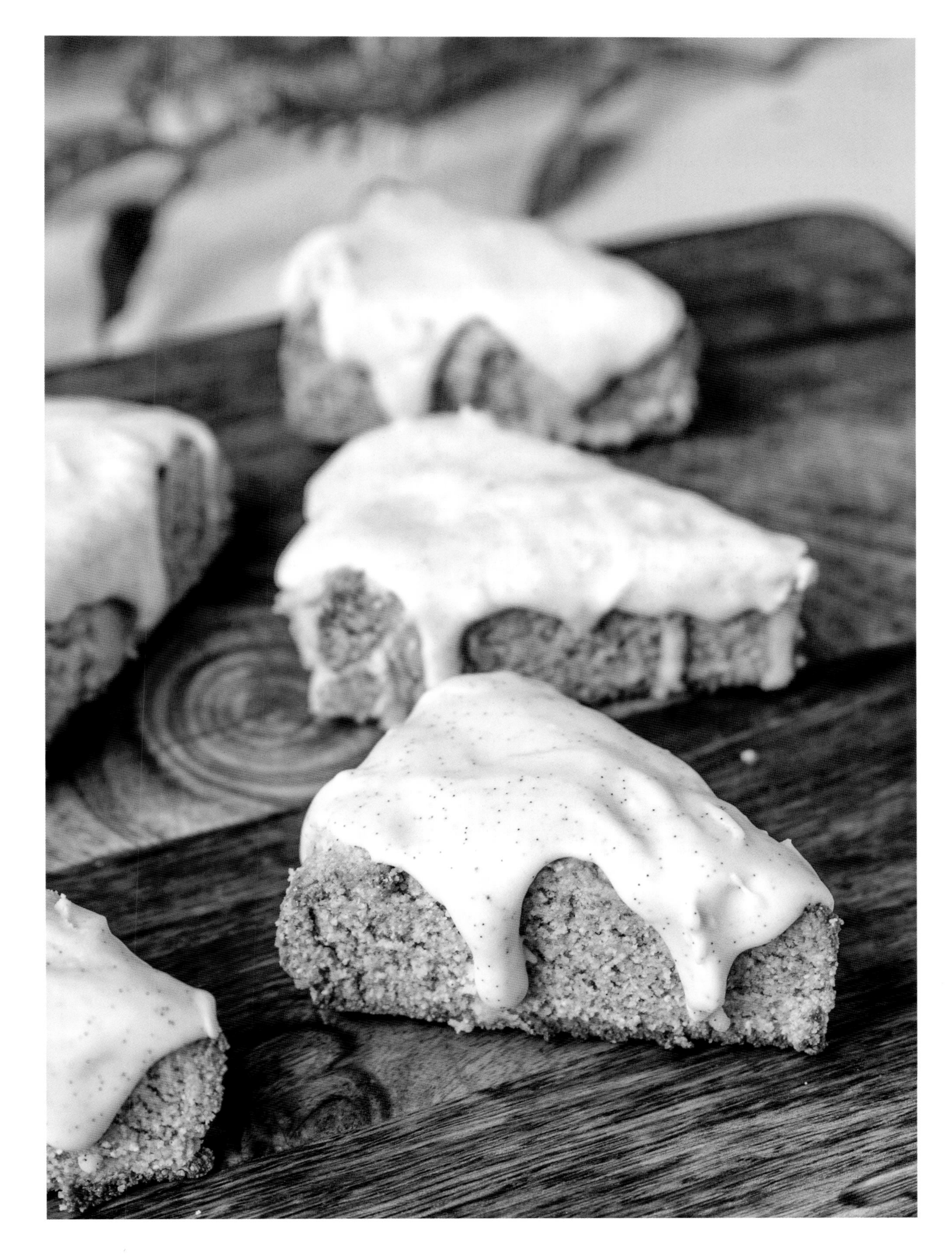

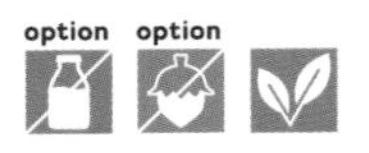

ZUCCHINI SPICE MUFFINS

YIELD: 12 muffins (1 per serving)

PREP TIME: 20 minutes

COOK TIME: 25 minutes

I suggest you try these muffins even if you're not a huge fan of zucchini: it gives them an unbeatable texture and moistness.

- 12 ounces zucchini (about 2 medium), shredded
- 1½ teaspoons fine sea salt, divided
- 4 large or 6 small eggs (about 1 cup; see Tip, page 82)
- ½ cup (1 stick) salted butter or coconut oil, softened
- ½ teaspoon cinnamon- or vanilla-flavored liquid stevia
- 1 cup (120g) coconut flour
- ½ cup (95g) packed Swerve brown sugar sweetener
- 2 teaspoons baking powder
- 1 teaspoon ground cinnamon
- ½ teaspoon ginger powder
- ½ teaspoon baking soda
- ¼ teaspoon ground cloves
- ½ cup chopped raw pecans or walnuts (optional)

Store in an airtight container in the refrigerator for up to 1 week.

1. Place the zucchini in a bowl and sprinkle with 1 teaspoon of the salt. Allow to sit for 15 minutes. Drain as much of the liquid as possible, then place the shredded zucchini on a clean dish towel. Wrap tightly and squeeze out as much liquid as you can.

2. Preheat the oven to 350°F.

3. Place the zucchini, eggs, butter, and stevia in the bowl of a stand mixer (or a large bowl if using an electric hand mixer). Add the remaining ingredients, except the nuts, and mix until combined.

4. Place a standard-size 12-well silicone muffin pan on a sheet pan for support or use a metal muffin pan lined with paper liners. Divide the batter evenly among the 12 muffin cups. If using the nuts, sprinkle them on top of the batter.

5. Bake for 25 minutes, or until a toothpick inserted in the center of a muffin comes out clean. Allow to cool for about 5 minutes before removing from the pan and serving.

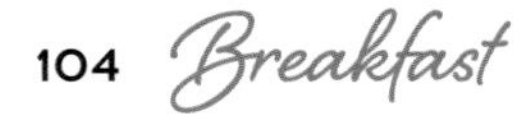

calories **144** | fat **11g** | protein **4g** | total carbs **6g** | dietary fiber **4g** | net carbs **2g**

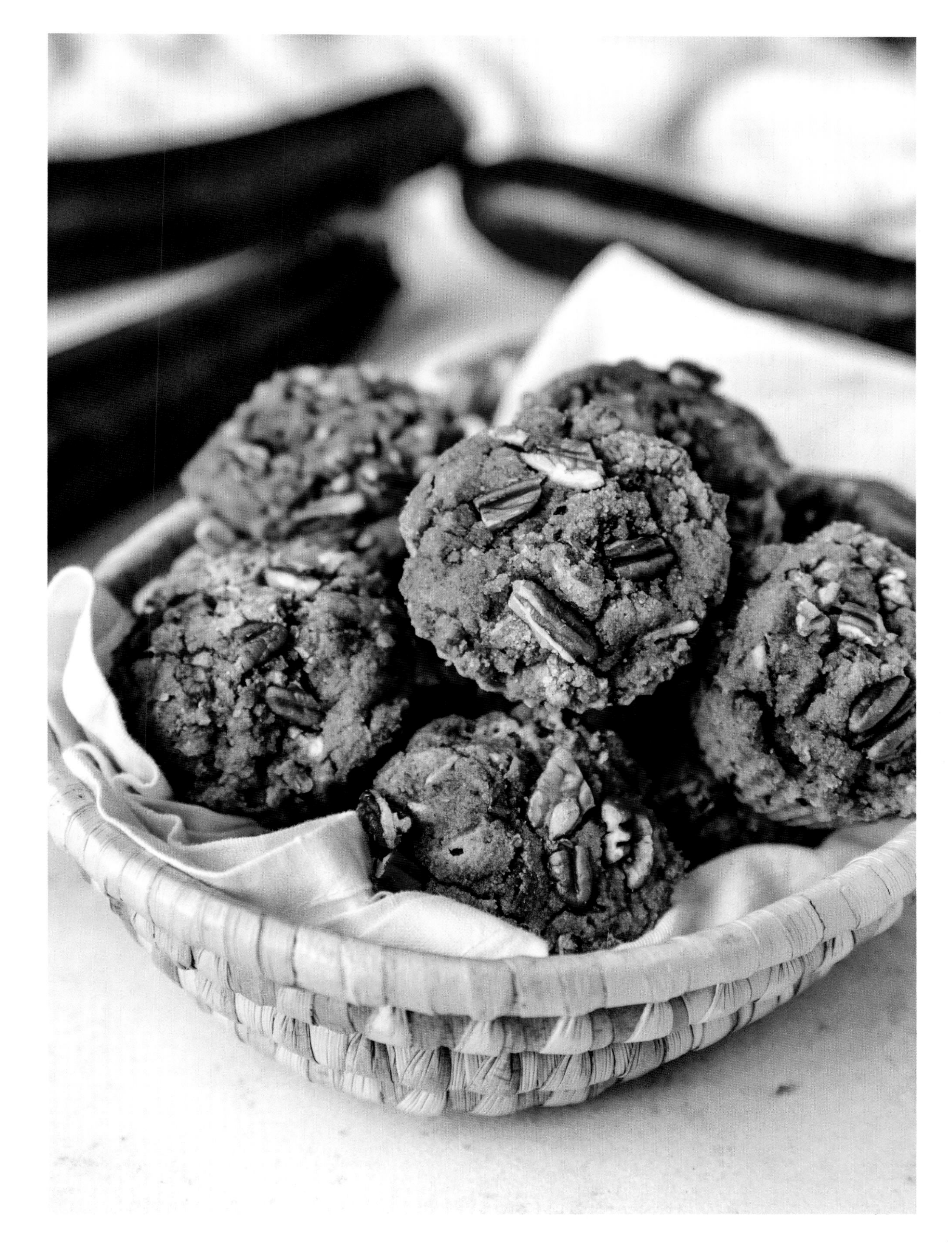

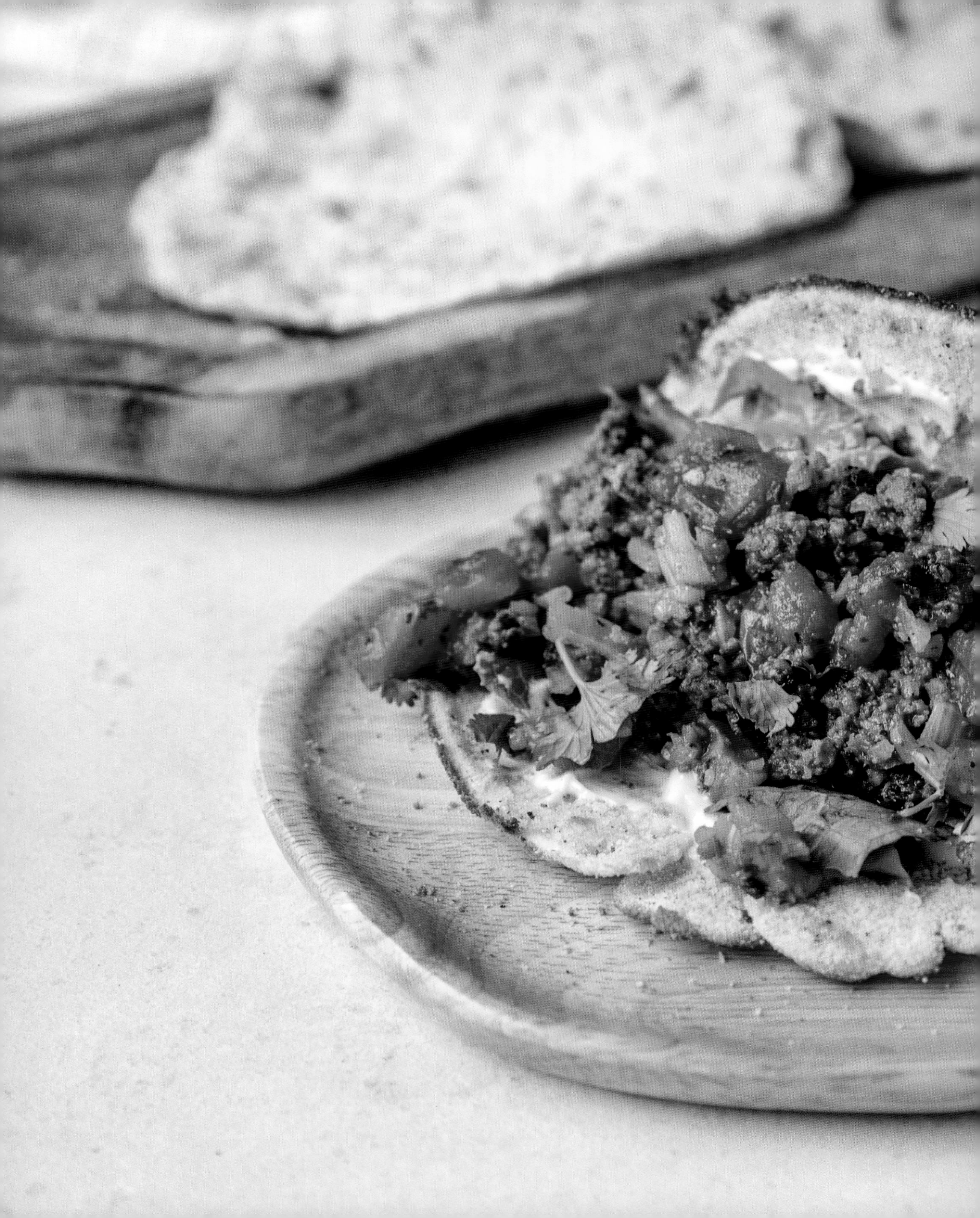

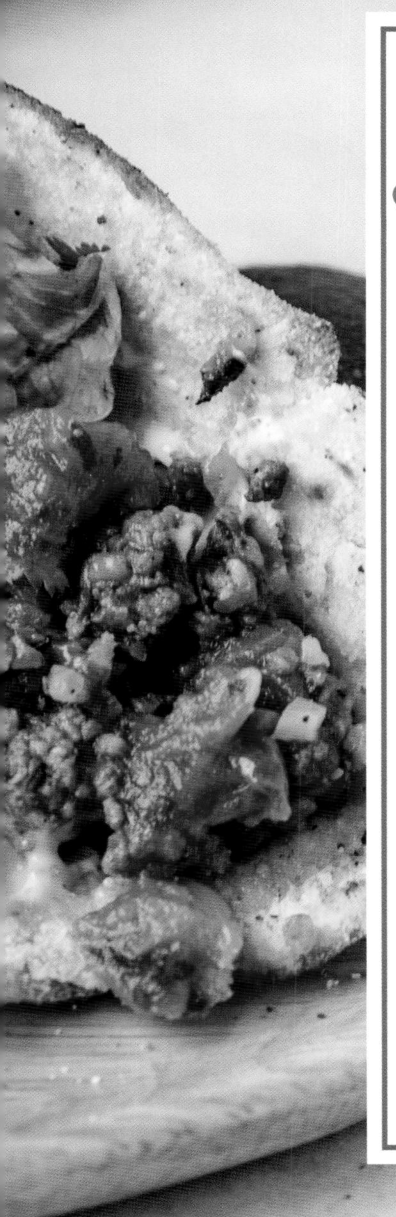

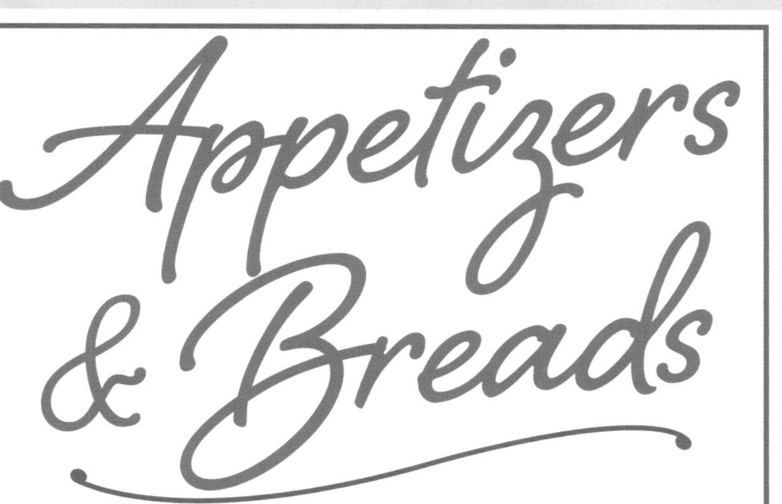
Appetizers & Breads

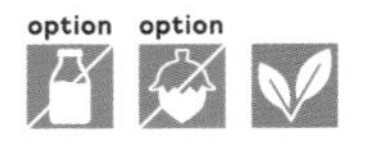

BANANA BREAD

YIELD: two 9 by 5-inch loaves (12 slices each, 1 slice per serving)

PREP TIME: 30 minutes

COOK TIME: 45 minutes

For years, I've received near-constant questions about adapting my popular Coconut Flour Bread recipe (page 114) into banana bread. Now, I've finally done it—for this cookbook! This recipe makes two 1-pound loaves of banana bread, so you can freeze one or share it. If you want only one loaf, just cut all of the ingredients in half.

12 large eggs (see Tip, page 82)

1 cup (2 sticks) melted salted butter or avocado oil

2/3 cup water

1 tablespoon plus 1 teaspoon banana extract

2 teaspoons maple extract

1/2 teaspoon vanilla-flavored liquid stevia

1 cup (190g) packed Swerve brown sugar sweetener

1 cup (120g) coconut flour

1 cup (112g) ground flaxseed

2 tablespoons baking powder

2 teaspoons ground cinnamon

2 teaspoons xanthan gum

1/2 teaspoon fine sea salt

1 cup sugar-free chocolate chips, store-bought or homemade (page 230), or chopped raw walnuts or pecans, divided (optional)

Wrap tightly in aluminum foil and refrigerate for up to 1 week or place in a zip-top freezer bag and freeze for up to 1 month.

1. Preheat the oven to 375°F. Line two 9 by 5-inch loaf pans with parchment paper, with the edges left hanging over the sides. Spray the parchment with cooking spray.

2. Place the eggs, butter, water, extracts, and stevia in the bowl of a stand mixer (or a large bowl if using an electric hand mixer) and mix until well combined.

3. In a large mixing bowl, whisk together the brown sugar sweetener, coconut flour, ground flaxseed, baking powder, cinnamon, xanthan gum, and salt. Pour the dry ingredient mixture into the wet ingredient mixture and blend until combined.

4. Divide the batter between two bowls and stir half of the chocolate chips or nuts, if using, into each bowl. Transfer the batter to the prepared loaf pans.

5. Bake for 40 to 45 minutes, or until a toothpick inserted in the center of a loaf comes out clean. Remove from the oven and allow to cool completely in the pans.

6. Once cool, remove from the pans by lifting up on the parchment paper. Slice and serve.

calories 158 | fat 13g | protein 5g | total carbs 5g | dietary fiber 3g | net carbs 2g

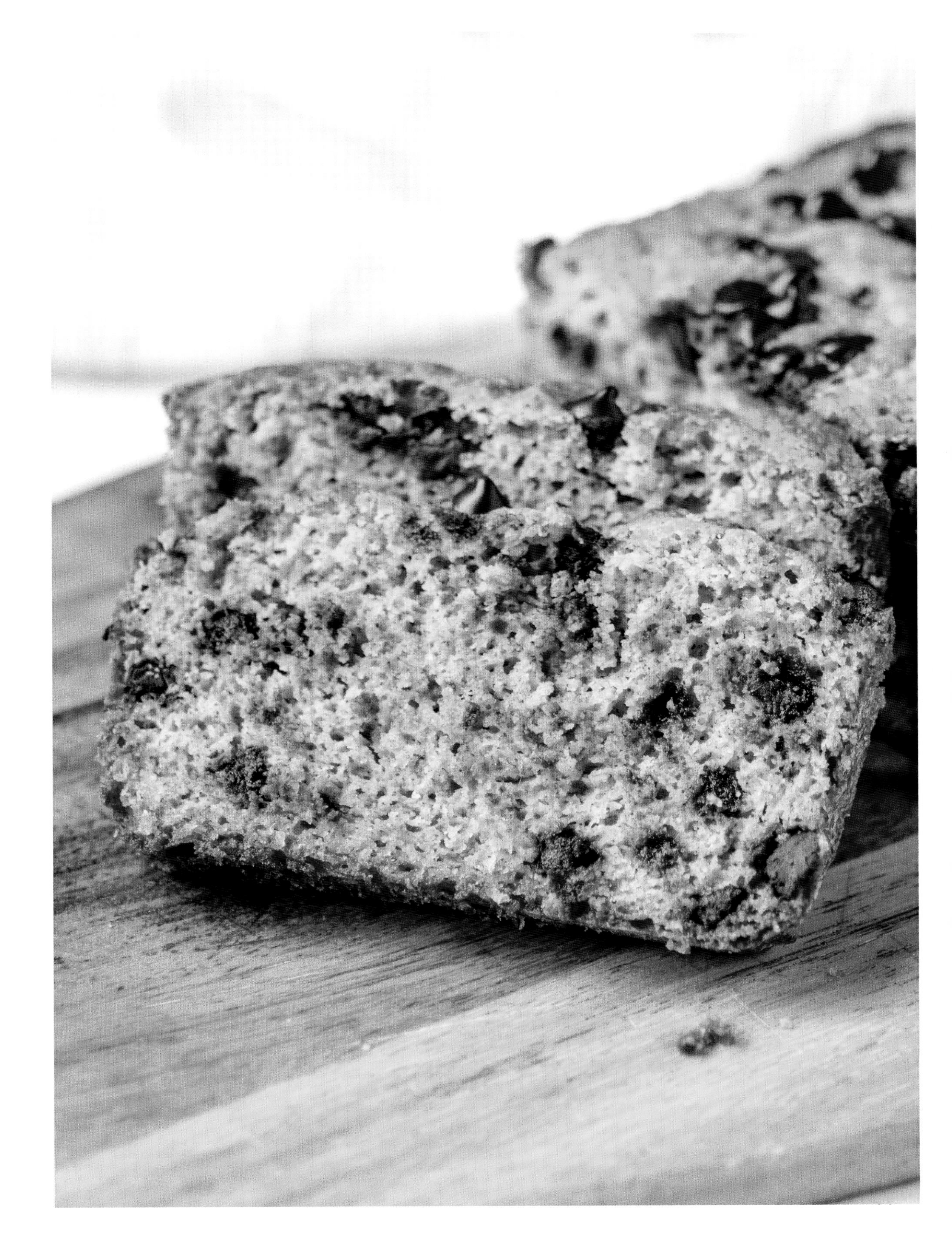

BUNLESS CHEESEBURGER BITES

YIELD: 48 bites (3 per serving)

PREP TIME: 30 minutes

COOK TIME: 15 minutes

These little cheeseburger bites are a fun appetizer for any party!

2 pounds grass-fed ground beef

1 teaspoon garlic powder

1 teaspoon fine sea salt

½ teaspoon freshly ground black pepper

½ teaspoon onion powder

8 ounces sliced cheddar cheese, cut into 48 (1-inch) squares

6 ounces bacon

24 cherry or grape tomatoes, halved

48 dill pickle slices (optional)

2 cups torn green or red leaf lettuce

1. Preheat the oven to 400°F. Line a sheet pan with aluminum foil.
2. Place the ground beef, garlic powder, salt, pepper, and onion powder in a mixing bowl and use your hands to combine.
3. Scoop out 1 tablespoon of the meat mixture and roll it into a ball or flatten it into a mini patty. Place on the prepared sheet pan. Repeat with the remaining meat mixture, making a total of 48 meatballs or mini patties.
4. Bake the mini burgers for 15 minutes. Remove from the oven and top each ball or patty with a slice of cheese. Turn off the heat and return the sheet pan to the oven for 2 to 3 minutes to melt the cheese.
5. While the mini burgers are in the oven, cook the bacon in a skillet over medium-high heat until it is fully cooked but not yet crisp. Remove the bacon from the skillet and set aside on a plate lined with paper towels. When cool enough to handle, break the bacon into 48 small pieces.
6. Assemble the burger bites by arranging them on 48 toothpicks in this order: 1 tomato half, 1 pickle slice (if using), 1 piece of bacon, 1 piece of lettuce, and 1 mini cheeseburger. Serve warm.

Store in an airtight container in the refrigerator for up to 3 days.

calories 251 | fat 20g | protein 14g | total carbs 1g | dietary fiber 0g | net carbs 1g

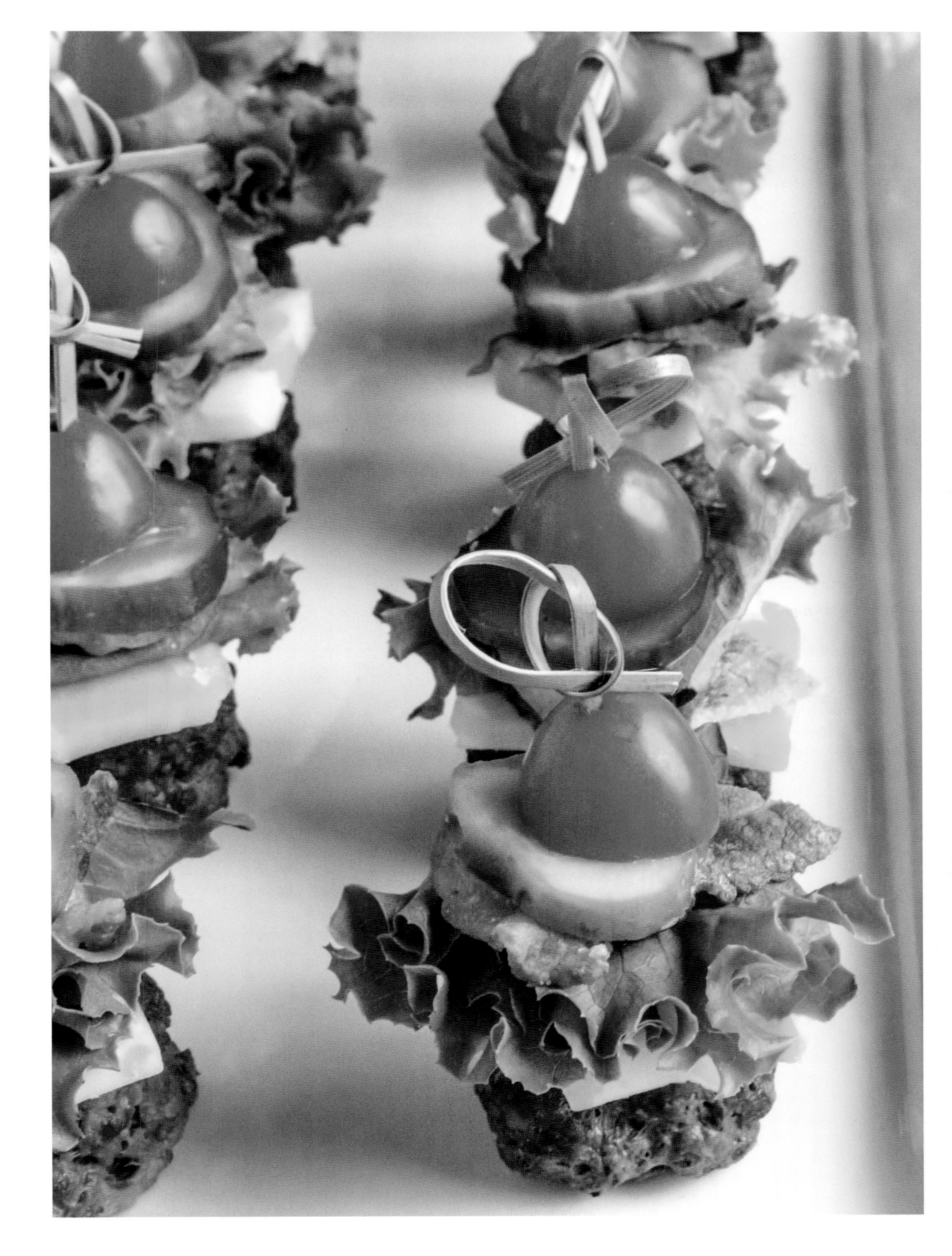

CLOUD BREAD LOAF

YIELD: one 9 by 5-inch loaf (12 slices, 1 slice per serving)

PREP TIME: 15 minutes

COOK TIME: 1 hour

You've probably made cloud bread before, but maybe you haven't tried making it as a loaf. Better yet, try this recipe, which has a few adaptations to make it even better. Switching out the usual cream cheese for sour cream helps prevent the cheese-sticking-to-the-roof-of-your-mouth problem, and adding protein powder gives the bread a little more substance. You'll really love this bread for Baked French Toast (page 78).

6 large eggs, separated (see Tip, page 82)

½ teaspoon cream of tartar

¾ cup sour cream (use dairy-free sour cream for dairy-free)

½ cup (50g) unflavored whey protein powder or egg white protein powder

½ teaspoon baking powder

¼ teaspoon garlic powder (optional)

¼ teaspoon onion powder (optional)

¼ teaspoon fine sea salt

1. Set a rack in the middle of the oven and preheat the oven to 300°F. Grease a 9 by 5-inch loaf pan with cooking spray.

2. Place the egg whites and cream of tartar in the bowl of a stand mixer (or a medium bowl if using an electric hand mixer) and whip until stiff peaks form. Set aside.

3. Place the egg yolks and the remaining ingredients in a mixing bowl and stir until well combined.

4. Fold a small amount of the whipped egg white mixture into the yolk mixture until it is fully incorporated. Repeat, adding a small amount of the egg white mixture at a time, until all of the egg white mixture has been incorporated.

5. Transfer the dough to the prepared loaf pan and bake on the middle rack of the oven for 50 minutes to 1 hour, or until a toothpick inserted in the center of the loaf comes out clean. Remove from the oven and let cool in the pan.

6. Once cool, loosen the edges of the loaf with a knife and remove the bread from the pan. Slice and serve.

Wrap tightly in aluminum foil and refrigerate for up to 1 week. If storing slices, place sheets of parchment paper between them, place in a zip-top freezer bag, and freeze for up to 3 months.

Tip: If you plan to use this bread for a sweet recipe, such as Baked French Toast, eliminate the garlic and onion powders.

calories 84 | fat 4.5g | protein 7.5g | total carbs 0.8g | dietary fiber 0g | net carbs 0.8g

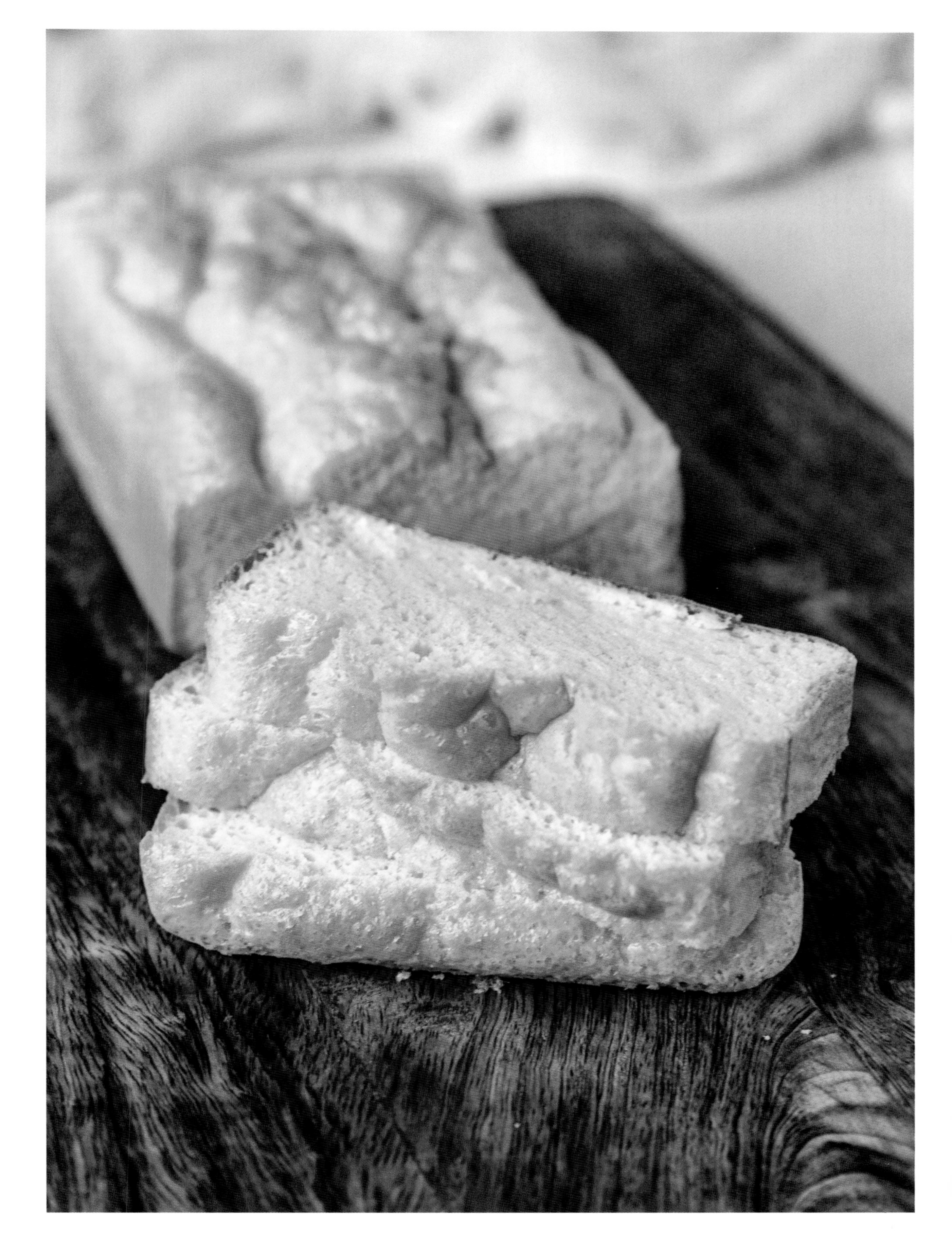

option

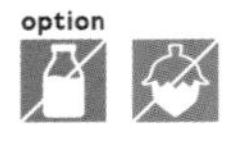

COCONUT FLOUR BREAD

YIELD: one 8 by 4-inch loaf (14 slices, 1 slice per serving)

PREP TIME: 15 minutes

COOK TIME: 45 minutes

This is one of the best breads I've ever made. The recipe took many attempts until I finally got the honeyed, wheatlike flavor and texture I was hoping for. Use this bread for Baked French Toast (page 78) or in sandwiches—even grilled cheese! Check out my website, SugarFreeMom.com, for a video tutorial.

6 large eggs (see Tip, page 82)

1/3 cup olive oil, melted coconut oil, or melted salted butter

1/3 cup water, heavy whipping cream, or coconut milk

1/2 cup (60g) coconut flour

1/2 cup (55g) ground flaxseed

2 tablespoons Swerve granular sweetener

1 tablespoon baking powder

1 teaspoon xanthan gum

1/2 to 1 teaspoon ground cinnamon

1/2 teaspoon fine sea salt

Sesame seeds, for topping (optional)

Wrap tightly in aluminum foil and refrigerate for up to 1 week. If storing slices, place sheets of parchment paper between them, place in a zip-top freezer bag, and freeze for up to 3 months.

1. Preheat the oven to 375°F. Line an 8 1/2 by 4 1/2-inch loaf pan with parchment paper, with the edges left hanging over the sides. Spray the parchment with cooking spray.

2. Place the eggs, oil, and water in the bowl of a stand mixer (or a medium bowl if using an electric hand mixer) and blend until combined. Add the coconut flour, ground flaxseed, sweetener, baking powder, xanthan gum, cinnamon, and salt and blend until well incorporated.

3. Transfer the dough to the prepared loaf pan. Sprinkle the sesame seeds on top of the dough, if desired. Bake for 40 to 45 minutes, or until a toothpick inserted in the center of the loaf comes out clean.

4. Remove from the oven and set aside to cool for 20 minutes, then remove the loaf from the pan by lifting up on the parchment paper. Place the loaf on a wire rack to cool completely.

5. Once cool, slice and serve.

calories 122 | fat 9g | protein 4g | total carbs 4g | dietary fiber 3g | net carbs 1g

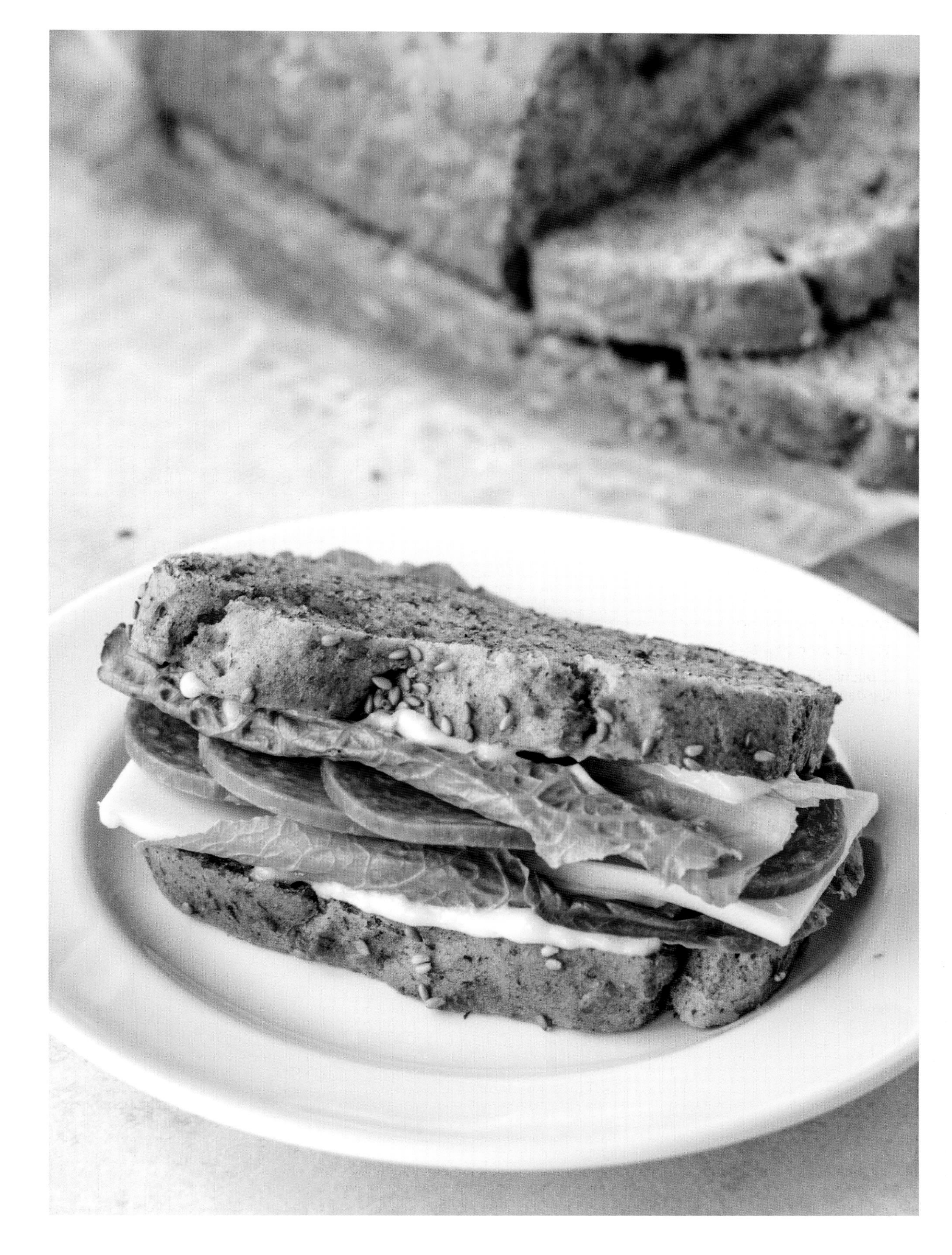

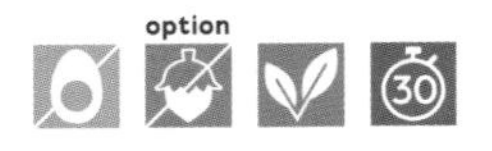

BURRATA PESTO CAPRESE STACKS

YIELD: 12 stacks (2 stacks per serving)

PREP TIME: 10 minutes (not including time to make pesto)

This pretty dish is great as an appetizer or a side. Even my kids will eat it!

4 large tomatoes (about 1 pound)

Fine sea salt and freshly ground black pepper

1 batch Pesto (page 54)

12 ounces Burrata cheese, cut into 12 slices

Chopped fresh flat-leaf parsley, for garnish

Extra-virgin olive oil, for drizzling

Store in an airtight container in the refrigerator for up to 3 days.

1. Slice the ends off of each tomato, then cut each tomato horizontally into 3 thick slices. Arrange on a platter and season with salt and pepper.

2. Cover each tomato slice with pesto, then top with a slice of the Burrata. Garnish with parsley, drizzle a little olive oil over the top, and serve.

calories 256 | fat 24g | protein 12g | total carbs 3g | dietary fiber 1g | net carbs 2g

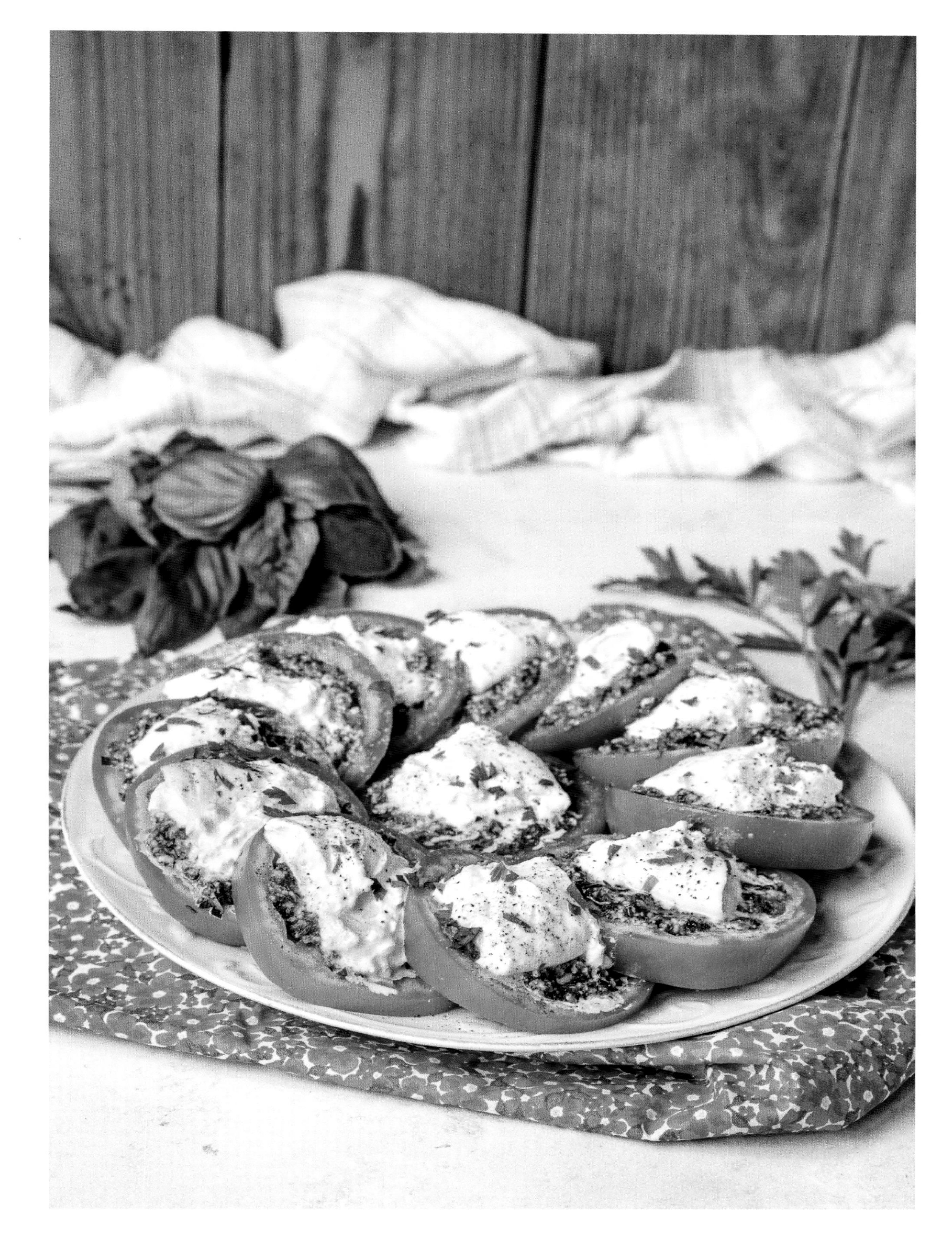

FOCACCIA

YIELD: one 9 by 6-inch flatbread (12 slices, 1 slice per serving)

PREP TIME: 25 minutes

COOK TIME: 15 minutes

When I'm throwing a party that includes non-keto family members and friends, I try to serve foods that I know they're used to eating. Bread is one of the most frequently eaten and enjoyed foods—especially in an Italian household! This focaccia is a favorite of my entire extended family. It works nicely on an antipasto platter with a selection of salami and cheese.

2 cups (225g) shredded part-skim mozzarella cheese

½ cup (60g) coconut flour

2 large eggs

2 ounces cream cheese (¼ cup), softened

1 tablespoon baking powder

1 teaspoon baking soda

1 teaspoon Italian seasoning

1 teaspoon xanthan gum

½ teaspoon garlic powder

½ teaspoon onion powder

½ teaspoon freshly ground black pepper

½ teaspoon fine sea salt

3 tablespoons extra-virgin olive oil, divided

FOR SERVING (OPTIONAL)

Lemon Aioli (page 51), Olive Sauce (page 57), or Pesto (page 54)

1. Preheat the oven to 400°F. Line a sheet pan with parchment paper.
2. Place all of the ingredients except 1 tablespoon of the oil in a food processor or stand mixer (or a medium bowl if using an electric hand mixer) and mix until a dough comes together. Remove the dough and form into 15 equal-sized balls.
3. Place the balls on the prepared sheet pan in 3 rows, making sure the balls are touching each other. Place another sheet of parchment paper on top of the balls and press down with your fingers until the dough is about ½ inch thick and all of the balls are stuck together, forming a rectangle measuring 9 by 6 inches. The top of the dough should appear dimpled, not flat.
4. Remove the top sheet of parchment and drizzle the remaining 1 tablespoon of olive oil over the dough. Bake for 15 minutes, or until browned. Remove from the oven and set aside to cool slightly.
5. Slice into 12 squares and serve with aioli, olive sauce, or pesto for dipping.

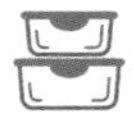

Wrap tightly in aluminum foil and refrigerate for up to 5 days.

Make-ahead tip: If you're making this recipe in advance, follow the directions through Step 3 and then cover the dough with plastic wrap. Refrigerate for up to 24 hours. Before baking, remove from the refrigerator and set out at room temperature for 1 hour. Follow the rest of the recipe as directed.

calories 144 | fat 11g | protein 4g | total carbs 6g | dietary fiber 4g | net carbs 2g

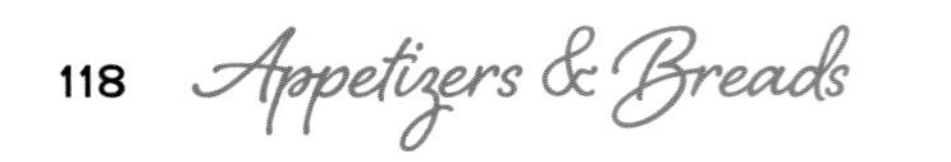

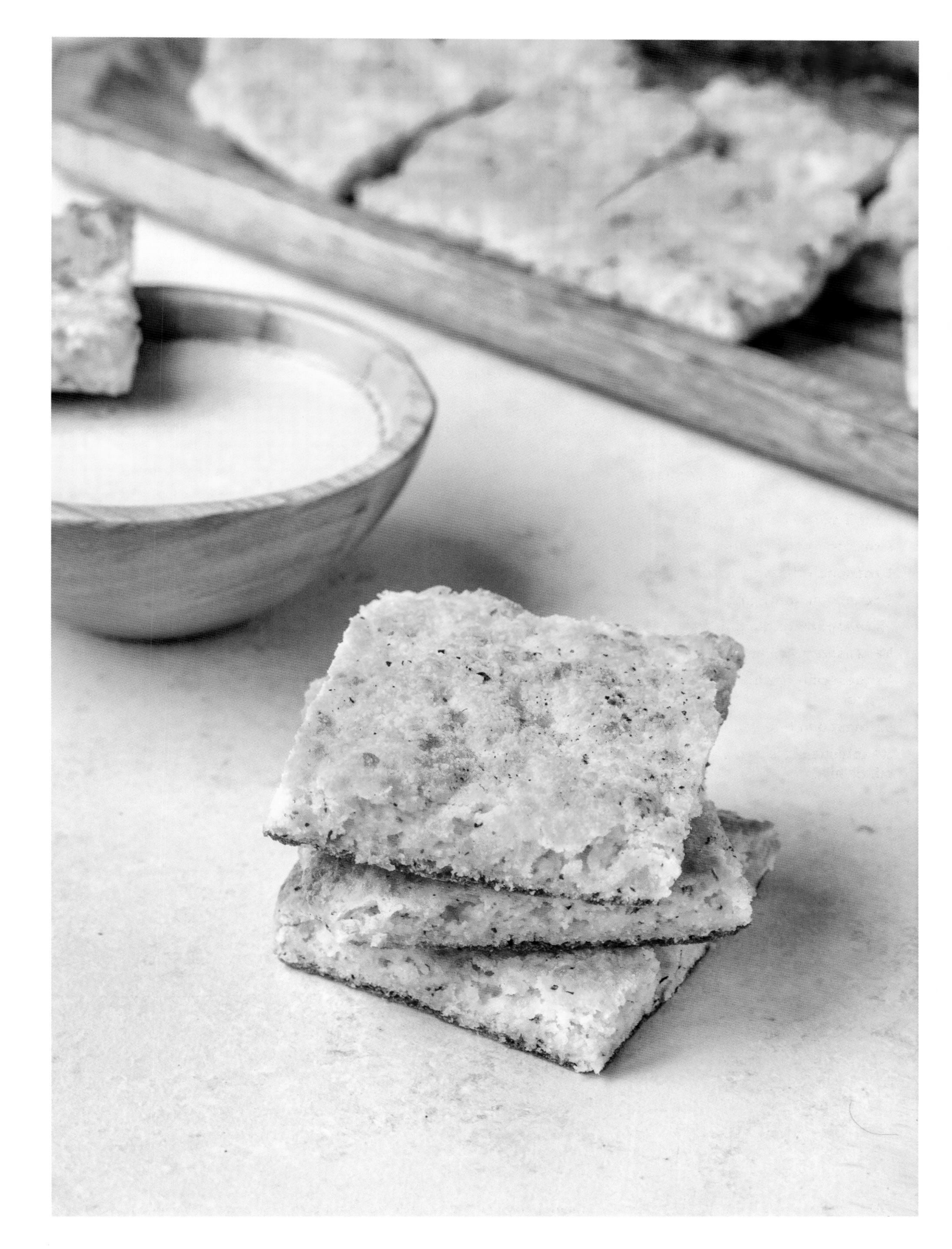

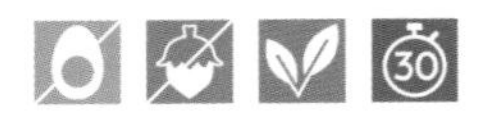

FRIED HALLOUMI STICKS

YIELD: 7 servings

PREP TIME: 2 minutes

COOK TIME: 12 minutes

Enjoy these sticks as an appetizer, a snack, or a side dish. They're tasty on their own but even better dipped in Quick Marinara Sauce (page 53).

14 ounces halloumi cheese

2 tablespoons unsalted butter, divided

Store in an airtight container in the refrigerator for up to 1 week. To reheat, microwave for 30 seconds or warm through in a dry skillet over medium heat.

1. Slice the cheese into sticks about ½ inch wide.
2. Melt 1 tablespoon of the butter in a medium skillet over medium-high heat. Place half of the cheese sticks in the skillet and fry for 2 to 3 minutes, or until browned on one side. Flip them over and fry for 2 to 3 minutes, or until browned on the other side. Transfer the fried sticks to a plate lined with a paper towel.
3. Melt the remaining 1 tablespoon of butter in the skillet and fry the remaining half of the cheese sticks as directed above. Serve immediately.

calories 207 | fat 17g | protein 12g | total carbs 0g | dietary fiber 0g | net carbs 0g

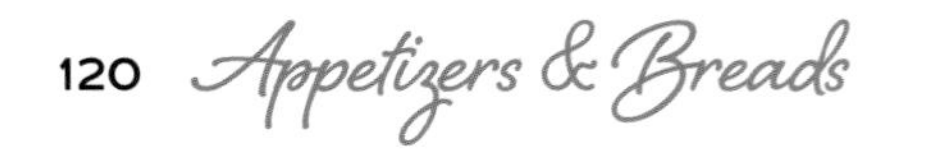

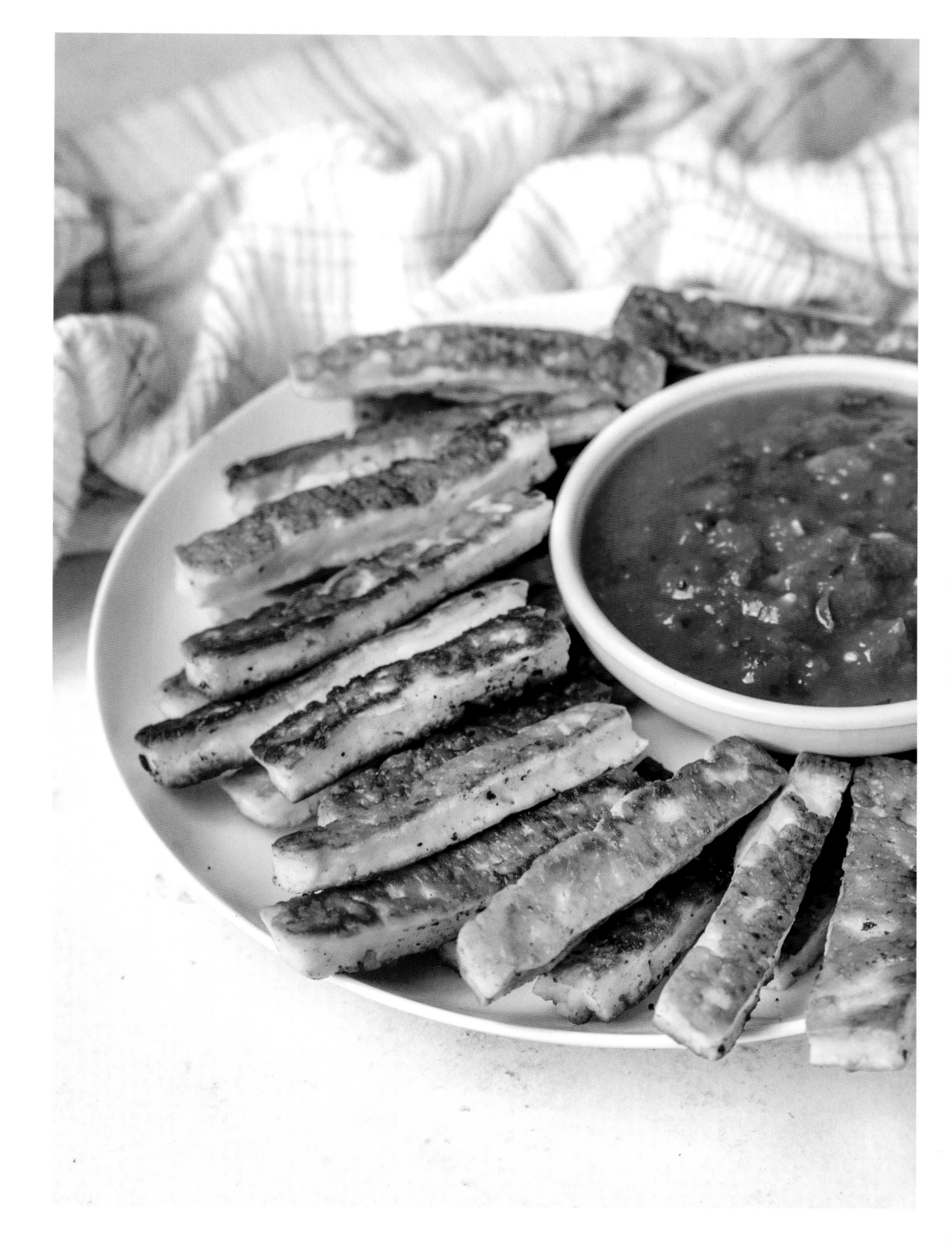

HAMBURGER ROLLS

YIELD: 8 rolls (1 per serving)

PREP TIME: 20 minutes

COOK TIME: 25 minutes

This recipe is adapted from my Coconut Flour Bread recipe (page 114), which went viral. I think the reason it did is that it doesn't require any special ingredients—almost everything is already on hand in a typical keto kitchen. I tried and tried, but the dough from that recipe just didn't work as a roll. It needed some tweaking in order to get a light, rather than dense, roll, and I worked for many, many hours to get this recipe just right for this cookbook.

- 3 large eggs (see Tip, page 82)
- 3 large egg whites
- ⅓ cup extra-virgin olive oil
- ⅓ cup water
- 1 tablespoon apple cider vinegar
- ½ cup (60g) coconut flour
- ½ cup (55g) ground flaxseed
- 1½ teaspoons Swerve granular sweetener
- 2 tablespoons baking powder
- 1 teaspoon baking soda
- 1 teaspoon xanthan gum
- ½ teaspoon fine sea salt
- ½ teaspoon garlic powder
- ½ teaspoon onion powder
- ¼ teaspoon freshly ground black pepper
- 1 tablespoon sesame seeds, for topping (optional)

1. Preheat the oven to 375°F. Line a sheet pan with parchment paper.
2. Place the whole eggs, egg whites, oil, water, and vinegar in the bowl of a stand mixer (or a medium bowl if using an electric hand mixer) and mix until combined. In a separate bowl, combine the remaining ingredients except the sesame seeds. Gradually add the dry ingredients to the wet ingredients and mix until fully incorporated.
3. Using a ⅓-cup measuring cup, scoop the dough onto the prepared sheet pan. You will have enough to make 8 rolls. (If you want more formed rolls that keep their shape, use a well-greased ramekin instead of a measuring cup. The rolls pictured were just scooped.) Top with the sesame seeds, if using.
4. Bake for 25 minutes, or until slightly browned. Remove from the oven and set aside to cool slightly.
5. Slice in half horizontally and serve.

If storing for the near term, allow the rolls to cool completely, transfer to a zip-top plastic bag, and refrigerate for up to 1 week. If storing for the long term, the rolls can be frozen: after cooling completely, wrap each roll in plastic wrap, place in a sealed zip-top freezer bag, and freeze for up to 2 months. Thaw in the refrigerator overnight before using. To rewarm the rolls, melt 1 tablespoon of butter in a skillet over medium heat. Slice the rolls in half and toast for 3 to 4 minutes on each side. Serve immediately.

Make-ahead tip: If you're making this recipe in advance, follow the directions through Step 3 and then cover the dough with plastic wrap. Refrigerate for up to 24 hours. Before baking, remove from the refrigerator and set out at room temperature for 1 hour. Follow the rest of the recipe as directed.

calories 199 | fat 15g | protein 6g | total carbs 9g | dietary fiber 5g | net carbs 4g

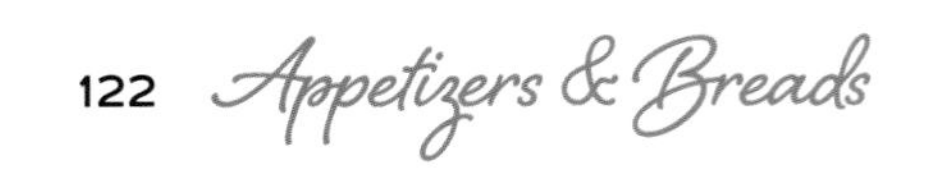

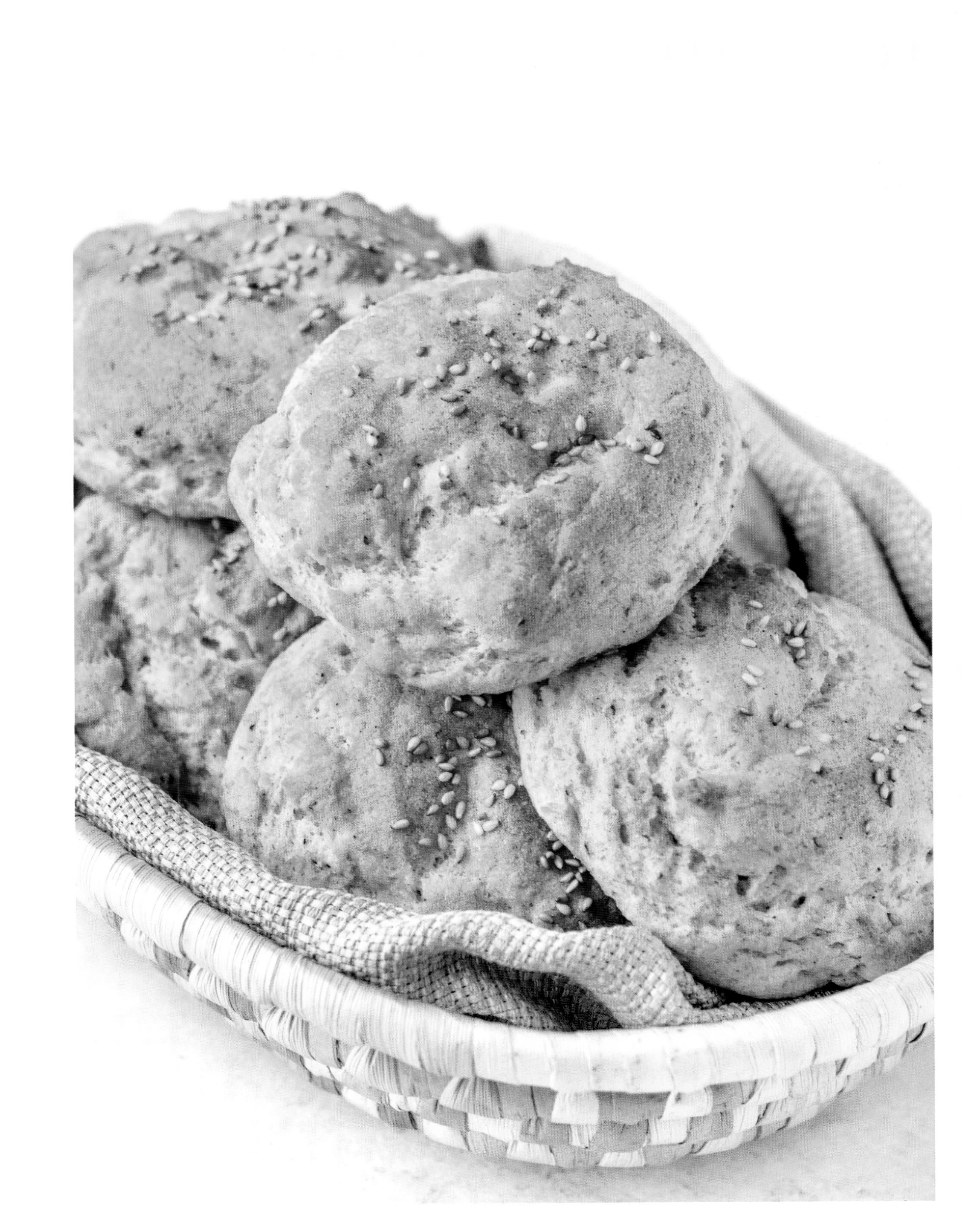

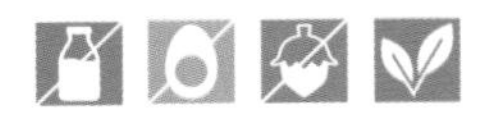

SALT AND VINEGAR ZUCCHINI CHIPS

YIELD: 8 servings (about 1/2 cup per serving)

PREP TIME: 15 minutes

COOK TIME: 3 hours or 8 to 14 hours, depending on method

I was a chipaholic before I started keto, and I still love a good crunchy snack. These zucchini chips are enough to satisfy me these days.

2 tablespoons extra-virgin olive oil

2 tablespoons white balsamic vinegar

4 cups thinly sliced zucchini (about 3 medium)

2 teaspoons coarse sea salt

Store in aluminum foil at room temperature for up to 2 days.

1. In a small bowl, whisk together the oil and vinegar.
2. Place the zucchini slices in a large bowl and pour the oil and vinegar mixture over them. Toss until well coated.

DEHYDRATOR DIRECTIONS:

1. Arrange the zucchini slices in even layers across the grates of a dehydrator and season with the salt.
2. Set the dehydrator to 135°F. Depending on how thinly sliced the zucchini is, the drying time will vary from 8 to 14 hours. Test for crispness and remove when the right texture is achieved. Serve.

OVEN DIRECTIONS:

1. Preheat the oven to 200°F. Line a sheet pan with parchment paper. (Use two sheet pans if needed.)
2. Arrange the zucchini slices evenly on the prepared sheet pan and sprinkle with the salt. Bake for 2 to 3 hours, rotating the pan halfway through the cooking time. Test for crispness and remove from the oven when the right texture is achieved. Serve.

calories 40 | fat 3.6g | protein 0.7g | total carbs 2.9g | dietary fiber 0.6g | net carbs 2.3g

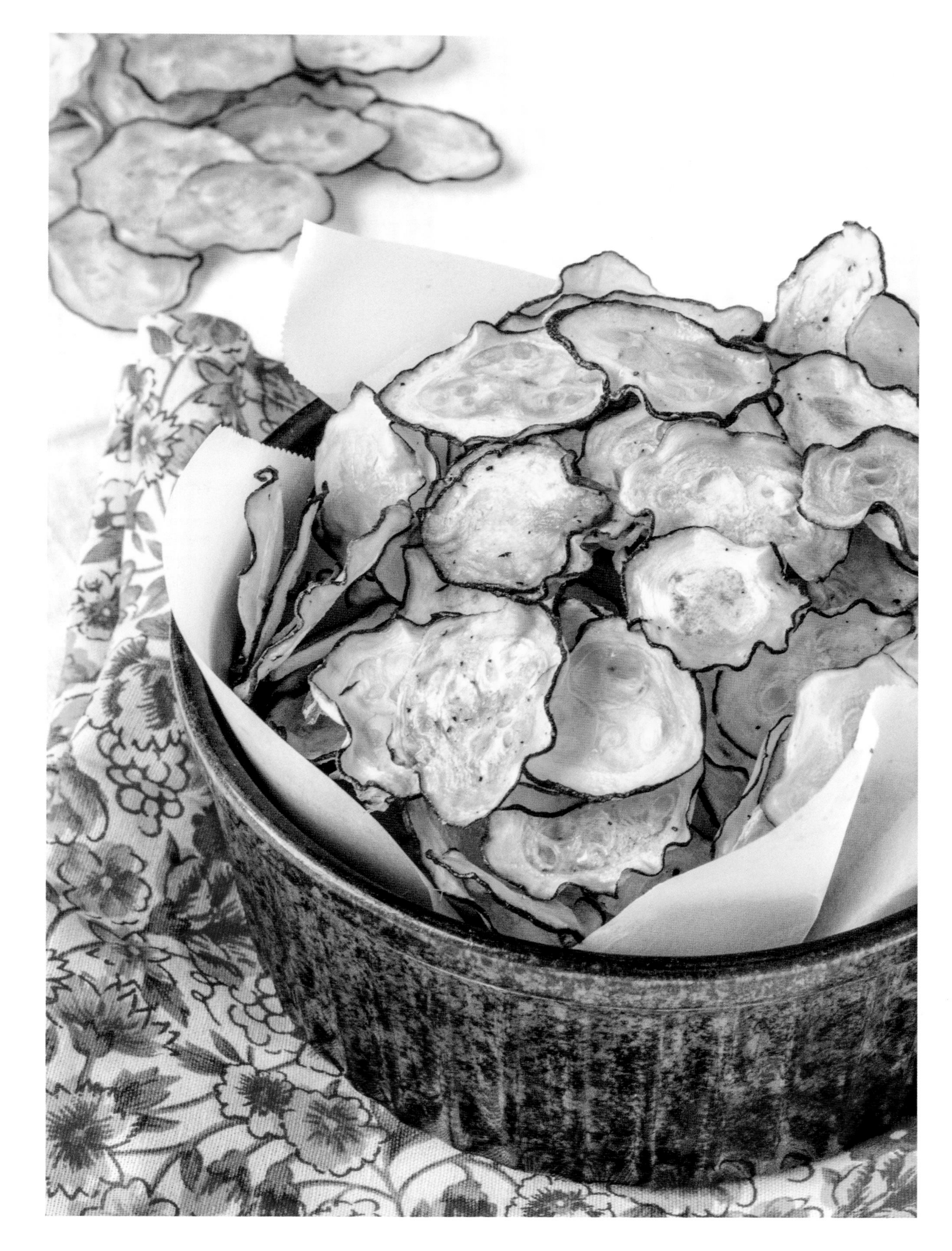

SESAME CRACKERS

YIELD: 48 crackers (4 per serving)
PREP TIME: 20 minutes
COOK TIME: 20 minutes

If you're a fan of sesame flavor, you'll love these crisp crackers. They are perfect for a charcuterie platter or with guacamole.

1 cup (120g) sesame flour
2 large eggs
1/2 cup avocado oil
1 teaspoon baking powder
1/2 teaspoon onion powder
1/2 teaspoon fine sea salt
1/4 teaspoon Italian seasoning

TOPPINGS
1 tablespoon sesame seeds
Pinch of fine sea salt

Wrap tightly in aluminum foil and store at room temperature for up to 1 week.

1. Preheat the oven to 350°F. Line a sheet pan with parchment paper.

2. Place the flour, eggs, oil, baking powder, onion powder, salt, and Italian seasoning in a food processor and process until well combined.

3. Transfer the dough to the prepared sheet pan and place another sheet of parchment paper on top. Using a rolling pin, roll the dough between the two sheets of parchment into a very thin rectangle, 12 by 10 inches. Remove the top sheet of parchment paper.

4. Cut along the edges of the dough to even out the rectangle. Using a greased pizza cutter or knife, score the dough into 48 squares.

5. Sprinkle on the sesame seeds and salt and press them into the dough. Bake for 20 minutes, or until lightly golden brown. Remove from the oven and set aside to cool on the pan for 5 minutes.

6. Gently separate the crackers along the scored lines. Let cool completely before serving.

calories 128 | fat 11g | protein 5g | total carbs 2g | dietary fiber 1g | net carbs 1g

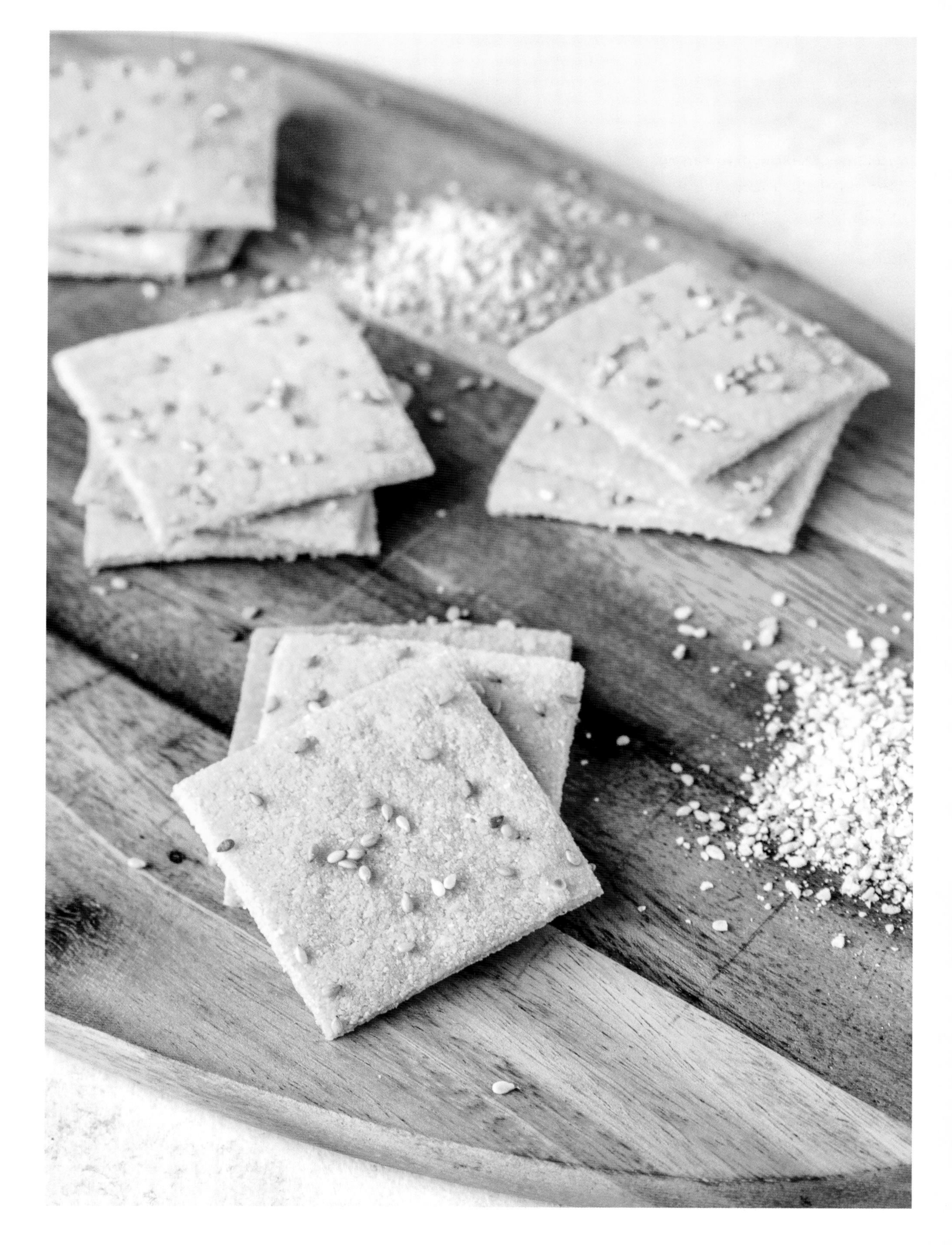

option

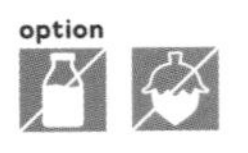

"FOR REAL" TORTILLAS

YIELD: 10 tortillas (1 per serving)

PREP TIME: 25 minutes

COOK TIME: 40 minutes

Finally, a real tortilla that's soft and pliable and won't break apart when you fill it, and it's not eggy tasting, either. I can't tell you how many attempts it took to perfect these. It was at least fifteen—no kidding! This recipe requires a bit of time in the kitchen, but it's worth the effort.

½ cup (60g) coconut flour, plus more for dusting

½ cup (60g) sesame flour

⅓ cup beef bone broth

2 large eggs

2 teaspoons xanthan gum

1 teaspoon onion powder

½ teaspoon garlic powder

½ teaspoon fine sea salt

Avocado oil, ghee, or unsalted butter, for the pan

Wrap tightly in aluminum foil and store in the refrigerator for up to 1 week, or place between sheets of parchment paper and freeze in a zip-top freezer bag for up to 1 month. Reheat in a skillet over low heat.

1. Place all of the ingredients except the oil in a food processor or blender and process until a smooth dough forms.

2. Separate the dough into 10 balls. Sprinkle some coconut flour on a sheet of parchment paper or other clean work surface. Place the dough balls on the parchment and dust with more coconut flour.

3. Using a rolling pin, flatten each ball into a 6-inch circle.

4. Warm 1 teaspoon of the oil in a small skillet over medium-high heat. Place 1 dough round in the skillet and cook for 1 to 2 minutes, or until the edges are browned. Carefully flip it over and cook for 1 to 2 more minutes, or until the edges are browned. Remove the cooked tortilla to a plate.

5. Repeat with the remaining dough rounds, oiling the skillet each time. Serve with the fillings of your choice.

calories 62 | fat 2g | protein 4g | total carbs 4g | dietary fiber 3g | net carbs 1g

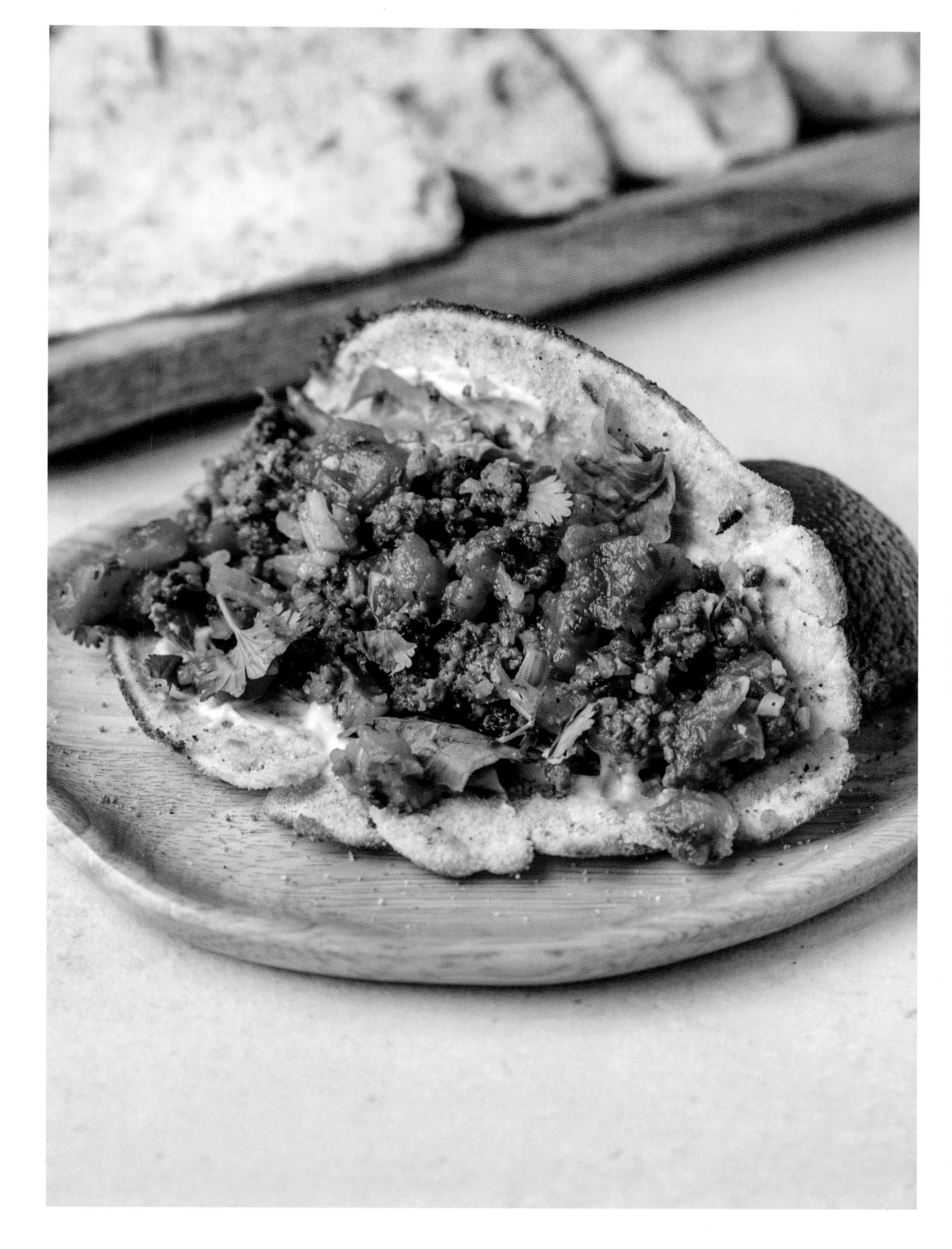

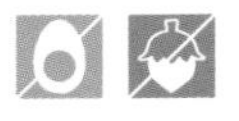

SPICY SAUSAGE-STUFFED MUSHROOMS

YIELD: 24 mushrooms (2 per serving)

PREP TIME: 20 minutes

COOK TIME: 35 minutes

This simple appetizer has lots of flavor but uses just a few ingredients.

24 baby bella mushrooms (about 1½ pounds), stems removed

12 ounces bulk pork sausage

2 to 3 teaspoons red pepper flakes, depending on heat preference, plus more for garnish if desired

1 teaspoon garlic powder

1 teaspoon dried basil

1 teaspoon dried parsley

1 (8-ounce) package cream cheese, softened

Chopped fresh flat-leaf parsley, for garnish

1. Preheat the oven to 350°F.
2. Scoop out and discard the insides of the mushrooms to make room for the stuffing. Place the mushrooms cavity side up in a 13 by 9-inch baking dish.
3. In a medium skillet over medium heat, cook the sausage, stirring often to crumble the meat, until it is no longer pink. Add the red pepper flakes, garlic powder, basil, and parsley and stir to combine. Remove from the heat.
4. Place the cream cheese in the bowl of a stand mixer (or a medium bowl if using an electric hand mixer) and add the cooked sausage. Blend until combined. Taste and adjust the seasonings, if desired.
5. Stuff the mushrooms with the sausage mixture.
6. Bake for 30 minutes, or until the mushrooms are tender.
7. Enjoy warm or at room temperature. Sprinkle with fresh parsley and additional red pepper flakes, if desired.

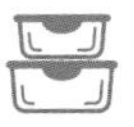

Store in an airtight container in the refrigerator for up to 2 days.

Make-ahead tip: After stuffing the mushrooms, cover and refrigerate for up to 2 days, then bake as directed.

calories 164 | fat 14g | protein 6g | total carbs 3g | dietary fiber 0g | net carbs 3g

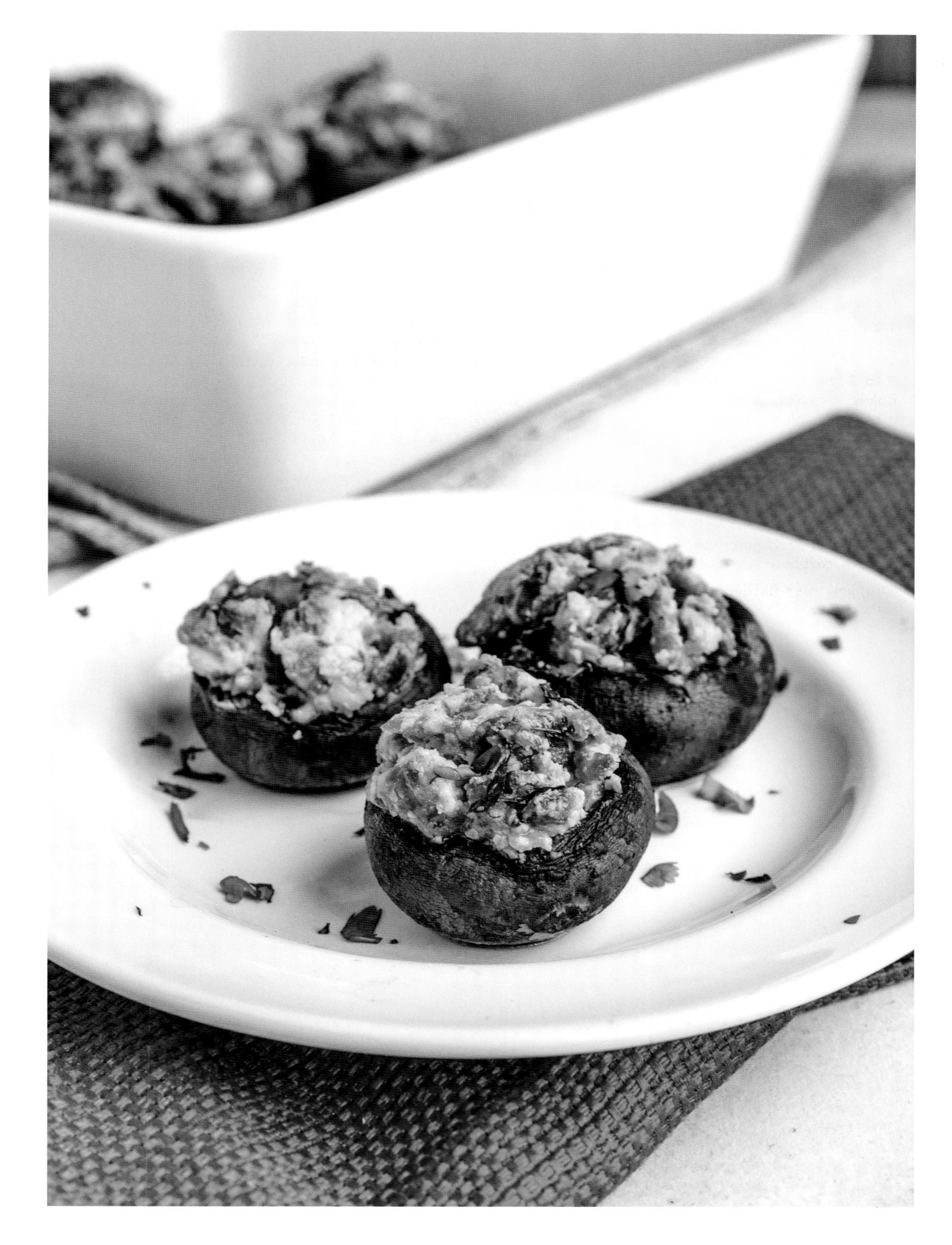

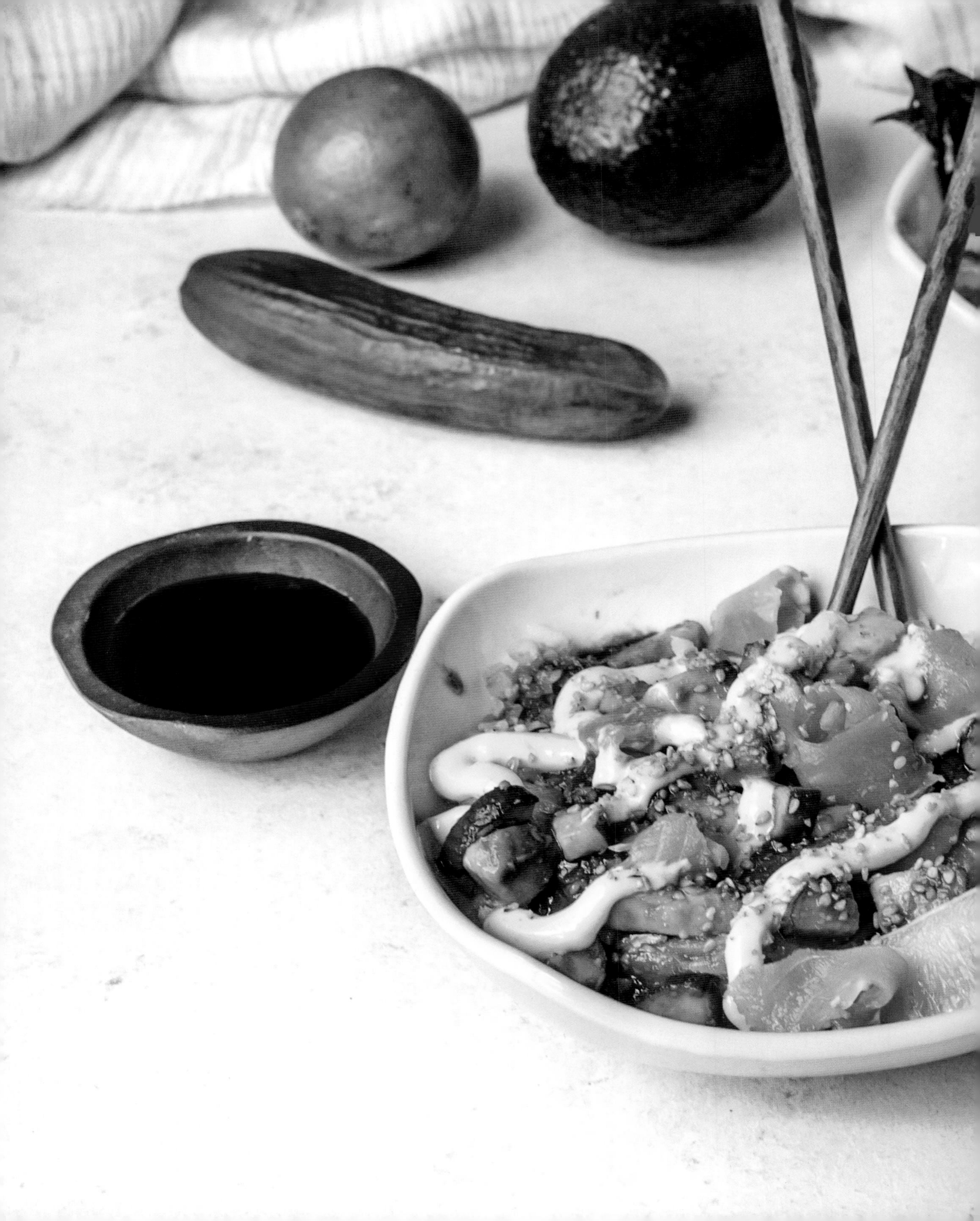

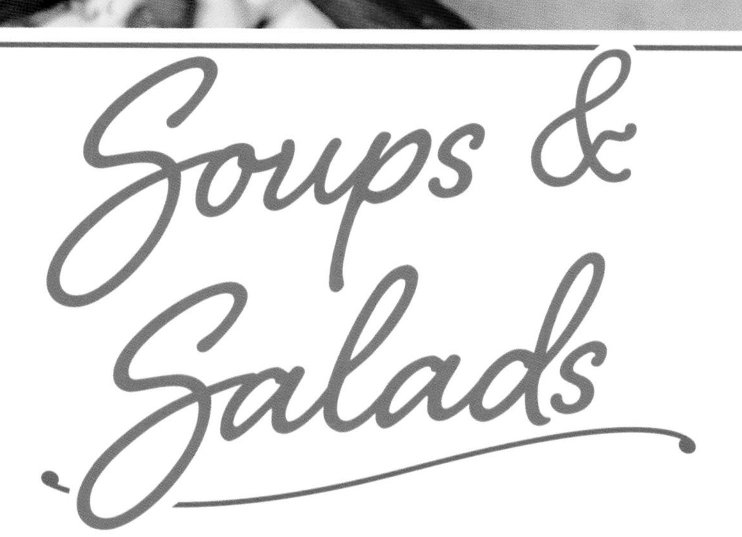
Soups &
Salads

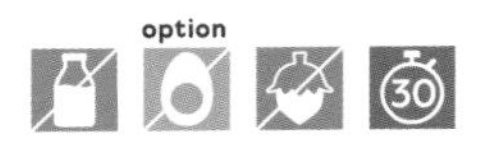

CRISPY BACON CHICKEN CABBAGE SALAD

YIELD: 8 servings

PREP TIME: 20 minutes

COOK TIME: 5 minutes

This recipe is a great use for rotisserie chicken, and dinner will be ready in a flash on a busy weeknight! Other than the task of pulling the chicken off the bones, this salad is a piece of cake to make and comes together in less than 30 minutes.

FOR THE DRESSING

1 cup avocado oil mayonnaise (for egg-free, use Egg-Free Mayo, page 48)

1/2 cup extra-virgin olive oil

2 tablespoons distilled vinegar

1 tablespoon freshly squeezed lemon juice

1 teaspoon prepared yellow mustard

1 teaspoon onion powder

1/2 teaspoon celery seed

1/2 teaspoon fine sea salt

1/4 teaspoon freshly ground black pepper

FOR THE SALAD

10 ounces bacon

4 cups shredded cooked chicken (from 1 rotisserie chicken)

2 teaspoons minced garlic

4 cups shredded green cabbage (about 1/2 medium head)

4 cups shredded red cabbage (about 1/2 medium head)

1/2 cup chopped green onions

1/2 cup chopped mixed fresh herbs (such as basil, chives, and/or flat-leaf parsley)

1. Make the dressing: Place all of the dressing ingredients in a blender and blend until smooth. Taste and adjust the seasonings as desired. Set aside.

2. Make the salad: Chop the bacon into bite-sized pieces. Place in a large skillet over medium-high heat and cook until crisp. Remove with a slotted spoon and set aside to cool on a plate lined with paper towels. Leave the bacon grease in the skillet.

3. Add the chicken to the skillet and reduce the heat to medium. Allow to sit for 2 minutes before tossing, which will give the chicken some crispness. Add the garlic and stir. Remove from the heat.

4. In a large serving bowl, toss together the cabbage, green onions, and herbs. Stir in the warm chicken and bacon. Pour the dressing over the salad, mix well, and enjoy!

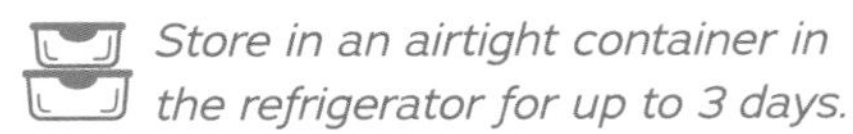
Store in an airtight container in the refrigerator for up to 3 days.

calories 665 | fat 58g | protein 25g | total carbs 11g | dietary fiber 3g | net carbs 7g

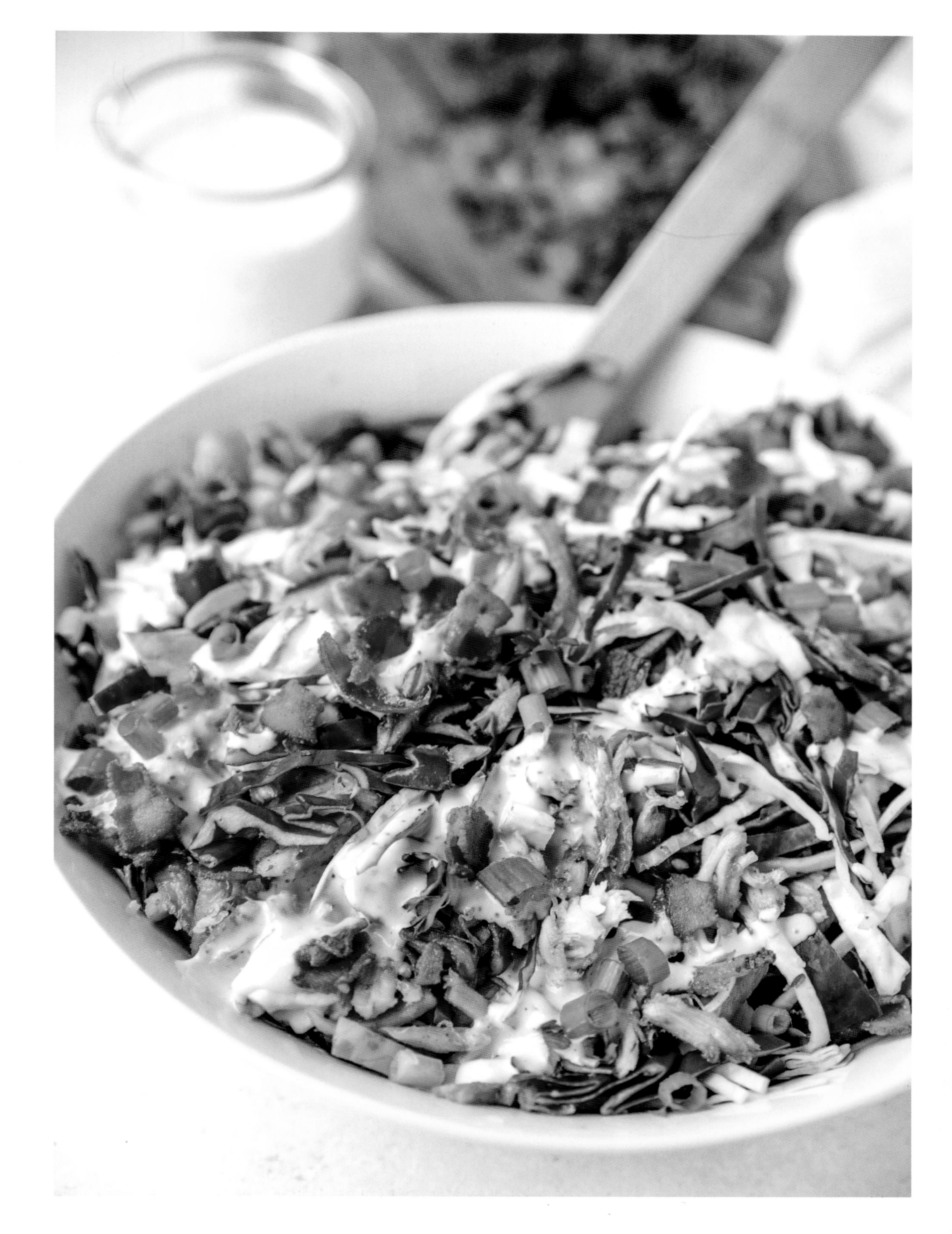

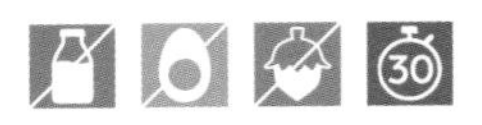

SMOKED SALMON AVOCADO FENNEL SALAD

YIELD: 4 servings

PREP TIME: 15 minutes

This fresh salad hits all the right notes! It's crunchy, creamy, hearty, and satisfying with healthy fats from the smoked salmon and avocado.

FOR THE SALAD

10 ounces fresh fennel bulbs (about 2 small)

¼ small red onion, sliced

2 tablespoons chopped fresh flat-leaf parsley

3 small or 2 large avocados (about 12 ounces), pitted, skinned, and diced

1 tablespoon freshly squeezed lemon juice

8 ounces smoked salmon, chopped

Fine sea salt and freshly ground black pepper

FOR THE DRESSING

3 tablespoons extra-virgin olive oil

2 tablespoons red wine vinegar

1 teaspoon minced garlic

Store in an airtight container in the refrigerator for up to 5 days.

1. Make the salad: Remove the stems and fronds from the fennel bulbs. Discard the stems and chop the fronds; set aside. Remove and discard the outer layer of the fennel bulbs, as they are very coarse. Use a mandoline to slice the bulbs, or slice them as thinly as you can by hand. Place the slices in a large bowl and add the fronds, red onion, and parsley.

2. Place the avocados in a small bowl, sprinkle with the lemon juice, and toss to coat. Set aside.

3. Make the dressing: In a small bowl, whisk together the oil, vinegar, and garlic. Pour the dressing over the salad. Season with salt and pepper to taste and toss until well combined.

4. Add the smoked salmon and avocado to the salad and serve.

calories 326 | fat 25g | protein 13g | total carbs 14g | dietary fiber 8g | net carbs 6g

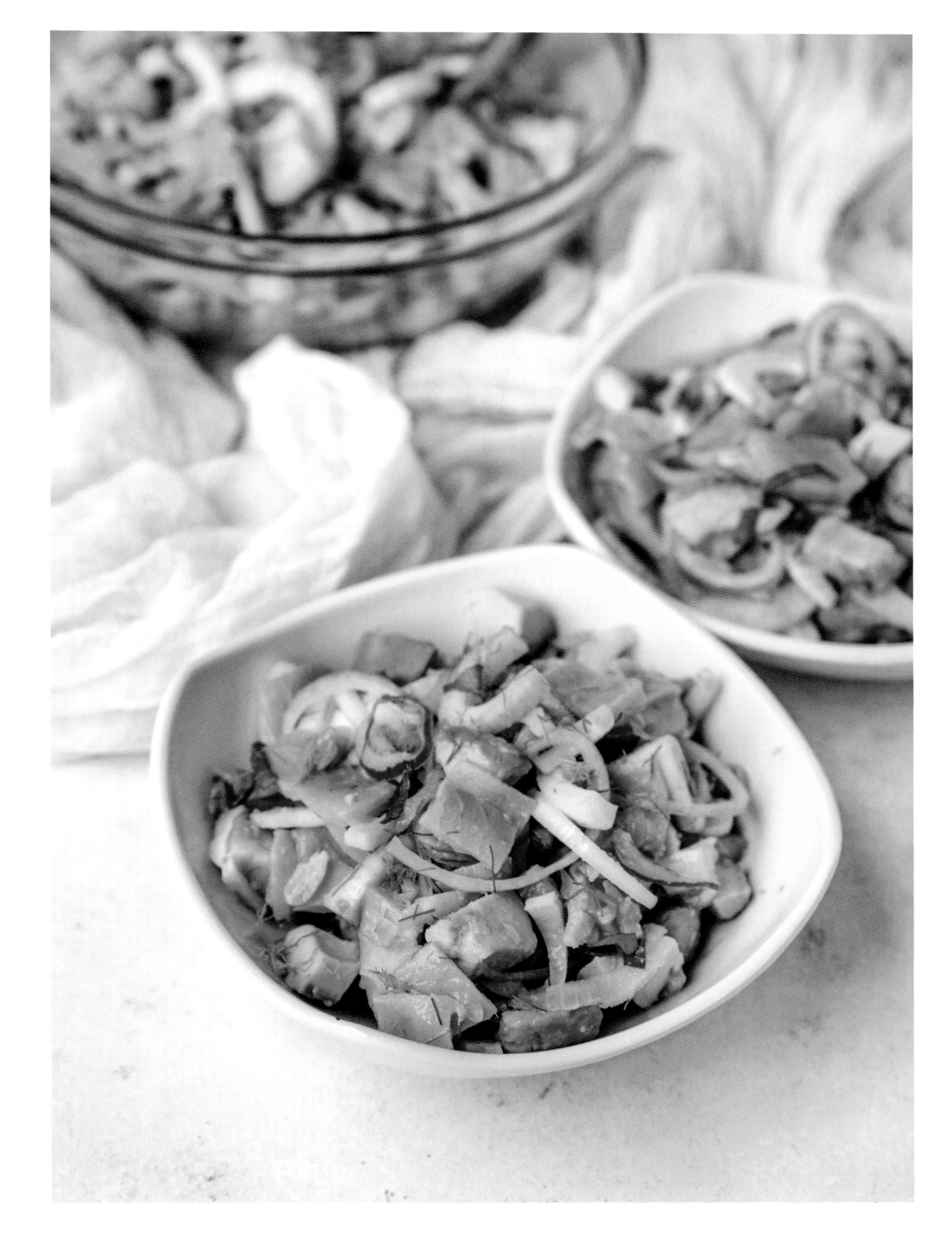

SLOW COOKER UNSTUFFED CABBAGE ROLL SOUP

YIELD: 9 servings

PREP TIME: 20 minutes

COOK TIME: 6 hours or 1 hour, depending on method

This is one of the most popular recipes on my blog, and for good reason—this soup is luscious! Non-keto family and friends will love it, too, and they'll never know that the "rice" in the soup is cauliflower.

2 tablespoons extra-virgin olive oil

2 cloves garlic, minced

½ cup chopped white onions

½ cup chopped shallots

2 pounds grass-fed ground beef

2 cups marinara sauce, store-bought or homemade (page 53)

1 teaspoon dried parsley

1 teaspoon fine sea salt

1 teaspoon freshly ground black pepper

½ teaspoon dried oregano leaves

2 cups fresh (not frozen) riced cauliflower (about ½ medium head)

8 cups shredded green cabbage (about 1 medium head)

5 cups beef bone broth

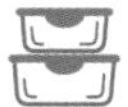

Store in an airtight container in the refrigerator for up to 3 days.

SLOW COOKER DIRECTIONS:

1. Heat the oil in a large skillet over medium-high heat. Add the garlic and cook for 1 minute. Add the onions and shallots and cook until softened.

2. Add the ground beef to the skillet and cook, stirring often to crumble the meat, until it is browned and no longer pink. Add the marinara sauce and season with the parsley, salt, pepper, and oregano. Add the riced cauliflower and stir until fully blended.

3. Transfer the contents of the skillet to a 6-quart slow cooker and add the cabbage and broth. Stir to combine well, cover, and cook on high for 3 hours or on low for 6 hours, or until the cabbage is tender. Serve hot.

STOVETOP DIRECTIONS:

1. Using a Dutch oven instead of a large skillet, follow Steps 1 and 2 above.

2. Add the cabbage and broth to the pot and bring to a boil. Reduce the heat to low and simmer, covered, for 1 hour, or until the cabbage is tender. Remove from the heat. Serve hot.

calories 356 | fat 26g | protein 20g | total carbs 8g | dietary fiber 2g | net carbs 6g

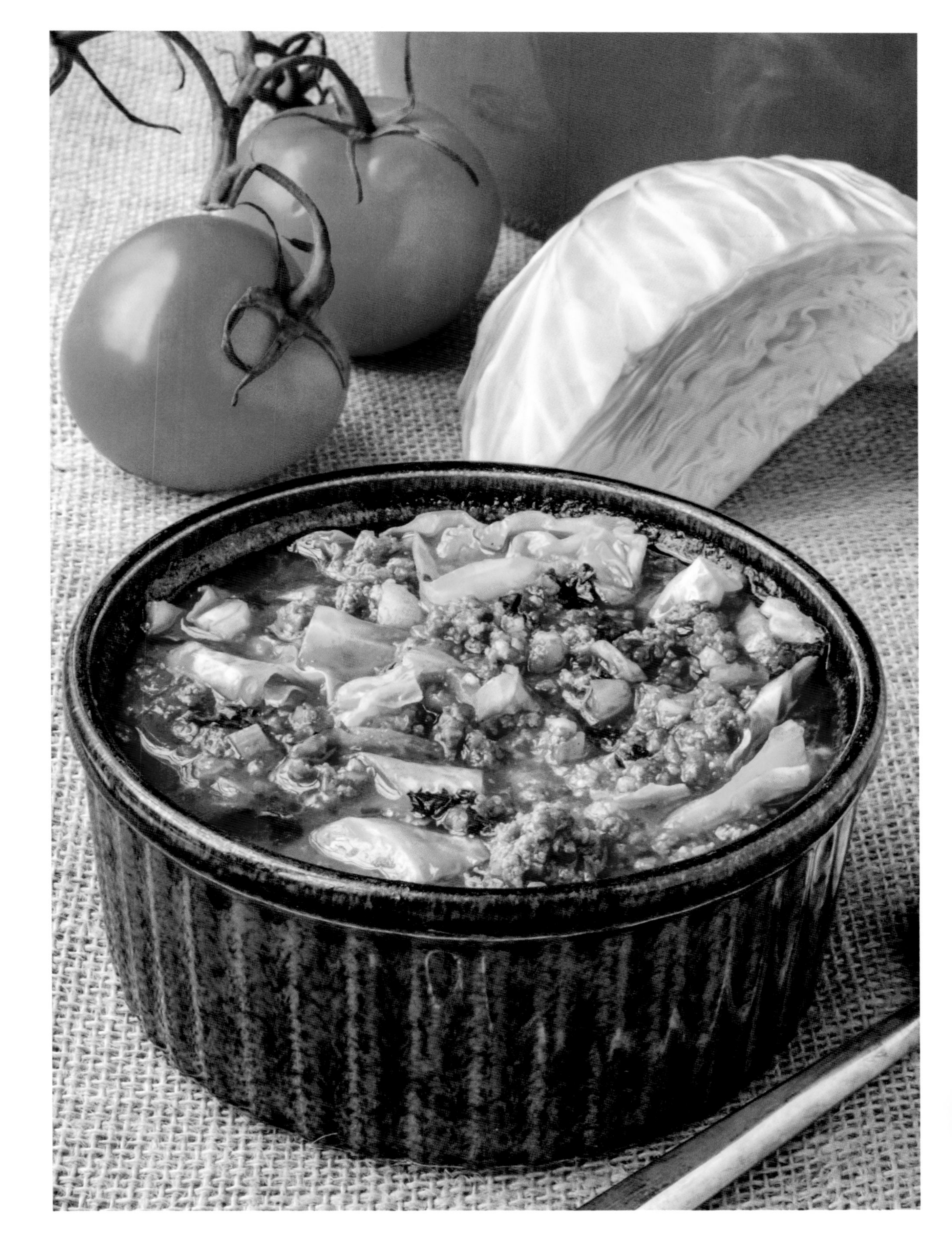

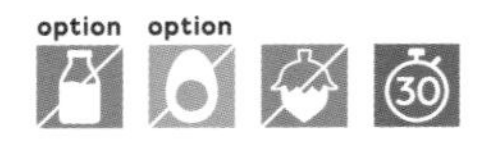

CHEESEBURGER SALAD BOWLS

YIELD: 4 servings

PREP TIME: 15 minutes (not including time to make spice rub or sauce)

COOK TIME: 10 minutes

If you're looking for a fairly easy meal for the whole family, consider this recipe, as these cheeseburger salad bowls come together fast. If you don't have Secret Burger Sauce on hand or don't feel like making it, use your favorite low-carb dressing instead—but note that the burger sauce really makes it taste like you're eating a messy, delicious cheeseburger!

1 pound grass-fed ground beef

2 teaspoons minced garlic

1 tablespoon Beef Spice Rub (page 46)

2 cups shredded or chopped romaine lettuce

½ cup chopped dill pickles or sliced cornichons

¼ cup halved cherry tomatoes

¼ cup sliced red onions

½ cup shredded or cubed cheddar cheese (optional; omit for dairy-free)

1 cup Secret Burger Sauce (page 55; for egg-free, make the sauce with egg-free mayo)

Tip: If you don't have any Beef Spice Rub on hand, you can use a combination of ½ teaspoon ground cumin, ½ teaspoon dried oregano leaves, ½ teaspoon smoked paprika, ¼ teaspoon chili powder, and ¼ teaspoon fine sea salt instead.

1. In a large skillet over medium-high heat, cook the ground beef until browned and no longer pink, stirring often to crumble the meat. Stir in the garlic and spice rub and remove from the heat.

2. Assemble the bowls: Place ½ cup of lettuce in each of four serving bowls. Top with equal portions of the pickles, tomatoes, red onions, and cheese, if using. Add equal portions of the ground beef mixture and sauce to each bowl and toss well. Serve immediately.

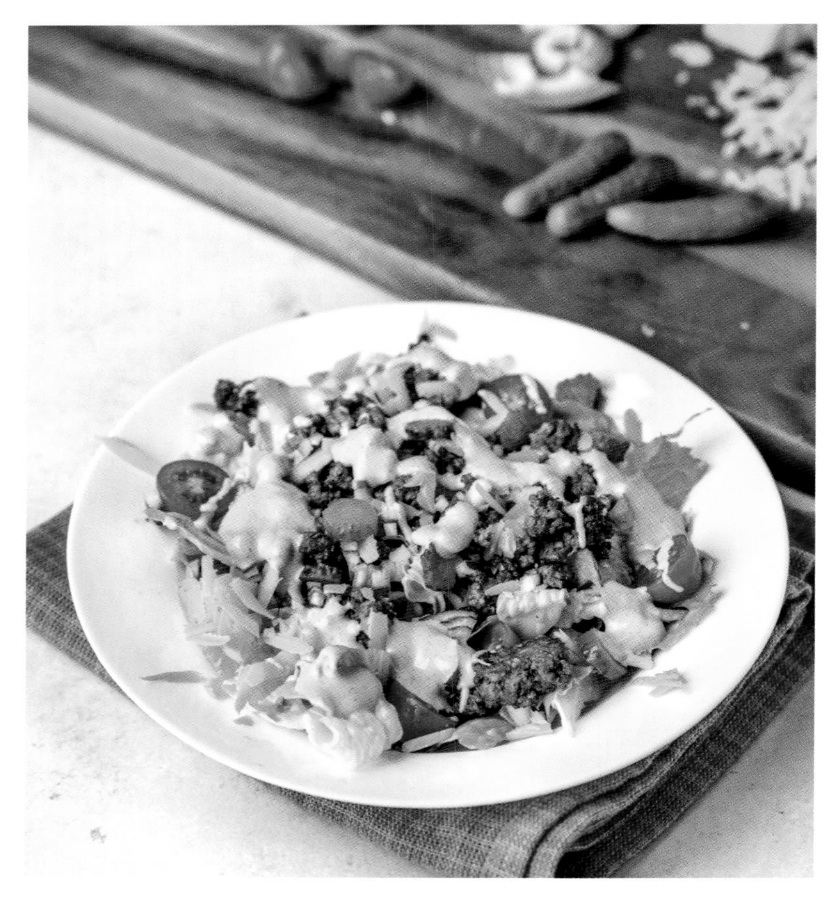

calories 657 | fat 58g | protein 24g | total carbs 6g | dietary fiber 1g | net carbs 5g

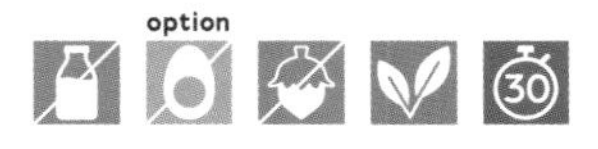

CREAMY CILANTRO LIME SLAW

YIELD: 8 servings

PREP TIME: 20 minutes, plus at least 1 hour to chill

This quick-and-easy side salad is so versatile that it goes with pretty much any entrée.

---

1 small head green cabbage (about 1 pound), cored and thinly sliced

1 small head red cabbage (about 1 pound), cored and thinly sliced

1 cup avocado oil mayonnaise (for egg-free, use Egg-Free Mayo, page 48)

1/4 cup white wine vinegar

1 teaspoon grated lime zest

1/4 cup freshly squeezed lime juice

1/2 teaspoon fine sea salt

1/4 teaspoon freshly ground black pepper

1/2 cup chopped fresh cilantro

Store in an airtight container in the refrigerator for up to 3 days.

1. Place the cabbage in a large bowl and set aside.
2. In a small bowl, whisk together the mayonnaise, vinegar, lime juice, lime zest, salt, and pepper. Stir in the cilantro.
3. Pour the dressing over the cabbage and toss until well combined. Taste and adjust the seasonings, if desired.
4. Refrigerate for at least 1 hour or up to 24 hours before serving. Serve chilled.

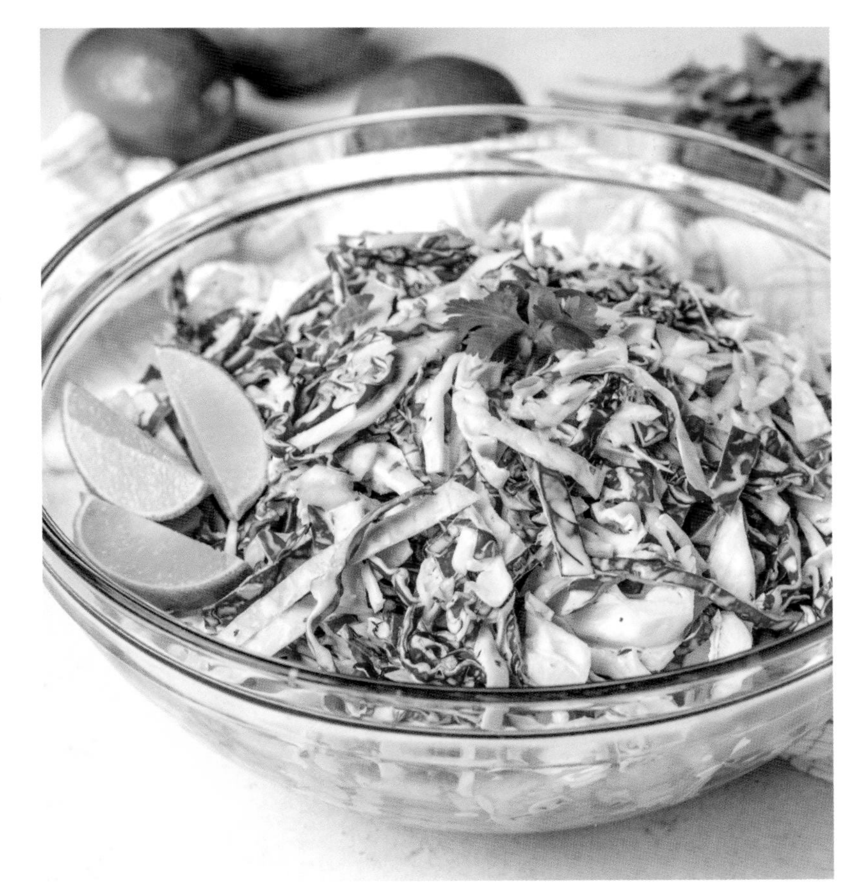

calories 235 | fat 24g | protein 1g | total carbs 8g | dietary fiber 2g | net carbs 6g

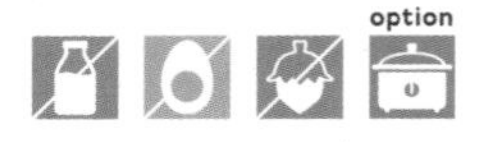

INSTANT POT (OR SLOW COOKER) CHILI

YIELD: 12 servings

PREP TIME: 10 minutes

COOK TIME: 36 minutes or 4 or 8 hours, depending on method

When I first made this chili, I tried to conceal the fact that it had no beans in it from my husband. After he finished his bowl, he looked at me and said, "No beans in this?" My reply, of course, was, "Nope." But he paused and said, "Still delicious! I didn't miss them!" I was shocked but thrilled: I knew that if he liked it, others would, too.

I often get asked why I add cocoa powder to my chili. I was inspired by my first encounter with Mexican mole sauce, which is spicy but includes chocolate to enhance the flavor. Ever since, I've always added cocoa powder to my chili.

2 tablespoons avocado oil

2 cups diced white onions

3 jalapeño peppers, seeded and finely chopped

¾ cup chopped bell peppers

3 pounds grass-fed ground beef

4 cloves garlic, minced

1 tablespoon ground cumin

1 teaspoon chili powder

1 teaspoon dried oregano leaves

1 teaspoon fine sea salt

1 teaspoon freshly ground black pepper

3 cups marinara sauce, store-bought or homemade (page 53)

3 cups beef bone broth

1 (14½-ounce) can diced tomatoes with green chilies

¼ cup tomato paste

2 tablespoons unsweetened cocoa powder

TOPPINGS (OPTIONAL)

Sour cream

Shredded cheddar cheese

Sliced avocado

Chopped fresh cilantro

INSTANT POT DIRECTIONS:

1. Set a 6-quart Instant Pot to the sauté mode and pour in the oil. Add the onions, jalapeños, and bell peppers and sauté for 4 to 6 minutes, or until tender.

2. Add the ground beef, garlic, and dry seasonings and cook until browned and no longer pink, stirring often to crumble the meat.

3. Stir in the marinara sauce, broth, tomatoes with green chilies, tomato paste, and cocoa powder. Cover and set the Instant Pot to the manual mode on high pressure for 20 minutes. Perform a quick release of the pressure. Remove the lid carefully, watching out for the steam.

4. Serve hot, with or without the optional toppings.

SLOW COOKER DIRECTIONS:

1. Heat the oil in a large skillet over medium-high heat. Add the onions, jalapeños, and bell peppers and sauté for 4 to 6 minutes, or until the onions are translucent and the peppers are tender.

2. Add the ground beef and cook until browned and no longer pink, stirring often to crumble the meat. Stir in the garlic and dry seasonings. Remove from the heat.

3. Transfer the contents of the skillet to a 6-quart slow cooker. Stir in the marinara sauce, broth, tomatoes with green chilies, tomato paste, and cocoa powder. Cover and cook on low for 8 hours or on high for 4 hours.

4. Serve hot, with or without the optional toppings.

Store in an airtight container in the refrigerator for up to 3 days or freeze for up to 4 months.

calories **363** | fat **26g** | protein **21g** | total carbs **9g** | dietary fiber **2g** | net carbs **7g**

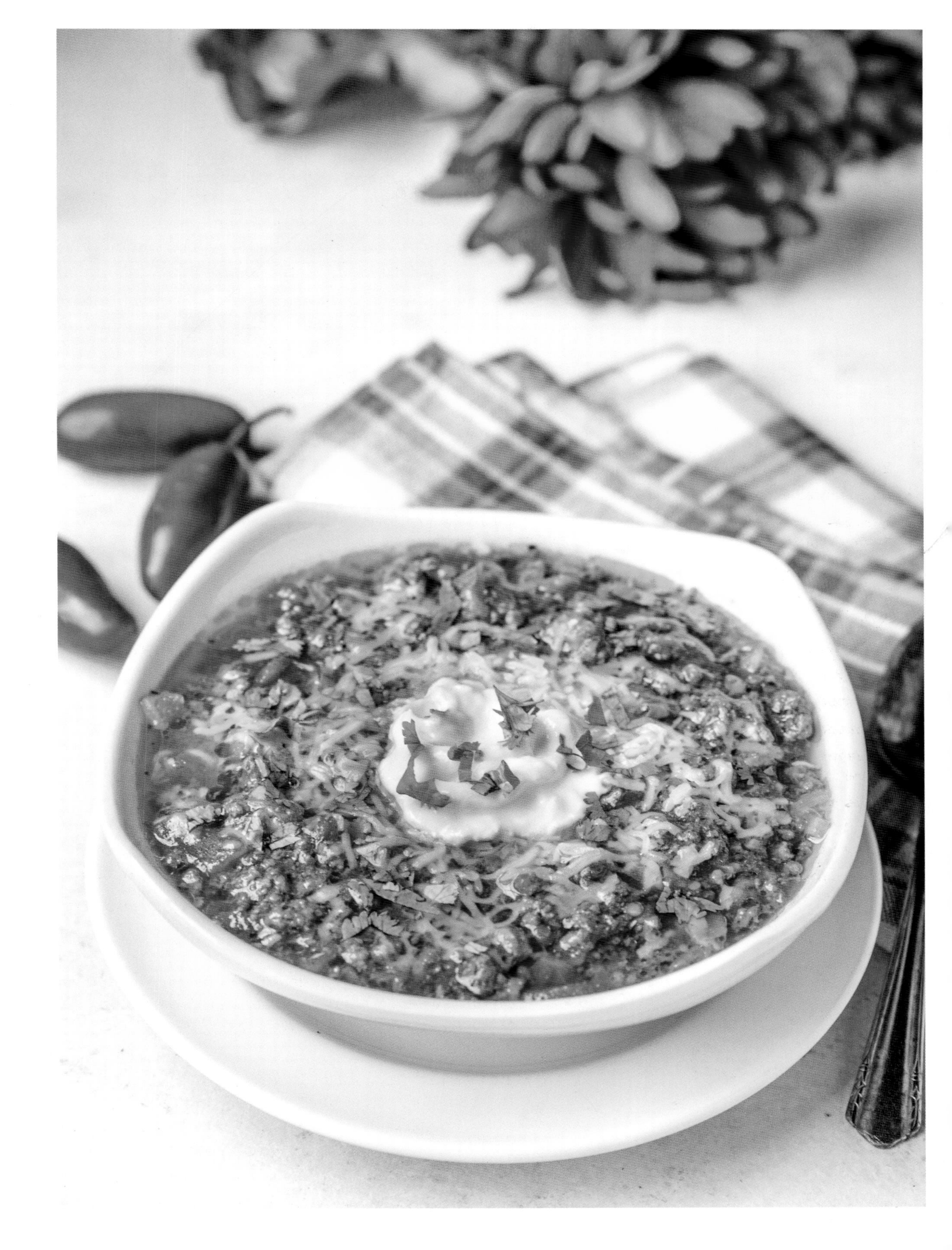

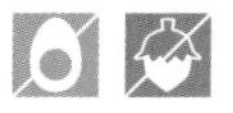

ITALIAN SEAFOOD SALAD

YIELD: 7 servings

PREP TIME: 25 minutes, plus at least 1 hour to chill

COOK TIME: 5 minutes

When you think of seafood salad, you probably think of the American version—something made with mayonnaise, right? But the classic seafood salads of Italy usually combine cooked or sometimes just marinated fish with olive oil, spices, and lemon juice. It's a light, bright, and refreshing combination, and it's a terrific starter for the Christmas Eve meal!

FOR THE SEAFOOD

- 2 tablespoons avocado oil
- 1 tablespoon salted butter
- 1 teaspoon minced garlic
- 1 pound raw medium shrimp, peeled, deveined, and tails removed
- 1 pound bay scallops
- 1 tablespoon freshly squeezed lemon juice
- ½ teaspoon fine sea salt
- ¼ teaspoon freshly ground black pepper

FOR THE SALAD

- 1 pound canned cooked crab meat
- ½ cup chopped celery
- ⅓ cup chopped red onions
- ¼ cup chopped fresh flat-leaf parsley
- ½ teaspoon garlic powder
- ½ teaspoon fine sea salt
- ¼ teaspoon freshly ground black pepper
- ⅓ cup freshly squeezed lemon juice
- ¼ cup extra-virgin olive oil

Store in an airtight container in the refrigerator for up to 2 days.

1. Make the seafood: Warm the avocado oil and butter in a large skillet over medium heat. Add the garlic and cook until the butter is melted and the garlic is fragrant.

2. Add the shrimp and scallops to the skillet and cook until the shrimp turn pink and the scallops are opaque. Stir in the lemon juice, salt, and pepper, remove from the heat, and set aside to cool.

3. Make the salad: Place the crab meat, celery, red onions, parsley, garlic powder, salt, and pepper in a large serving bowl. Drizzle the lemon juice and olive oil over the mixture and toss until all of the ingredients are thoroughly coated. Toss in the cooled shrimp and scallops and stir until combined.

4. Cover and refrigerate for 1 to 2 hours, or until ready to serve. Serve cold.

calories 292 | fat 15g | protein 33g | total carbs 4g | dietary fiber 0g | net carbs 4g

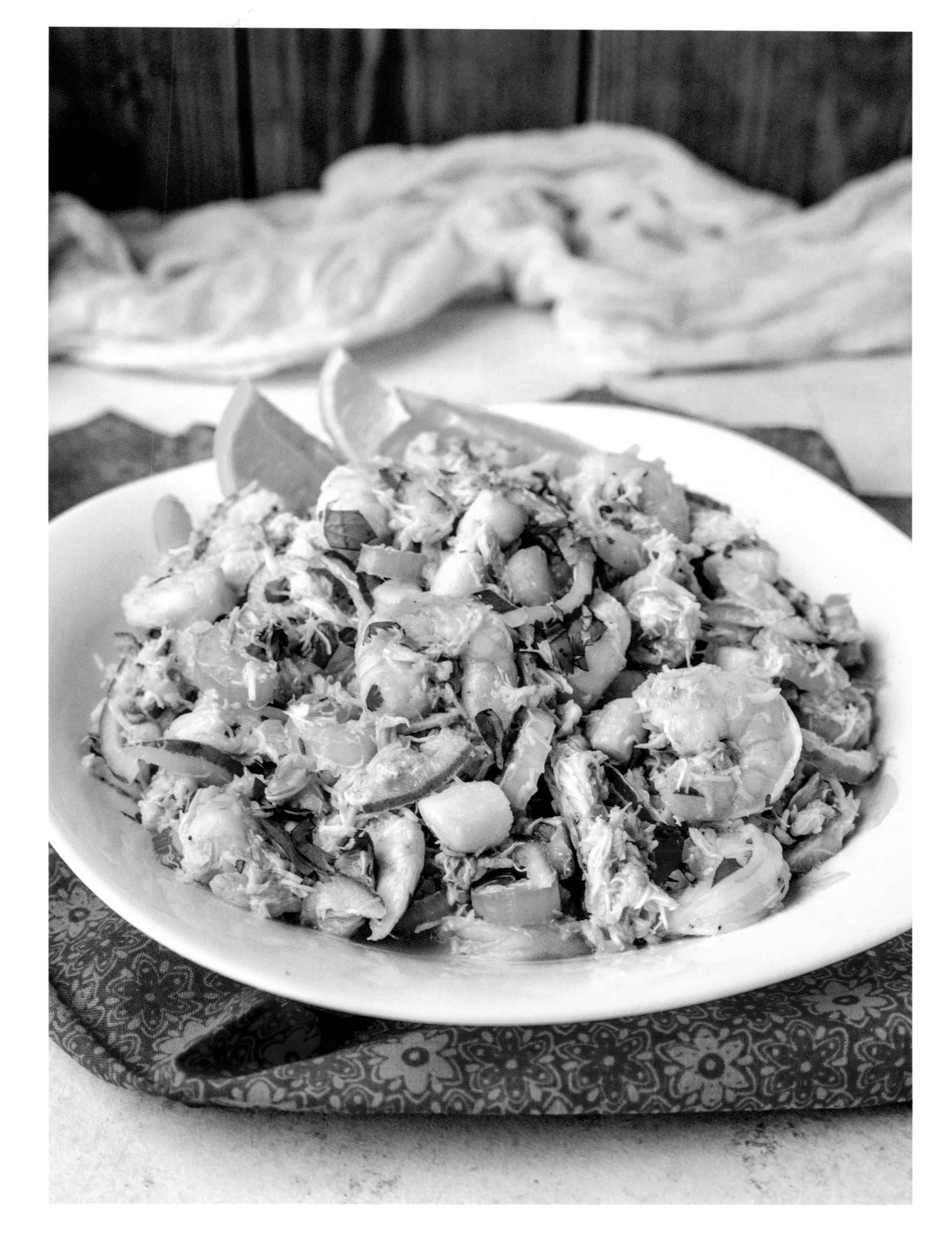

KALE CAESAR SALAD WITH GARLIC CROUTONS

YIELD: 8 servings

PREP TIME: 20 minutes (not including time to make bread or dressing)

COOK TIME: 5 minutes

Massaging kale with lemon juice softens the leaves a bit, which makes the kale more enjoyable to eat raw. Try not to over-massage it; you don't want it to get mushy. Make sure there's still a nice bite to it. To make this salad a meal, top it with a protein such as cooked bacon or shrimp, drained canned tuna, shredded cooked chicken, or smoked salmon.

8 ounces curly kale, stems and stalks removed, chopped

2 tablespoons freshly squeezed lemon juice

2 (1-inch-thick) slices Coconut Flour Bread (page 114), cut into 1-inch cubes (omit for egg-free)

2 tablespoons extra-virgin olive oil

2 cloves garlic, minced

1 cup Caesar Dressing (page 60; for egg-free, make the dressing with egg-free mayo)

TOPPINGS (OPTIONAL)

Shaved Parmesan cheese

Sliced avocado

Store the salad in an airtight container in the refrigerator for up to 3 days. Wrap the croutons tightly in aluminum foil and store on the counter for up to 2 days.

1. Place the kale and lemon juice into a large zip-top plastic bag and seal it. Massage the kale, allowing it to absorb the lemon juice. Set aside while you prepare the rest of the salad.

2. Toast the bread cubes in a toaster oven or in a preheated 350°F oven, for 5 minutes, or until browned and crisp.

3. Heat the oil in a large skillet over medium heat. Add the garlic and cook for 2 to 3 minutes, or until fragrant. Toss the toasted bread cubes into the skillet and cook, stirring frequently, until the cubes are golden and all of the oil is absorbed. Remove from the heat and set aside.

4. Transfer the kale to a large bowl and add the toppings of your choice. Top with the croutons and toss with the Caesar dressing. Enjoy!

calories 188 | fat 18g | protein 3g | total carbs 4g | dietary fiber 0g | net carbs 4g

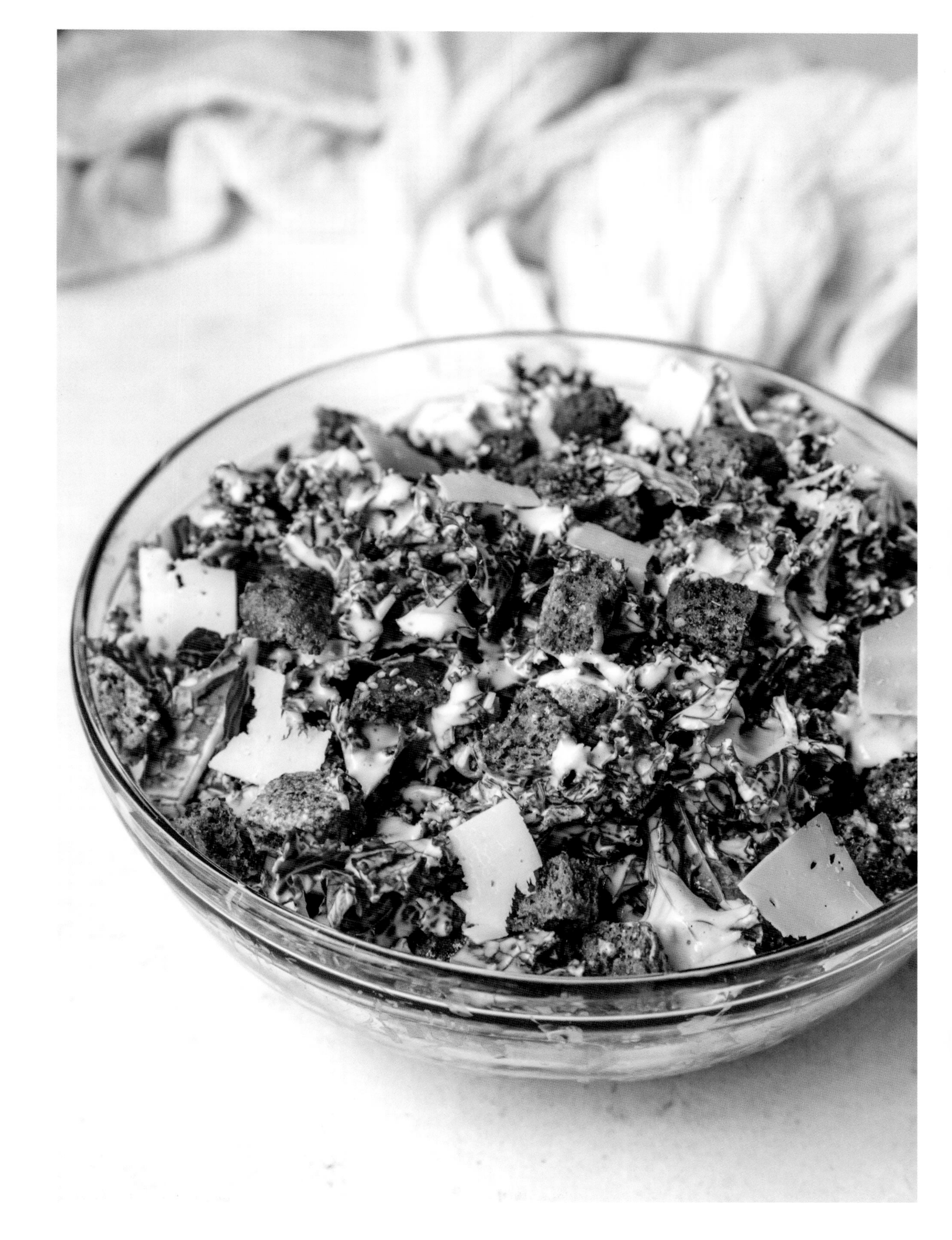

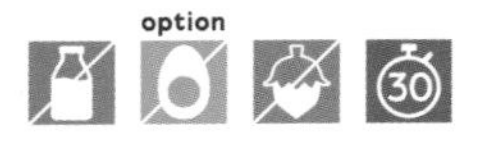

LAZY SUSHI BOWLS

YIELD: 4 servings

PREP TIME: 20 minutes

COOK TIME: 5 minutes

I've always wanted to make my own sushi at home, but I've never wanted to do the work. In my opinion, these lazy sushi bowls are way easier and way better—all of the flavors with little of the effort!

2 large avocados (about 12 ounces), pitted, skinned, and diced

1/2 cup diced cucumbers

1/4 cup chopped green onions

1/4 cup coconut aminos

3 tablespoons apple cider vinegar, divided

12 ounces riced cauliflower

2 tablespoons Swerve granular sweetener

2 teaspoons freshly squeezed lime juice

1/2 teaspoon fine sea salt

1/2 cup avocado oil mayonnaise (for egg-free, use Egg-Free Mayo, page 48)

1 teaspoon Sriracha sauce

1 pound smoked salmon or sushi-grade salmon or tuna, chopped

2 pieces nori (dried seaweed), cut into pieces

1 tablespoon sesame seeds, for topping (optional)

Wasabi, for topping (optional)

4 lime wedges, for serving (optional)

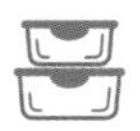
Store in an airtight container in the refrigerator for up to 3 days.

1. In a mixing bowl, stir together the avocados, cucumbers, green onions, coconut aminos, and 1 tablespoon of the vinegar. Set aside.

2. In a large skillet over medium heat, stir-fry the riced cauliflower with the remaining 2 tablespoons of vinegar, the sweetener, lime juice, and salt until fragrant and lightly browned. Remove from the heat and divide the cooked cauliflower evenly among four serving bowls.

3. In a zip-top plastic bag or squeeze bottle, combine the mayonnaise and Sriracha sauce. If using a plastic bag, cut off one corner of the bag.

4. Top the cauliflower in the bowls with equal portions of the avocado mixture, smoked salmon, and nori. Drizzle the Sriracha mayo over the bowls.

5. If desired, top the bowls with the sesame seeds and wasabi and serve with lime wedges. Serve immediately.

calories 469 | fat 37g | protein 23g | total carbs 13g | dietary fiber 5g | net carbs 8g

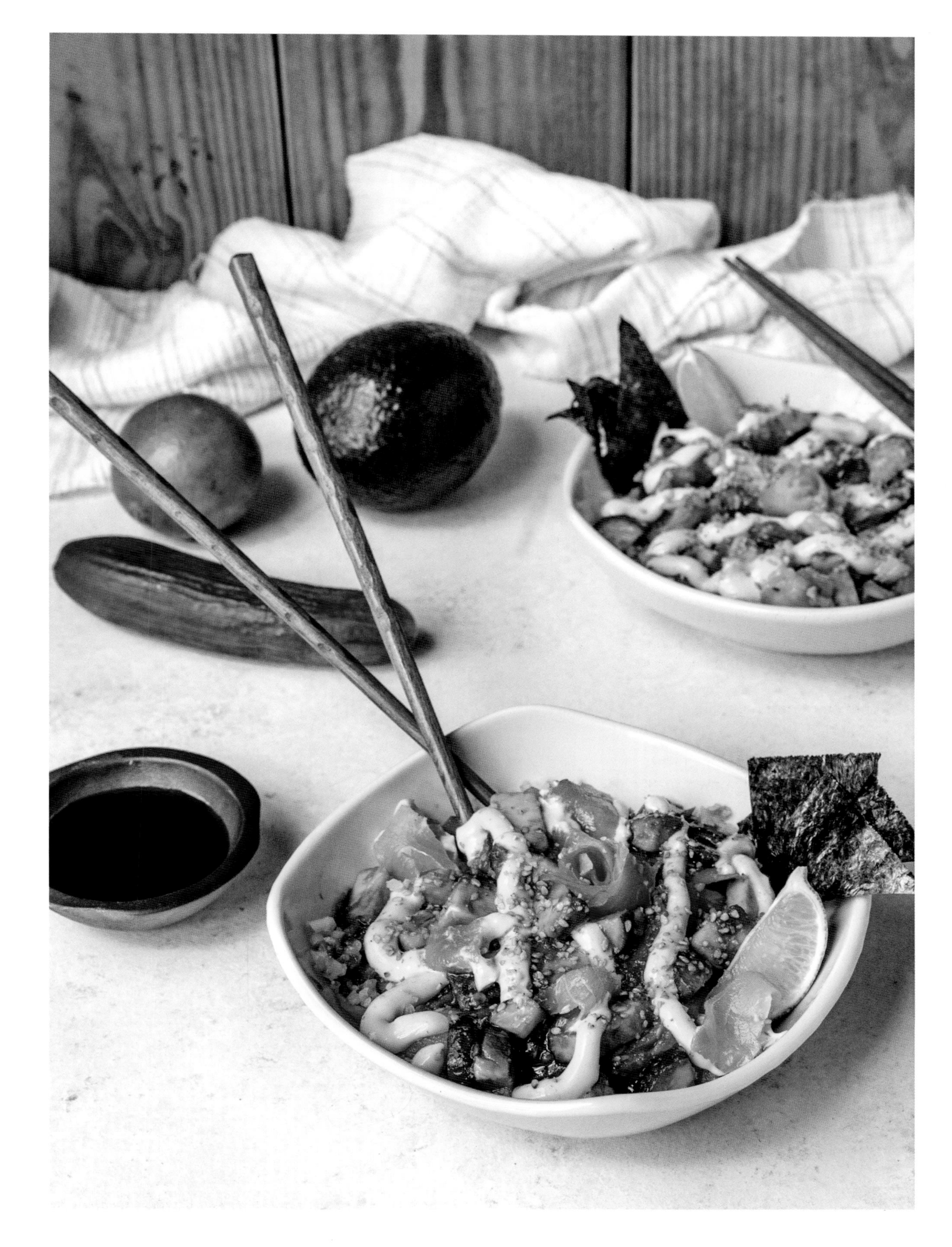

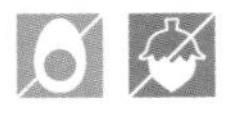

NEW ENGLAND CLAM CHOWDER

YIELD: 10 servings

PREP TIME: 30 minutes

COOK TIME: 40 minutes

In many recipes, especially this one, radishes make a great replacement for potatoes. My children were shocked after I told them they'd eaten radishes in this chowder, and even my picky hubby was surprised. When boiled in broth, radishes become very mild and absorb the flavors of this delicious chowder.

2 tablespoons salted butter, ghee, or avocado oil

6 ounces no-sugar-added salt pork, chopped

1½ cups diced celery

1 cup chopped white onions

2 cloves garlic, minced

2 cups peeled and diced red radishes

2 cups chicken bone broth

1 cup canned clam juice

1 teaspoon chopped fresh thyme leaves

½ teaspoon ground white pepper

1 bay leaf

5 (6½-ounce) cans minced clams, undrained

2 cups heavy whipping cream

2 tablespoons unflavored gelatin, or 1 teaspoon xanthan gum

Store in an airtight container in the refrigerator for up to 2 days.

1. Melt the butter in a large Dutch oven or other heavy pot over medium-high heat. Add the salt pork and cook until crisp.

2. Add the celery, onions, and garlic to the pot and stir until combined. Cover and cook for 5 minutes, or until the celery and onions are tender.

3. Uncover and stir in the radishes, broth, clam juice, thyme, and pepper. Add the bay leaf and bring to a boil.

4. Reduce the heat to low and simmer, covered, for 20 to 25 minutes, or until the radishes are tender. Uncover and remove and discard the bay leaf.

5. Stir in the clams, cream, and gelatin. Raise the heat to medium and bring to a boil.

6. Reduce the heat to low and simmer for 3 to 5 minutes, or until the chowder has thickened. Enjoy!

calories **351** | fat **32g** | protein **4g** | total carbs **6g** | dietary fiber **1g** | net carbs **5g**

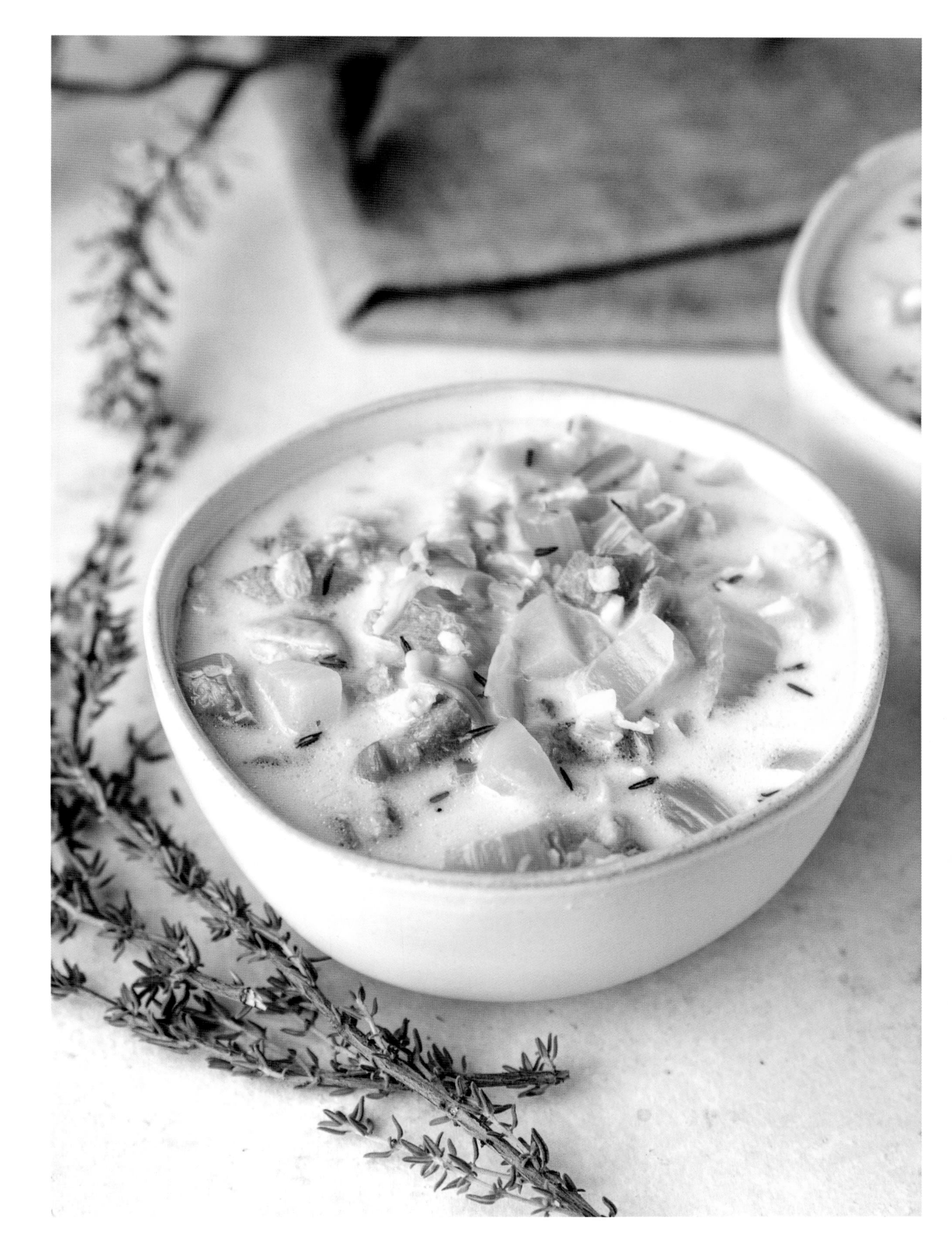

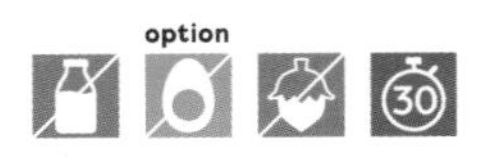

SHRIMP AVOCADO TACO SALAD

YIELD: 8 servings

PREP TIME: 20 minutes (not including time to make seasoning or dressing)

COOK TIME: 5 minutes

Whether you want a quick lunch or a light dinner, this tasty meal comes together in less than half an hour!

- 2 pounds raw small shrimp, peeled, deveined, and tails removed
- 4 tablespoons Taco Seasoning (page 62), divided
- 1 cup Ranch Dressing (page 61)
- 3 tablespoons avocado oil
- 2 tablespoons freshly squeezed lime juice, divided
- 1 avocado (about 5 ounces), pitted, skinned, and diced
- 8 ounces romaine lettuce, chopped
- 4 ounces cherry tomatoes, halved
- 1/2 cup sliced red onions
- 1/4 cup chopped fresh cilantro

Store in an airtight container in the refrigerator for up to 3 days. (The avocado tends to turn brown, so you may want to leave it off the salad until just before serving.)

1. Place the shrimp in a large bowl and sprinkle 3 tablespoons of the taco seasoning over them. Toss until nicely coated, then set aside.
2. Stir the remaining 1 tablespoon of taco seasoning into the ranch dressing and refrigerate until ready to use.
3. Heat the oil in a large nonstick skillet over medium-high heat. Add the shrimp and cook until they turn pink. Remove the pan from the heat.
4. Pour 1 tablespoon of the lime juice over the cooked shrimp. Pour the remaining 1 tablespoon of lime juice over the diced avocado.
5. Place the lettuce, tomatoes, and red onions in a large serving bowl. Add the shrimp, avocado, and cilantro and toss well. Drizzle the dressing over the salad and serve immediately.

calories 365 | fat 27g | protein 24g | total carbs 6g | dietary fiber 2g | net carbs 4g

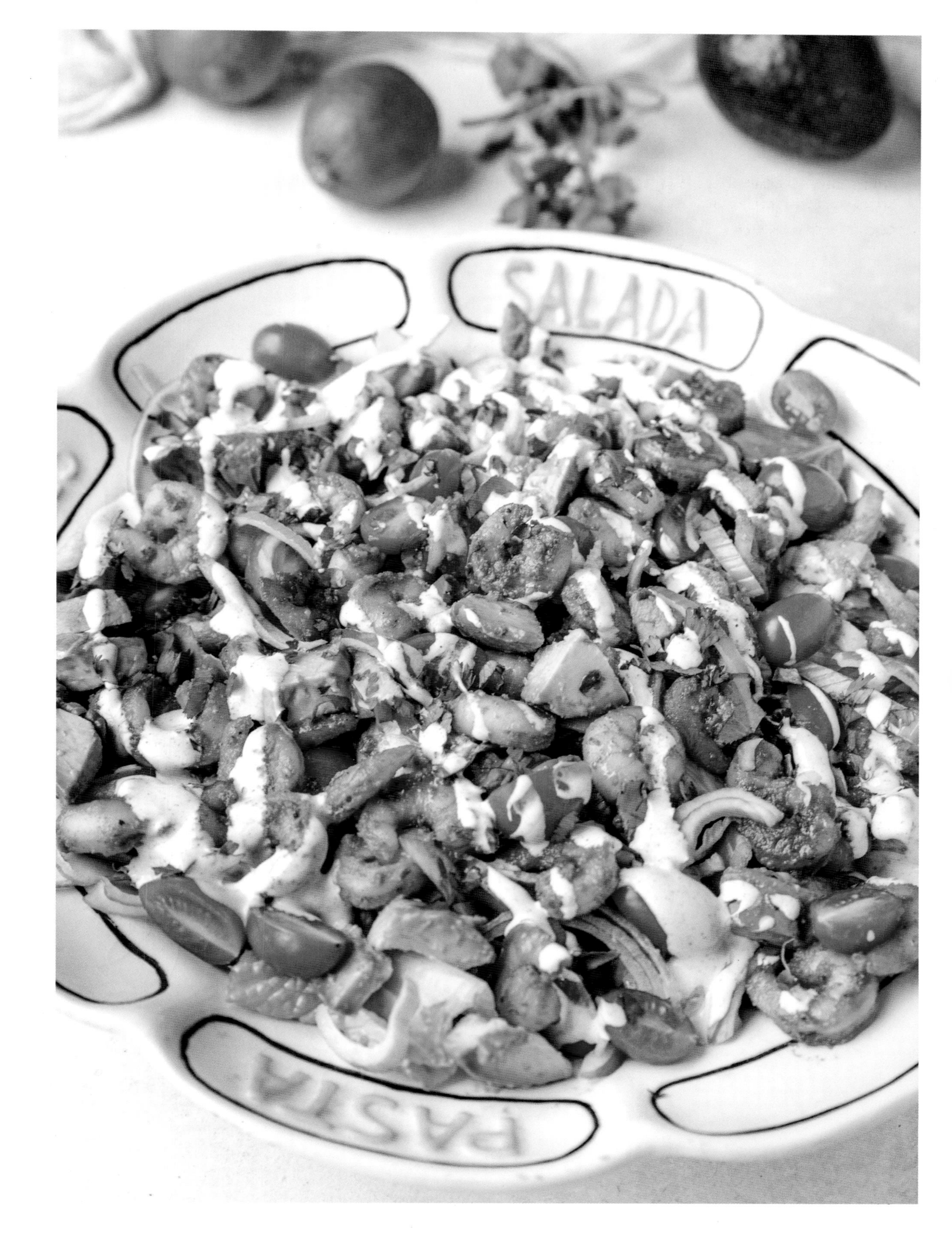
SALADA
PASTA

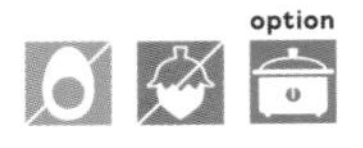

ZUPPA TOSCANA

YIELD: 8 servings

PREP TIME: 45 minutes

COOK TIME: 1 hour or 4 hours, depending on method

The first time I made this soup for my husband, he fell in love with me all over again. He couldn't believe there were radishes in it. After my youngest son tried and loved it, he suggested using radishes in New England Clam Chowder (page 150), too. Don't knock radishes 'til you try them—I think you'll be surprised at how much you like them in this recipe.

8 ounces pancetta or bacon, diced

2 pounds bulk Italian sausage

1 cup diced white onions

1 tablespoon minced garlic

1½ cups peeled and diced daikon radishes

4 cups chicken bone broth

3 cups water

1 cup heavy whipping cream

4 ounces curly kale, stems and stalks removed, chopped

Fine sea salt and freshly ground black pepper

Chopped fresh flat-leaf parsley, for garnish (optional)

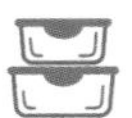

Store in an airtight container in the refrigerator for up to 3 days.

STOVETOP DIRECTIONS:

1. In a Dutch oven over medium heat, cook the pancetta until crisp. Remove with a slotted spoon and set aside on a plate lined with paper towels. Leave about 2 tablespoons of the drippings in the pot and drain the rest.

2. Add the sausage to the pot and cook until browned, stirring often to crumble the meat. Remove from the pot and set aside.

3. Add the onions and garlic to the pot and sauté for 5 minutes, or until soft.

4. Add the radishes, broth, and water to the pot. Cover and bring to a boil. Cook at a low boil for about 20 minutes, or until the radishes are fork-tender.

5. Reduce the heat to low. Return the sausage and pancetta to the pot. Stir in the cream and kale, cover, and simmer for 20 minutes.

6. Season with salt and pepper to taste, garnish with parsley (if using), and serve hot.

SLOW COOKER DIRECTIONS:

1. In a large skillet over medium heat, cook the pancetta until crisp. Remove with a slotted spoon and set aside on a plate lined with paper towels. Leave about 2 tablespoons of the drippings in the skillet and drain the rest.

2. Add the sausage to the skillet and cook until browned, stirring often to crumble the meat. Transfer the sausage to a 6-quart slow cooker.

3. Add the onions and garlic to the skillet and sauté for 5 minutes, or until soft. Transfer the onions and garlic to the slow cooker.

4. Add the radishes, broth, and water to the slow cooker. Cover and cook on high for 3 to 4 hours, or until the radishes are fork-tender. About 30 minutes before the end of the cooking time, stir in the cream, kale, and pancetta.

5. Season with salt and pepper to taste, garnish with parsley (if using), and serve hot.

calories 636 | fat 57g | protein 21g | total carbs 6g | dietary fiber 0g | net carbs 6g

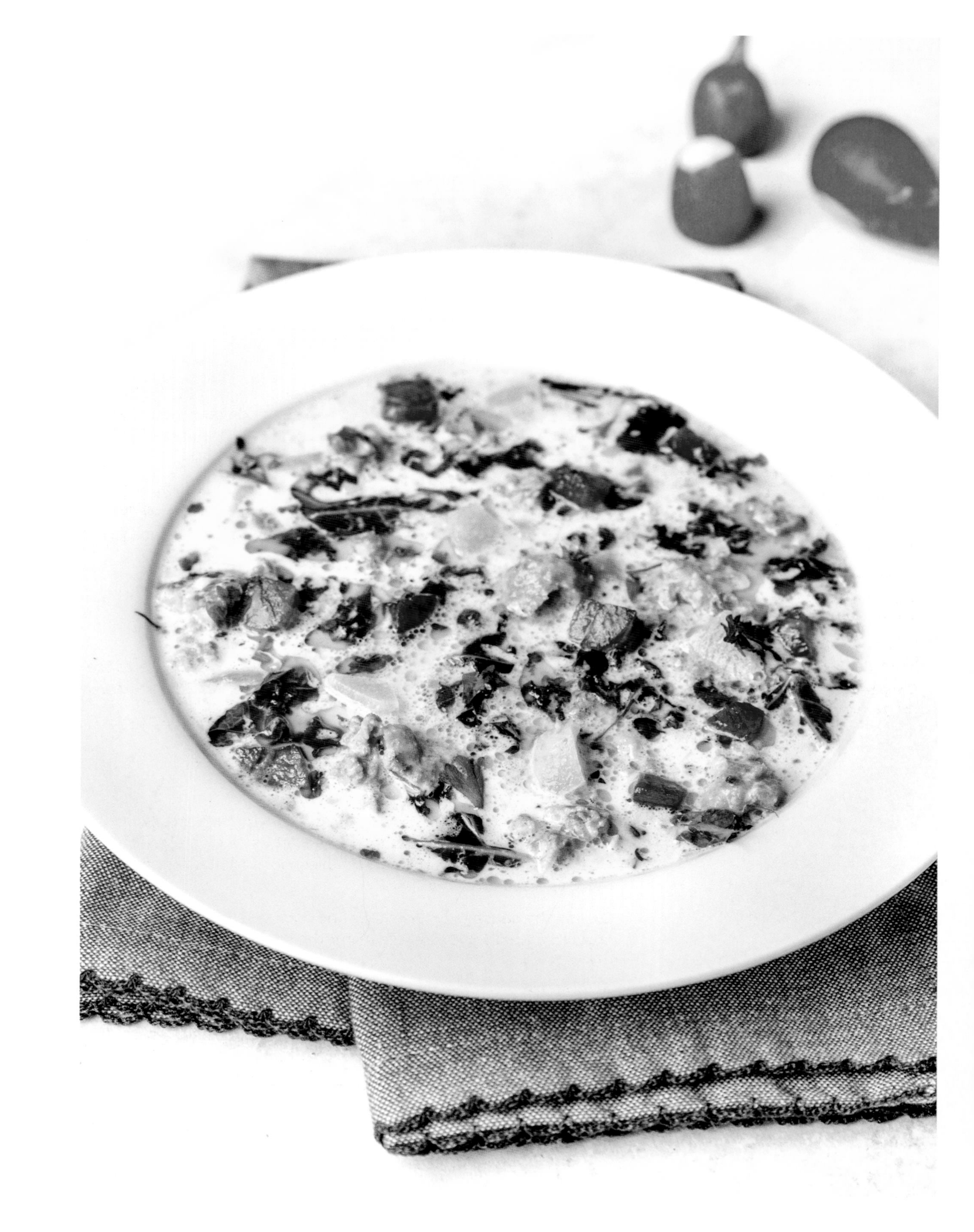

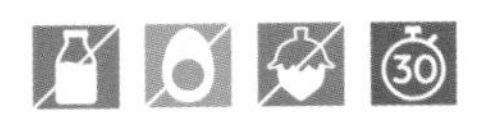

WARM BRUSSELS BACON SHRIMP SALAD

YIELD: 6 servings

PREP TIME: 10 minutes

COOK TIME: 15 minutes

Some days, a cold salad just doesn't sound appealing to me, so I created this warm Brussels sprouts and bacon salad for a nice change of pace. It takes little time to make and provides some nice leftovers—unless you're like me and have teenagers in the house, in which case nothing will ever be left over.

10 ounces bacon, chopped

1½ pounds raw medium shrimp, peeled, deveined, and tails removed

Fine sea salt and freshly ground black pepper

¼ cup freshly squeezed lime juice

1 pound Brussels sprouts, ends trimmed, thinly sliced

1 teaspoon minced garlic

1 avocado, pitted, skinned, and diced

1. In a large skillet over medium-high heat, cook the bacon until crisp. Remove the bacon to a plate lined with paper towels, leaving the grease in the pan.

2. Add the shrimp to the skillet and cook for about 2 minutes on each side, or until they turn pink. Season with salt and pepper. Remove from the skillet and keep warm.

3. Place the empty skillet over medium heat and deglaze it with the lime juice, scraping the bottom of the pan to release all of the bacon bits. Add the Brussels sprouts and garlic and cook for 2 minutes, or until the garlic is fragrant. (The Brussels sprouts should still have a good bite to them and should not be too soft and tender.)

4. Return the shrimp and bacon to the skillet and stir until just combined.

5. Transfer the salad to a serving bowl. Top with the avocado and enjoy immediately.

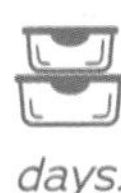

Store in an airtight container in the refrigerator for up to 3 days.

Note: The bacon grease and lime juice coat this warm salad nicely and act as the dressing, but if you feel you need more fat, feel free to drizzle the salad with 1 tablespoon of extra-virgin olive oil.

calories 252 | fat 10g | protein 29g | total carbs 10g | dietary fiber 5g | net carbs 5g

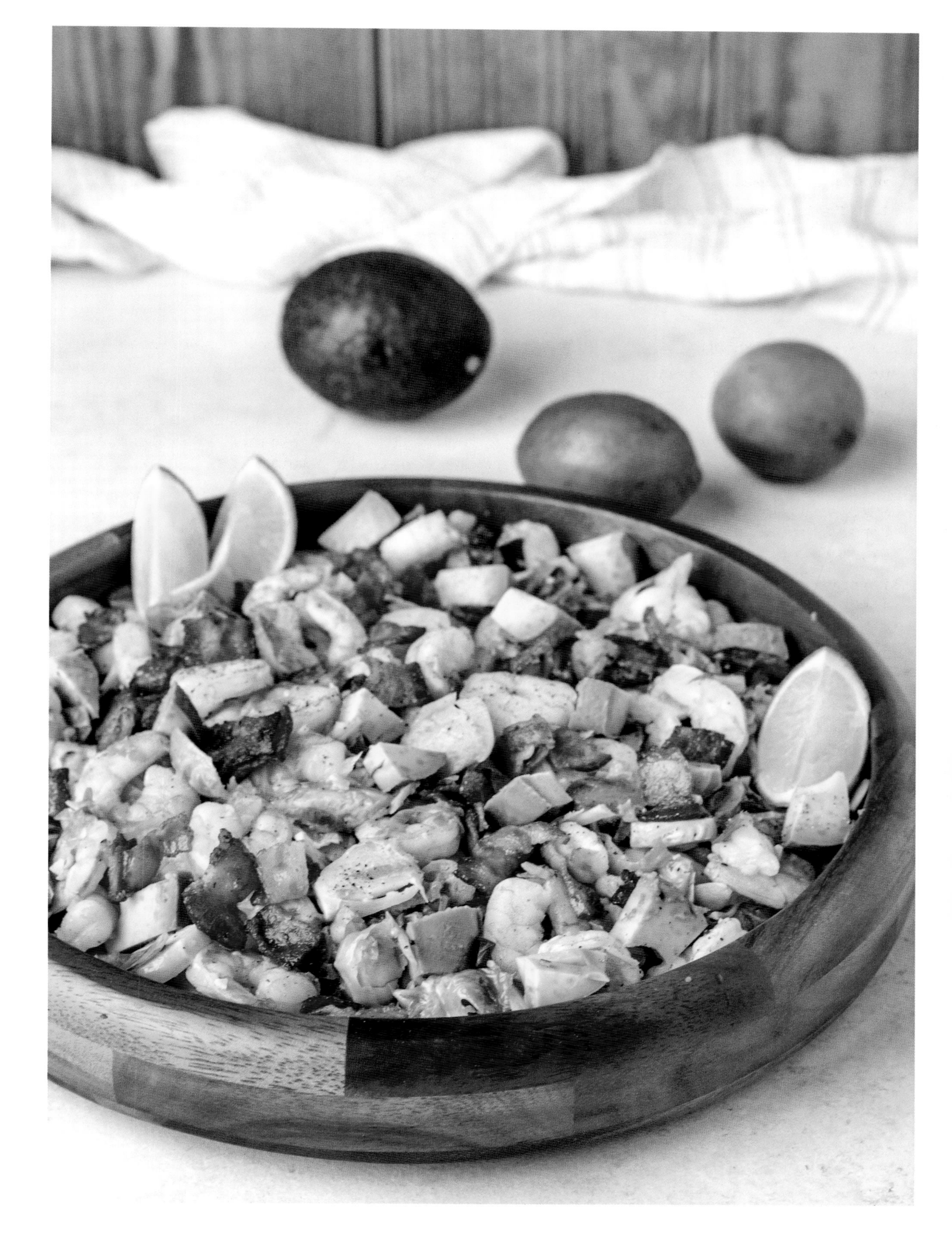

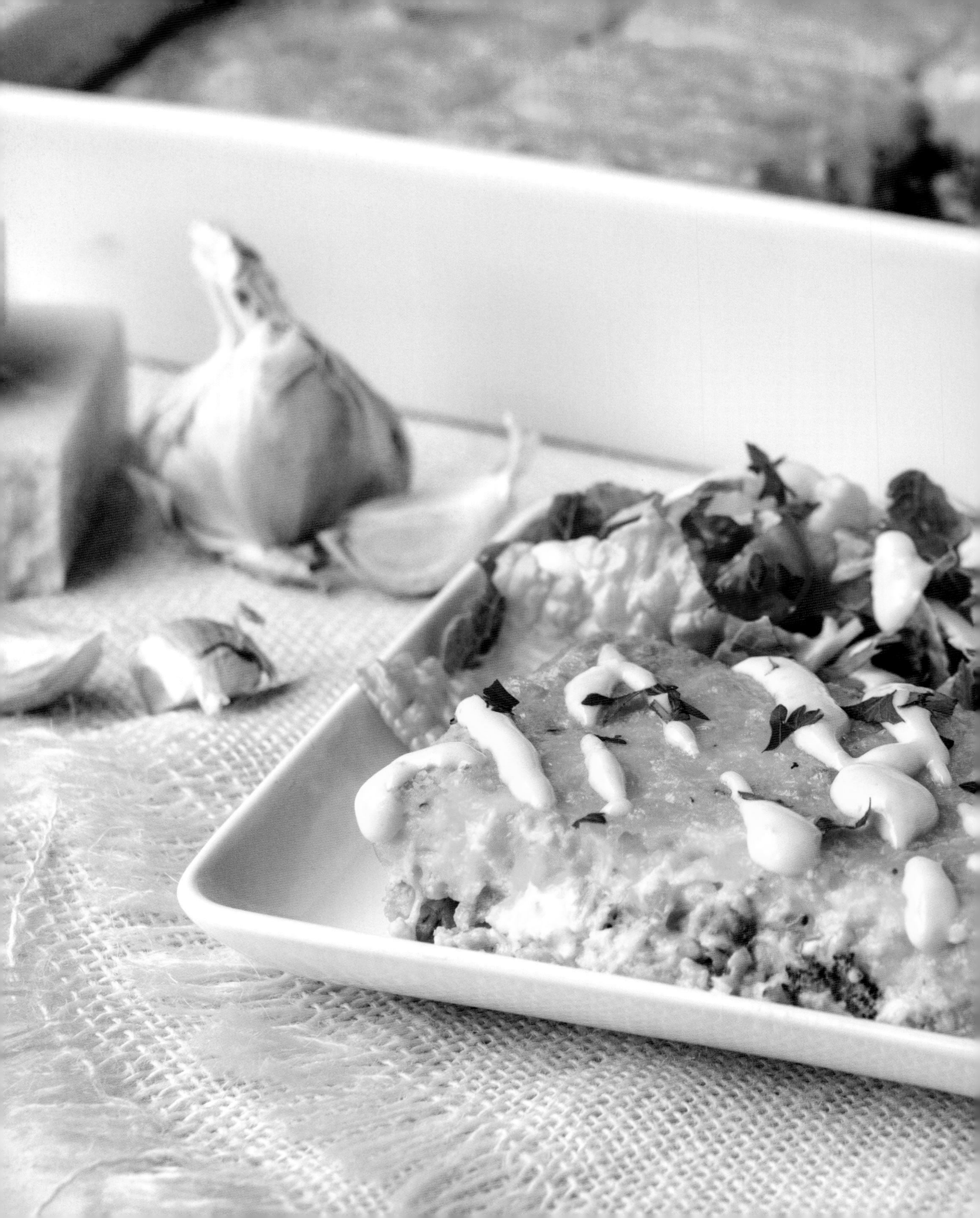

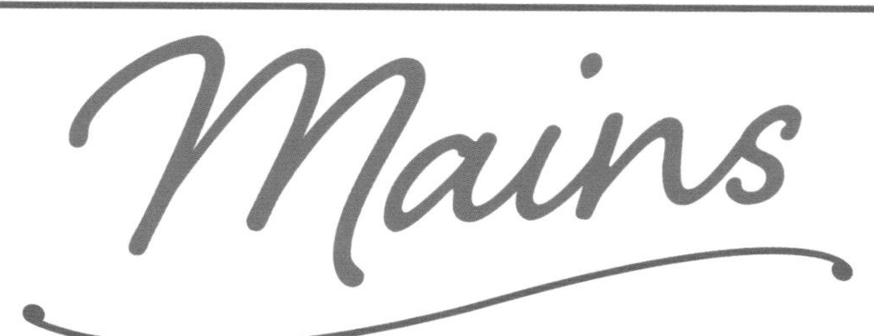

Mains

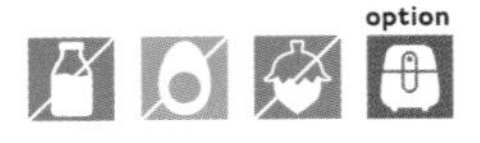

OVEN-FRIED (OR AIR FRYER) CHICKEN WINGS

YIELD: 8 servings

PREP TIME: 10 minutes, plus at least 1 hour to chill and 20 minutes to rest

COOK TIME: 20 minutes or 50 minutes, depending on method

This recipe guarantees you crispy chicken wings! There's no flour in sight, but the coating is outstanding: crispy and flavorful. This is yet another recipe that never gives me leftovers—because my family devours these wings!

- 3 pounds chicken wings
- 1 tablespoon baking powder
- 2 teaspoons smoked paprika
- 1 teaspoon dried parsley
- 1 teaspoon onion powder
- 1 teaspoon fine sea salt
- 1 teaspoon freshly ground black pepper

1. Pat dry the wings and refrigerate, uncovered, for at least 1 hour or up to overnight to dry out the skin for extra crispness.

2. Allow the wings to sit out at room temperature for 20 to 30 minutes before cooking.

3. In a wide, shallow bowl, combine the baking powder, paprika, parsley, onion powder, salt, and pepper. Toss the wings in the mixture until well coated.

OVEN DIRECTIONS:

1. Preheat the oven to 425°F. Line a sheet pan with aluminum foil or parchment paper.

2. Arrange the coated wings on the prepared sheet pan and bake for 25 minutes. Turn the wings over and bake for 25 more minutes. If you prefer extra crispy wings, broil for 2 to 3 minutes. Serve hot.

AIR FRYER DIRECTIONS:

1. Set the air fryer to 400°F.

2. Arrange as many of the coated wings as you can standing upright around the edges of the air fryer basket. Then arrange the others standing upright against the ones on the edges until all of the wings are standing upright in the air fryer. (This arrangement helps to crisp the wings evenly, as 3 pounds of wings is a lot for an air fryer.) If you do not have a large air fryer, you will need to cook the wings in batches.

3. Set the air fryer to cook for 20 minutes. Check the wings for crispness. If you prefer them to be very crispy, cook for an additional 5 minutes. Serve hot.

calories 208 | fat 14g | protein 16g | total carbs 1g | dietary fiber 0g | net carbs 1g

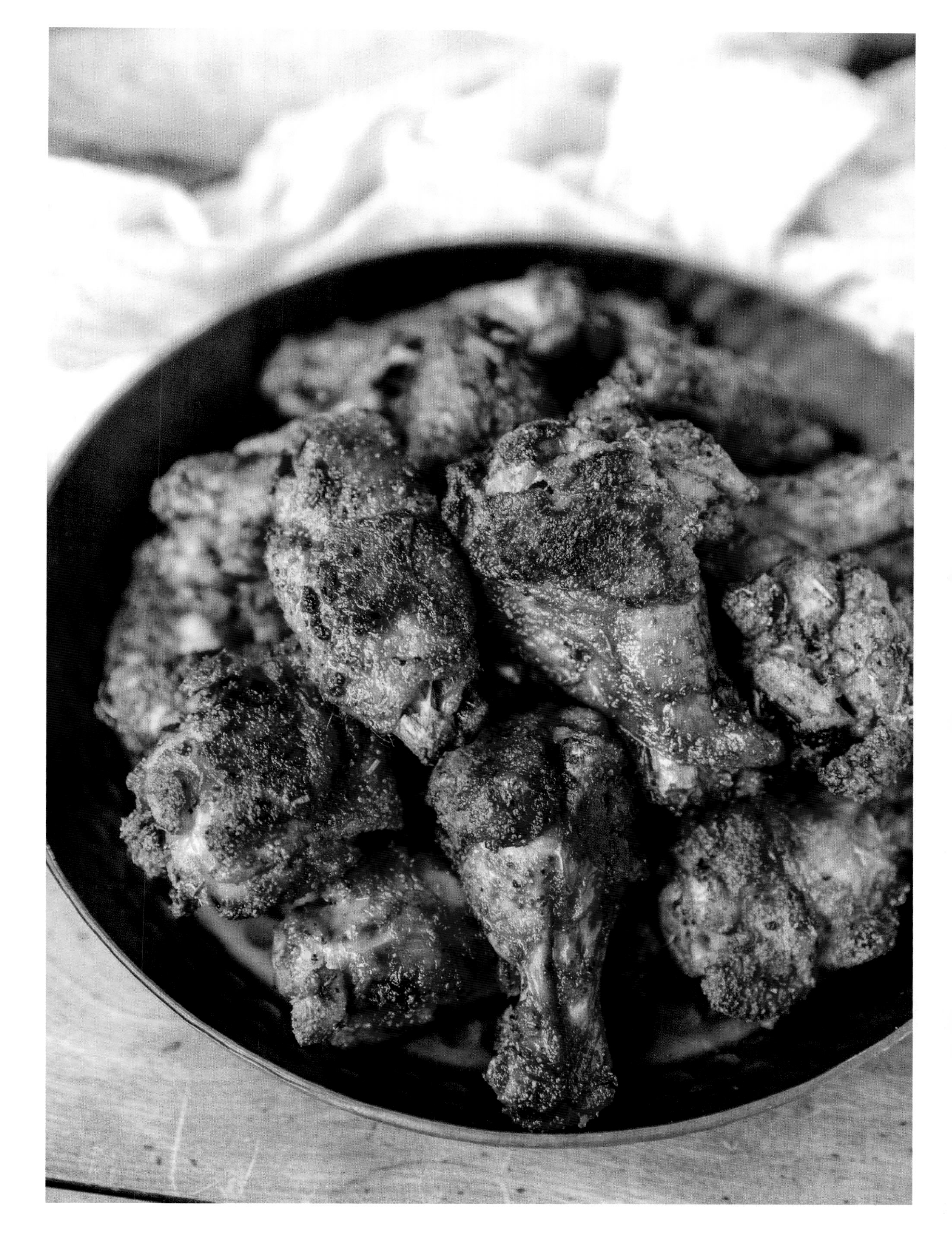

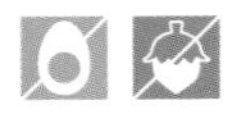

BACON CHEESEBURGER CAULIFLOWER CASSEROLE

YIELD: 10 servings

PREP TIME: 10 minutes, plus at least 15 minutes to cool

COOK TIME: 1 hour 5 minutes

If you're a lover of cheeseburgers and also appreciate a casserole that includes hidden veggies, this recipe is for you! It takes a few steps, but the casserole is very satisfying, and your family and friends may be shocked when they learn they've just eaten cauliflower. This dish has been a family favorite for years, and it's a big hit among the followers of my blog, too.

1 large head cauliflower, cored and cut into florets (about 6 cups)

6 ounces bacon

1/3 cup coconut flour

1 1/4 teaspoons fine sea salt, divided

1 1/2 pounds grass-fed ground beef

1 teaspoon garlic powder

1 teaspoon onion powder

1 teaspoon dried oregano leaves

1/2 teaspoon freshly ground black pepper

8 ounces cheddar cheese, sliced or shredded

Sliced green onions, for garnish

FOR THE SAUCE

1 tablespoon unsalted butter

1 tablespoon coconut flour

1 1/2 cups heavy whipping cream

2 tablespoons prepared yellow mustard

1. Set a large pot with a steamer insert over medium heat. Pour 1 inch of water into the pot and bring to a boil. Add the cauliflower and steam for 10 minutes, or until fork-tender. Remove the pot from the heat.

2. Meanwhile, in a large skillet over medium heat, cook the bacon until it is fully cooked but not yet crisp, about 10 minutes. Remove the bacon from the skillet and set aside to drain on a plate lined with paper towels. Leave the bacon grease in the skillet.

3. When the cauliflower is done, place it in a food processor and pulse until it resembles grains of rice. Transfer the riced cauliflower to a bowl and set aside to cool.

4. Add the flour and 1/4 teaspoon of the salt to the bowl with the riced cauliflower and mix well. Set aside.

5. Once the bacon is cool, chop it into bite-sized pieces. Set aside.

6. Place the skillet with the bacon grease over medium-high heat and add the ground beef. Cook, stirring often to crumble the meat, for about 10 minutes, or until it is browned and no longer pink. Remove the pan from the heat and drain some of the grease, if desired.

7. Season the beef with the garlic powder, onion powder, oregano, the remaining 1 teaspoon of salt, and the pepper. Mix well, then use a slotted spoon to transfer the meat to a bowl, leaving the grease in the skillet.

8. Preheat the oven to 350°F.

9. Make the sauce: Return the skillet to low heat and add the butter. Once it is melted, stir in the flour and cook until the flour has absorbed the butter.

10. While whisking constantly to remove any lumps, slowly pour in the cream and mustard. Cook for about 10 minutes, or until the sauce thickens.

calories **444** | fat **34g** | protein **27g** | total carbs **6g** | dietary fiber **2g** | net carbs **4g**

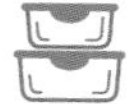

Store in an airtight container in the refrigerator for up to 3 days.

Tips: You can swap out the coconut flour with any keto flour of your choice. You can also replace the ground beef with ground turkey or pork if you like. If you have 1 pound of frozen riced cauliflower on hand and prefer to use that instead having to steam and rice a head of cauliflower, skip Steps 1 and 3; just be sure to thaw the frozen cauliflower before using. (The microwave is fine.)

11. Assemble and finish the dish: Spread ½ cup of the sauce in a 13 by 9-inch baking dish. Place the cauliflower mixture on top of the sauce, spreading it as evenly as possible. Place half of the cheese over the cauliflower. Evenly spread the ground beef over the cheese. Pour half of the remaining sauce over the beef. Place the remaining cheese over the sauce and pour the remaining sauce over the top. Sprinkle with the chopped bacon, cover, and bake for 30 minutes. Remove from the oven.

12. Uncover and bake for 5 more minutes, or until the casserole is bubbling around the edges and the cheese is nicely melted. Allow to cool for 15 to 20 minutes.

13. Garnish with the green onions, slice, and serve.

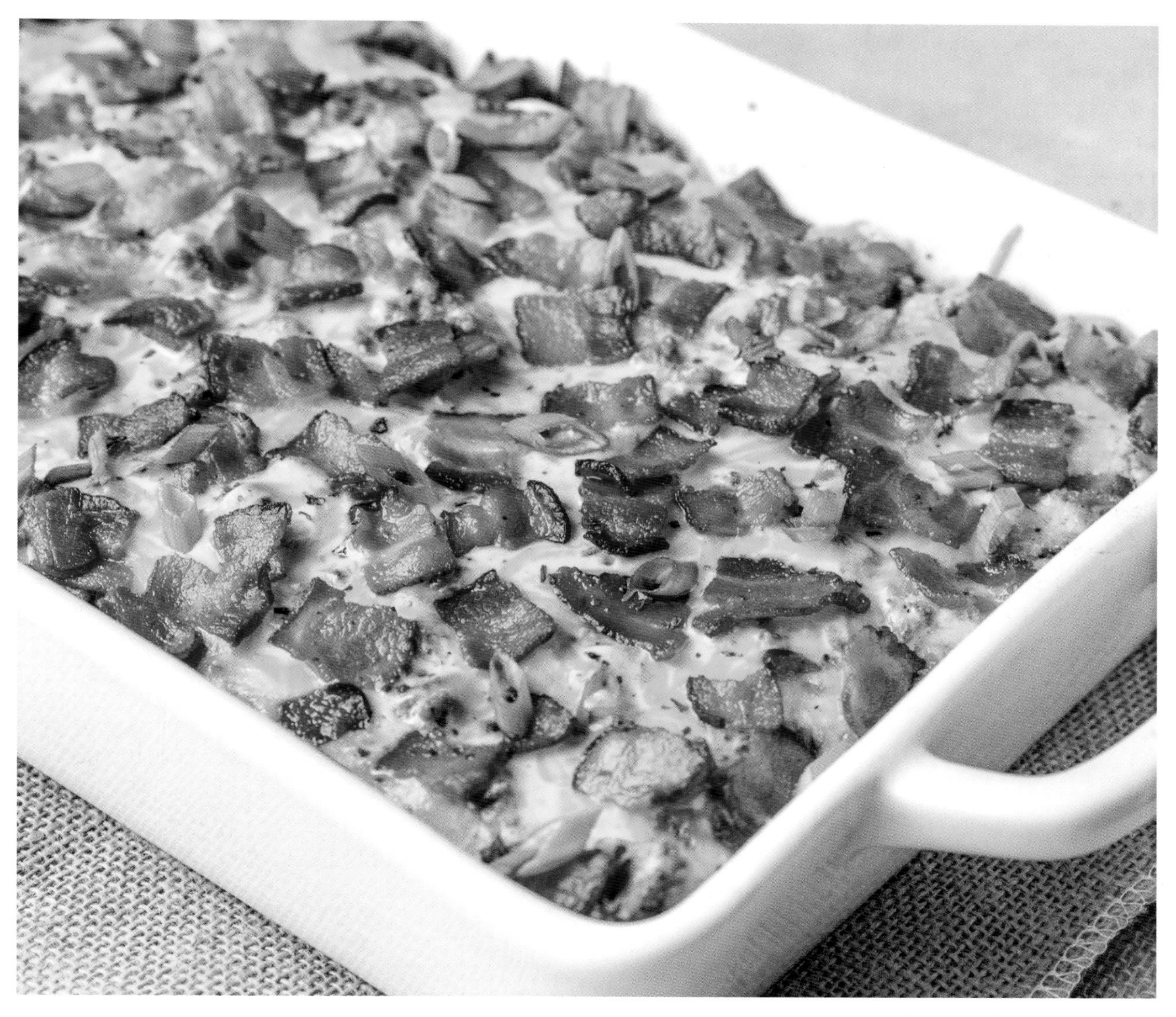

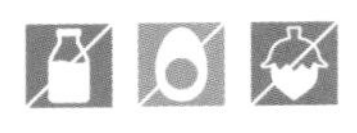

BARBECUE RIBS

YIELD: 10 servings

PREP TIME: 10 minutes, plus 1 hour to chill

COOK TIME: 3 hours

My family would eat these fall-off-the-bone ribs every night if I made them that often. There are never any leftovers with this recipe—it's finger-licking good!

4 pounds baby back ribs

1/2 cup Beef Spice Rub (page 46)

Store in an airtight container in the refrigerator for up to 3 days.

1. Using a knife, peel away the thin membrane from the back of the ribs. It should come off in one sheet, but if it breaks, start again in another section and pull until you can grab it with a paper towel and pull it off.

2. Line a sheet pan with aluminum foil or parchment paper.

3. Sprinkle the spice rub all over both sides of the ribs. Set the ribs, curved side down, on the prepared sheet pan. Cover and refrigerate for 1 hour.

4. Preheat the oven to 250°F.

5. Uncover the ribs and bake for 2 hours. Remove from the oven and flip the ribs over.

6. Raise the oven temperature to 325°F. Bake the ribs for 1 more hour, or until the meat is falling off the bone. If desired, broil the ribs for 2 to 4 minutes for more crispness. Serve.

calories 355 | fat 21g | protein 35g | total carbs 2g | dietary fiber 0g | net carbs 2g

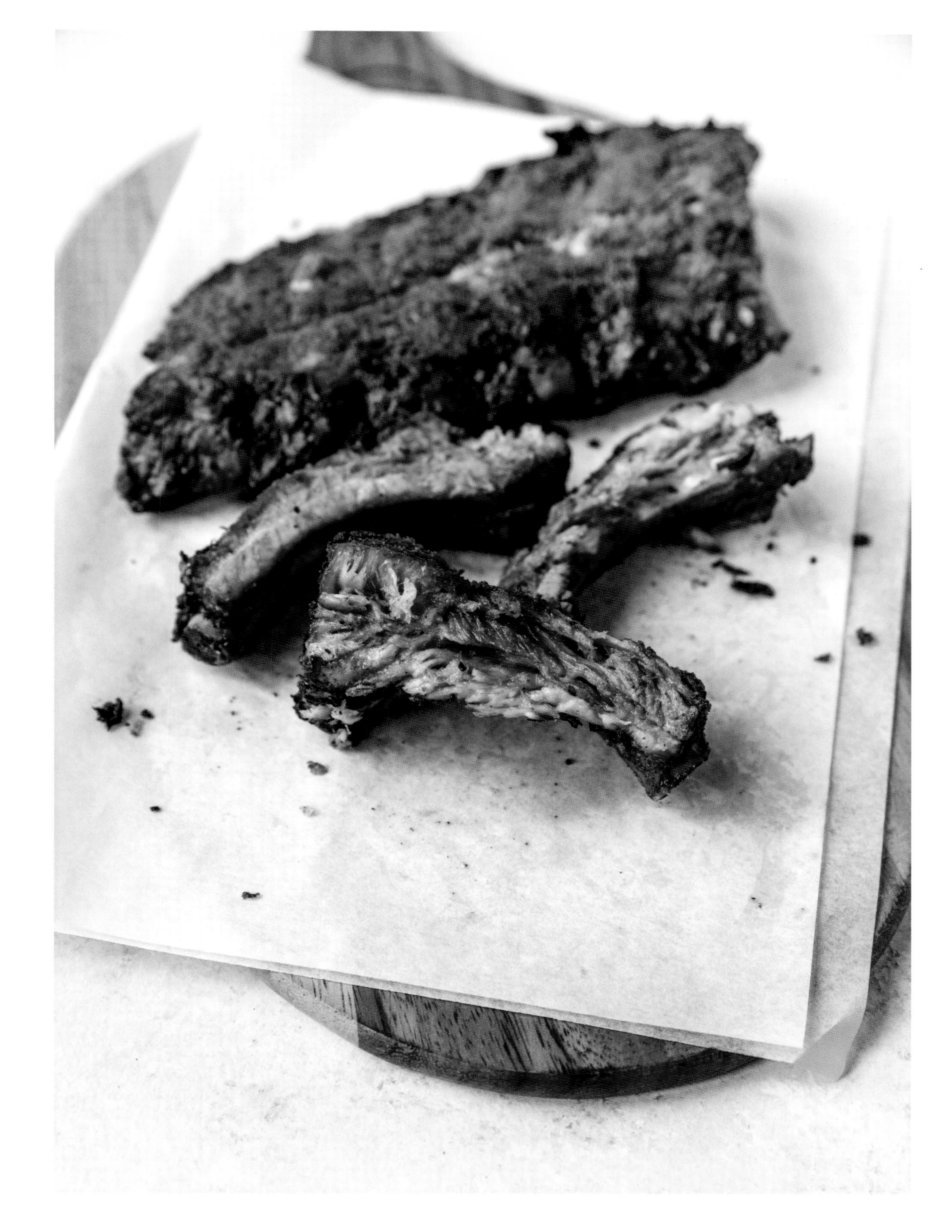

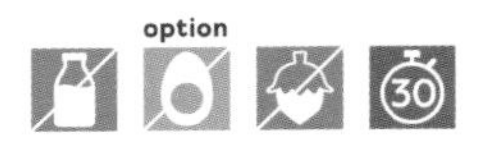

BEST KETO BURGERS

YIELD: 8 burgers (1 per serving)

PREP TIME: 15 minutes (not including time to make spice rub or rolls)

COOK TIME: 10 minutes

When you're in the mood for a juicy burger, this recipe will knock your socks off. It's hard not to love a good burger. I've had success grilling these, but they're also great when pan-fried in a skillet on the stovetop. Keep them dairy-free by topping them with my Secret Burger Sauce (page 55), or add cheese and other toppings of your choice, and use my Hamburger Rolls to make the ultimate burger!

2 pounds grass-fed ground beef

¼ cup avocado oil mayonnaise (for egg-free, use Egg-Free Mayo, page 48)

1 tablespoon prepared yellow mustard

1½ tablespoons Beef Spice Rub (page 46)

Burger toppings of choice, for serving (optional)

8 Hamburger Rolls (page 122), for serving

Store in an airtight container in the refrigerator for up to 3 days.

1. Place the ground beef, mayonnaise, mustard, and spice rub in a bowl and mix with your hands until fully combined. Form the mixture into 8 equal-sized patties.

2. Preheat a grill to medium-high heat, or preheat a skillet over medium-high heat. Cook the patties for 4 to 5 minutes with the grill open or the skillet uncovered. Flip the patties over, cover, and cook for 5 minutes for medium-done burgers, or until they reach the desired doneness. Remove from the heat.

3. Top the burgers as desired and serve on the rolls.

| BURGERS ONLY, WITHOUT TOPPINGS OR ROLLS |

calories 339 | fat 27g | protein 19g | total carbs 0g | dietary fiber 0g | net carbs 0g

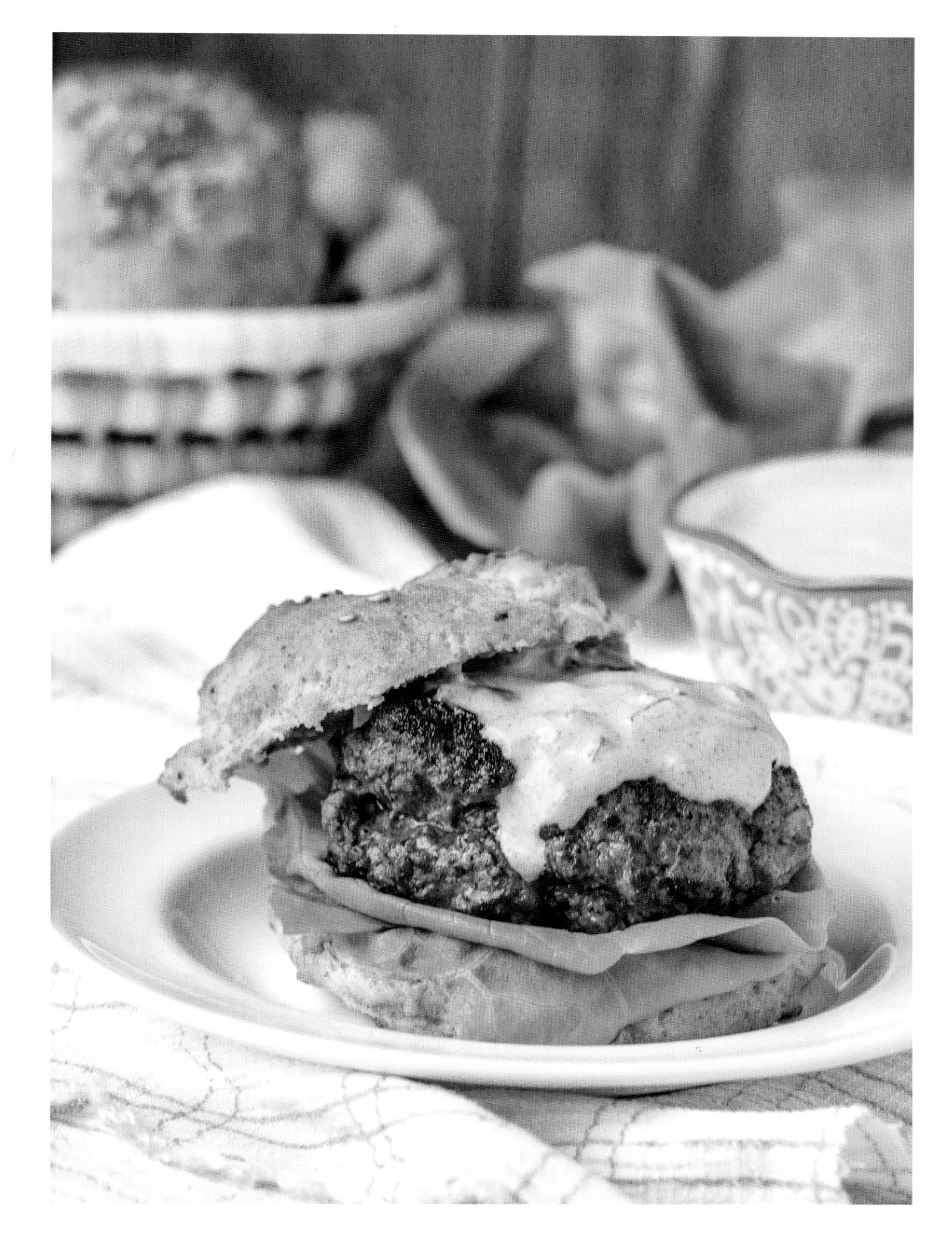

PAN-SEARED CILANTRO LIME CHICKEN THIGHS

YIELD: 6 servings

PREP TIME: 10 minutes, plus at least 30 minutes to marinate

COOK TIME: 15 minutes

This quick and tasty chicken pairs nicely with my Cilantro Lime Cauliflower Rice (page 208).

- ½ cup chopped fresh basil
- ½ cup chopped fresh cilantro, plus more for garnish
- ¼ cup avocado oil
- ¼ cup freshly squeezed lime juice
- 2 cloves garlic
- 2 teaspoons fine sea salt
- ½ teaspoon freshly ground black pepper
- 2 pounds boneless, skinless chicken thighs
- 2 tablespoons extra-virgin olive oil, for the pan

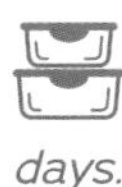

Store in an airtight container in the refrigerator for up to 3 days.

1. Place the basil and cilantro in a blender. Add the avocado oil, lime juice, garlic, salt, and pepper and puree until smooth.

2. Transfer the herb mixture to a zip-top plastic bag and add the chicken thighs. Seal the bag and massage the chicken until it is thoroughly coated with the marinade. Refrigerate for at least 30 minutes or up to 24 hours.

3. Heat the oil in a large skillet over medium-high heat. Add the marinated chicken thighs and cook without disturbing them for 5 minutes. Turn the chicken over and cook for 5 minutes, then turn the chicken over again.

4. Reduce the heat to medium, cover, and cook for 5 minutes, or until the chicken is no longer pink in the center and an instant-read thermometer inserted in the thickest part of a thigh registers 165°F. Remove from the heat.

5. Serve immediately, garnished with extra cilantro.

calories 457 | fat 39g | protein 25g | total carbs 2g | dietary fiber 0g | net carbs 2g

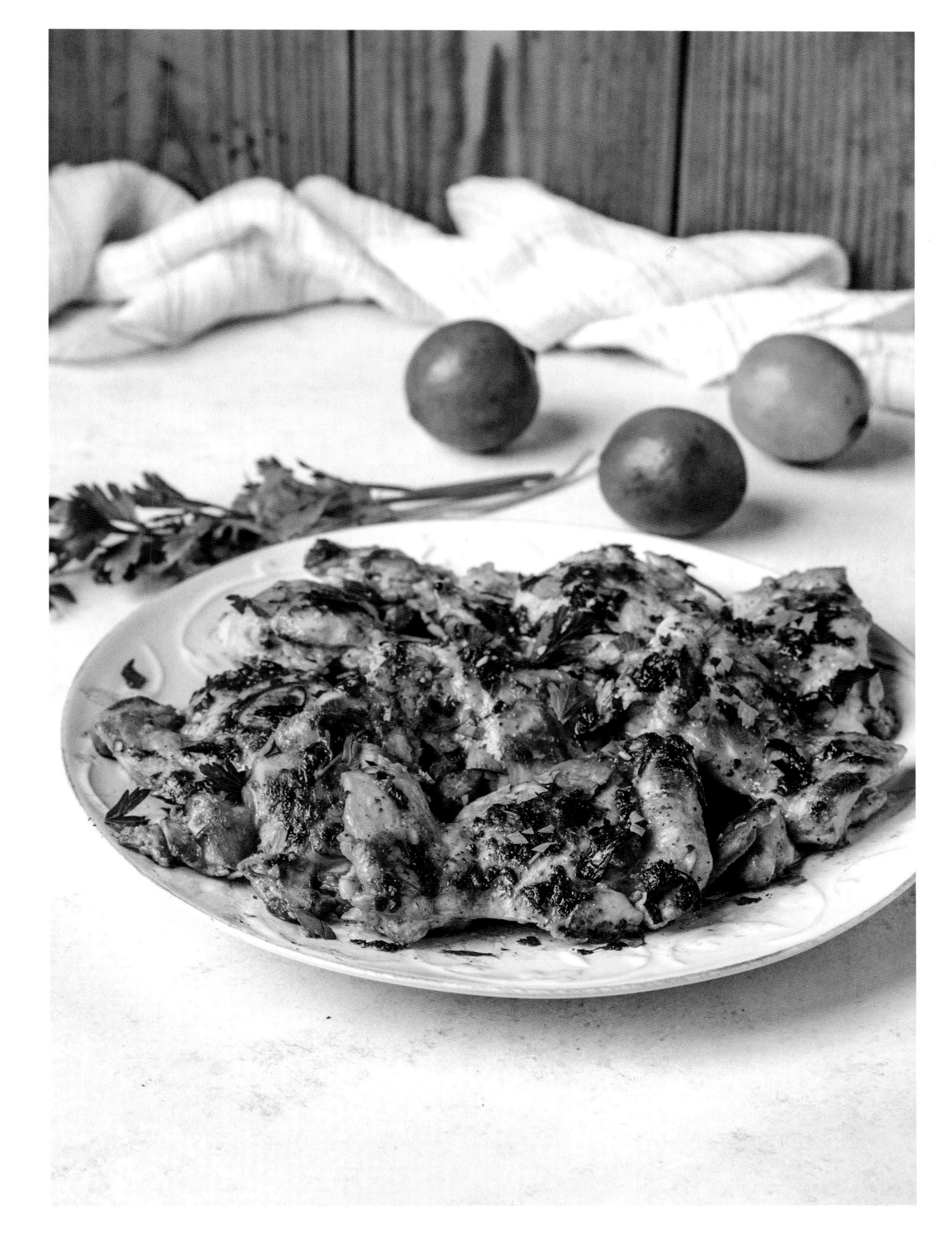

CABBAGE LASAGNA

YIELD: 12 servings

PREP TIME: 30 minutes

COOK TIME: 50 minutes

Cooked cabbage leaves as a replacement for traditional lasagna noodles are a lot less work than using zucchini or than making fathead dough. Even my kids and non-keto family members eat this up without complaint.

- 1 small head green cabbage (about 1 pound), cored and quartered
- Kosher salt
- 1 tablespoon avocado oil
- 2 pounds grass-fed ground beef
- 2 cups marinara sauce, store-bought or homemade (page 53), divided
- 1 clove garlic, minced
- 1 teaspoon fine sea salt, divided
- ½ teaspoon freshly ground black pepper
- 2 cups ricotta cheese
- 2 cups shredded mozzarella cheese, divided
- 2 large eggs
- ⅓ cup grated Parmesan cheese
- 1 teaspoon dried basil
- ½ teaspoon dried oregano leaves
- ½ teaspoon dried parsley
- ½ teaspoon garlic powder
- ½ teaspoon onion powder
- ½ teaspoon fine sea salt
- ¼ teaspoon red pepper flakes

Store in an airtight container in the refrigerator for up to 3 days. You can also freeze the lasagna before baking: Follow the recipe through Step 7, then tightly cover the baking dish and freeze for up to 6 months. Thaw in the refrigerator overnight before baking.

1. Bring a large pot of water to a boil. After it reaches a boil, add the cabbage quarters and season generously with kosher salt. Boil for 10 minutes, or until the outer leaves look translucent and tender. Once done, remove from the heat, drain, and set aside to cool.

2. Meanwhile, heat the oil in a large skillet over medium-high heat. Add the ground beef and cook, stirring often to crumble the meat, until it is browned and no longer pink.

3. Add 1 cup of the marinara sauce, the garlic, ½ teaspoon of the salt, and the pepper and stir to combine. Remove from the heat and set aside.

4. In a mixing bowl, combine the ricotta, 1 cup of the mozzarella, the eggs, Parmesan, basil, oregano, parsley, garlic powder, onion powder, red pepper flakes, and remaining ½ teaspoon of salt and set aside.

5. Preheat the oven to 375°F.

6. Assemble the lasagna: Cover the bottom of a 13 by 9-inch baking dish with a layer of cabbage leaves. Spread half of the ricotta mixture over the cabbage, then spread half of the meat mixture over the ricotta mixture. Place another layer of cabbage leaves over the meat and repeat the process until all of the ricotta and meat mixtures have been used. Top with the rest of the cabbage leaves.

7. Pour the remaining 1 cup of marinara sauce over the lasagna and top with the remaining 1 cup of mozzarella cheese.

8. Cover and bake for 30 minutes, then uncover and bake for 10 minutes. If you prefer a crispy top, broil for 5 minutes. Serve hot.

calories 384 | fat 29g | protein 24g | total carbs 5g | dietary fiber 1g | net carbs 4g

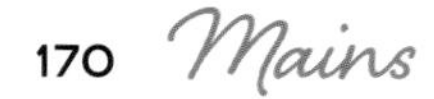

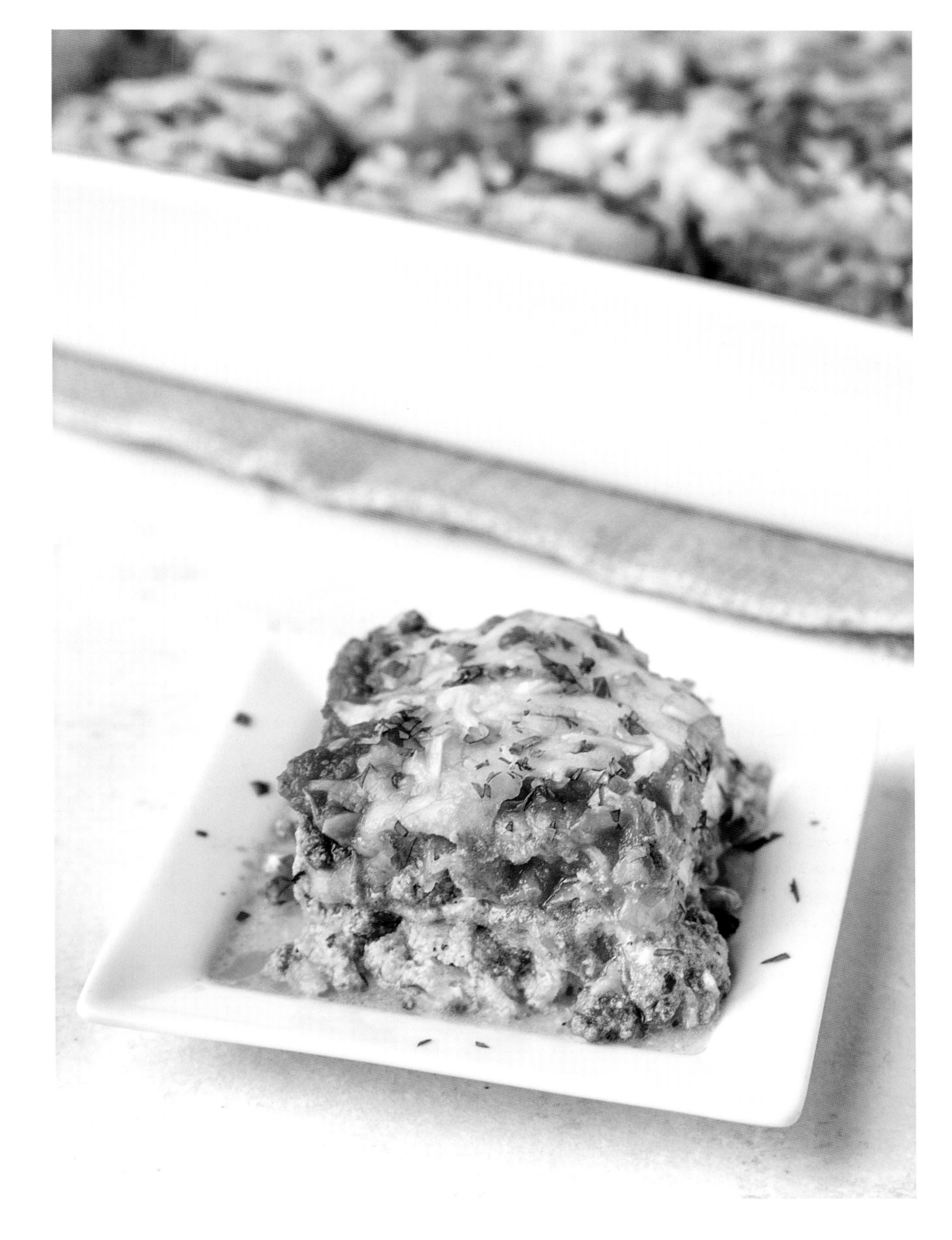

CHICKEN BACON RANCH CALZONE

YIELD: 12 servings

PREP TIME: 40 minutes (not including time to make dressing)

COOK TIME: 25 minutes

A calzone is a hot Italian sandwich stuffed with any kind of filling you like. My bacon cheeseburger calzone has been incredibly popular on my website, and it inspired me to create a new version for this cookbook. On my site, you'll also find other delicious calzone options: chicken Parmesan, Reuben, and sausage and peppers.

FOR THE DOUGH

2 cups (225g) shredded part-skim mozzarella cheese

2 ounces cream cheese (1/4 cup)

2 large eggs

1/2 cup (60g) coconut flour

1/4 teaspoon dried basil

1/4 teaspoon dried oregano leaves

1/4 teaspoon dried parsley

1/4 teaspoon garlic powder

1/4 teaspoon onion powder

1/4 teaspoon fine sea salt

FOR THE FILLING

4 ounces bacon, chopped

2 cups shredded rotisserie chicken

2 cups shredded mozzarella cheese

1/2 cup Ranch Dressing (page 61)

1/4 cup chopped green onions

2 tablespoons chopped fresh flat-leaf parsley

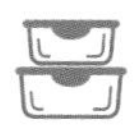

Wrap tightly in aluminum foil and refrigerate for up to 3 days.

1. Preheat the oven to 425°F. Line a sheet pan with parchment paper.

2. Make the dough: Place all of the dough ingredients in a food processor and process until well combined.

3. Transfer the dough to a microwave-safe bowl and microwave for 2 minutes, or until melted. Stir to combine well.

4. Place the dough on the prepared sheet pan and place another sheet of parchment paper on top of it. Using a rolling pin, roll the dough into a 12 by 10-inch rectangle. Remove the top sheet of parchment and set the dough aside.

5. Make the filling: Cook the bacon in a small skillet over medium-high heat until crisp. Remove from the skillet and allow to drain on a plate lined with paper towels.

6. Place the cooked bacon, chicken, mozzarella cheese, ranch dressing, green onions, and parsley in a large mixing bowl and stir together. Spread the filling mixture down the middle of the longer length of the dough.

7. Grasp the parchment paper on the long end and use it to fold one side of the dough over the filling; it will reach only about halfway. Turn the pan around and lift the other side of the parchment paper to fold the other side of the dough over the filling. Wet your fingers and use them to connect the dough ends together; the moistness will help the dough stick together. Roll the calzone over so that it is seam side down on the sheet pan.

8. Bake for 20 minutes, or until golden brown. Remove from the oven and set aside to rest for 10 to 15 minutes. Slice and serve warm.

calories 286 | fat 22g | protein 16g | total carbs 4g | dietary fiber 1g | net carbs 3g

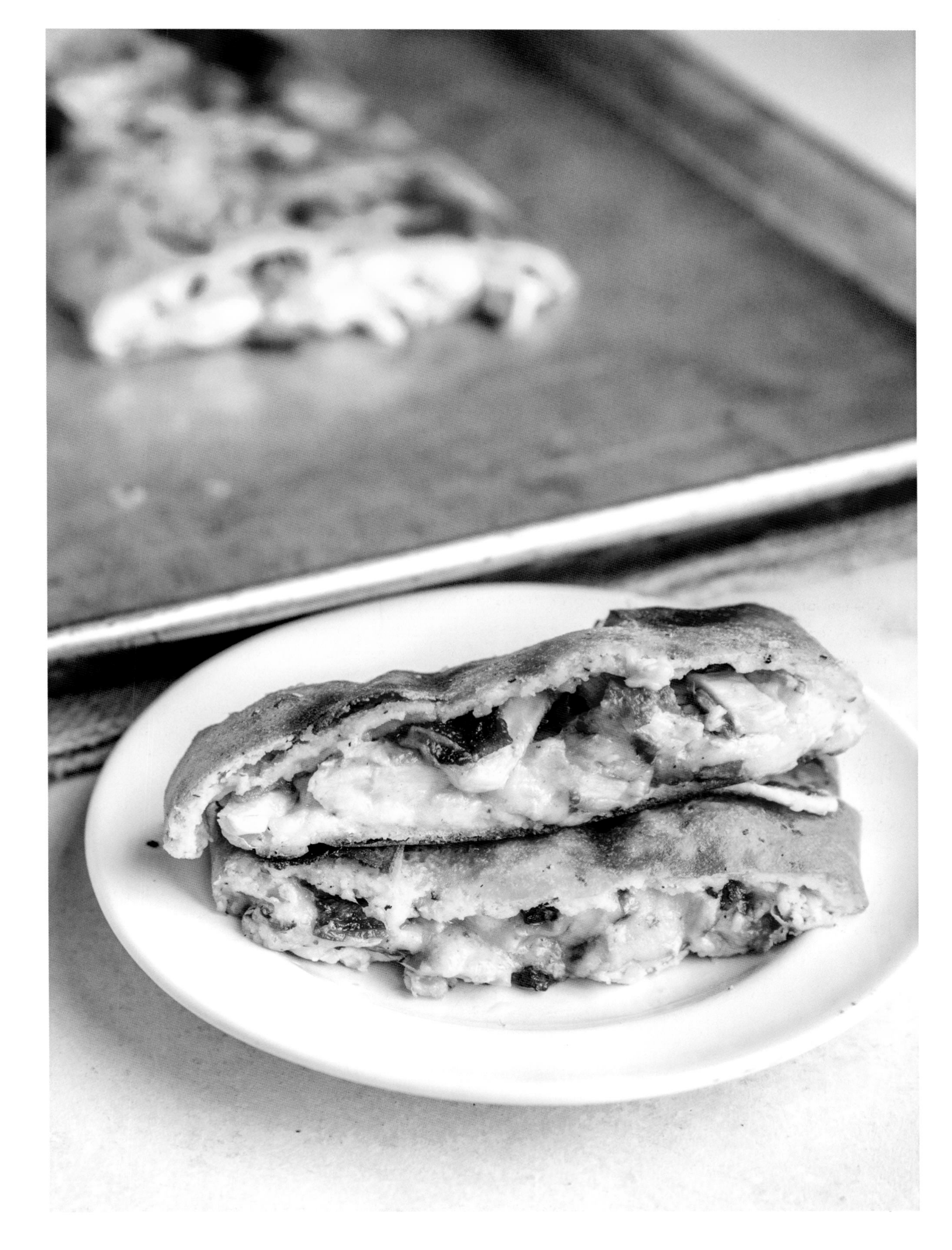

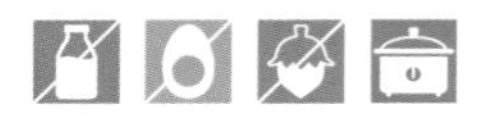

SLOW COOKER PORK CARNITAS

YIELD: 12 servings

PREP TIME: 15 minutes

COOK TIME: 12 hours

The convenience of slow cooker meals can't be denied. If you've had bad experiences with dry slow cooker meals in the past, you might be hesitant to try again, but I promise this will be the best pork you've ever tasted! Use it to make tacos or burritos with my "For Real" Tortillas (page 128) or in a salad with Mexican-inspired toppings.

3 tablespoons extra-virgin olive oil

2 teaspoons dried oregano leaves

1 teaspoon ground cumin

1 teaspoon smoked paprika

1 teaspoon garlic powder

1 teaspoon onion powder

1 teaspoon fine sea salt

½ teaspoon freshly ground black pepper

4 pounds boneless pork butt or shoulder

1 cup beef bone broth

1 cup chopped white onions

4 cloves garlic, minced

1 jalapeño pepper, sliced or chopped (optional)

Juice of 2 limes, plus more for serving

Chopped fresh cilantro, for garnish

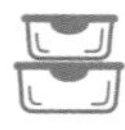

Store in an airtight container in the refrigerator for up to 3 days.

1. In a small bowl, combine the oil and dry seasonings. Rub the mixture all over the pork.

2. Place the broth, onions, garlic, and jalapeño pepper, if using, in a 6-quart slow cooker. Add the seasoned pork and pour the lime juice over the meat. Cover and cook on low for 10 to 12 hours, or until you can easily shred the pork.

3. Using two forks, shred the pork while still in the slow cooker.

4. Set the oven to broil.

5. Arrange the shredded pork on a sheet pan and pour 2 cups of the liquid from the slow cooker over it. Broil for 8 to 10 minutes, or until some of the pieces are browned and crispy.

6. Immediately before serving, pour more of the juices from the slow cooker over the pork, if desired. Squeeze more lime juice over the top, garnish with the cilantro, and serve.

calories **245** | fat **12g** | protein **28g** | total carbs **3g** | dietary fiber **0g** | net carbs **3g**

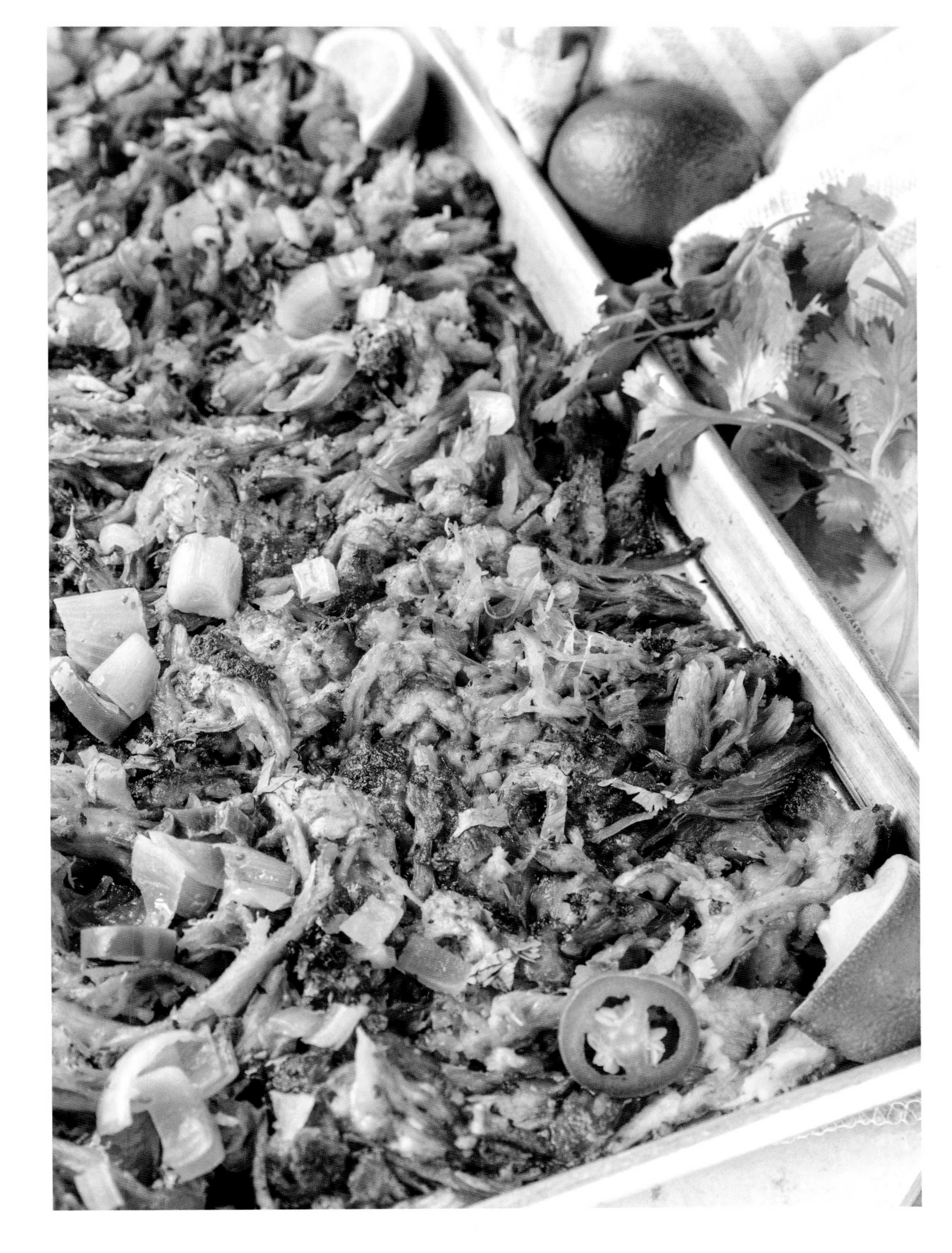

CHICKEN CRUST PIZZA

YIELD: 4 servings

PREP TIME: 20 minutes

COOK TIME: 20 minutes

Don't knock pizza crust made out of chicken until you try it! Of course, you shouldn't expect it to taste like a Miracle Dough Pizza Crust (page 58), but it sure is tasty when you want to skip the time and effort of making miracle dough or you just want pizza that has only 1 gram of carbs per serving. I have provided two sauce-and-topping combinations below, but you can top this crust however you like.

3 cups shredded cooked chicken (about 1 pound)

2 large eggs

2 cloves garlic, minced

½ teaspoon Italian seasoning

½ teaspoon fine sea salt

½ teaspoon freshly ground black pepper

½ cup shredded part-skim mozzarella cheese

TOPPINGS FOR CHICKEN PARMESAN PIZZA *(pictured)*

½ cup marinara sauce, store-bought or homemade (page 53)

¼ cup grated Parmesan cheese

1 cup shredded mozzarella cheese

Chopped fresh basil (optional)

TOPPINGS FOR CHICKEN ALFREDO PIZZA

½ cup Alfredo Sauce (page 44)

½ cup sliced red onions

Chopped fresh flat-leaf parsley (optional)

Store in an airtight container in the refrigerator for up to 3 days. Reheat slices by placing them on a parchment-lined sheet pan in a preheated 350°F oven for about 5 minutes.

1. Preheat the oven to 400°F. Grease a 12-inch round pizza pan.
2. Place the chicken, eggs, garlic, Italian seasoning, salt, and pepper in a large bowl and mix until well combined. Stir in the mozzarella cheese until just combined.
3. Place the mixture on the prepared pizza pan and cover with parchment paper. Using a rolling pin or your hands, flatten the mixture to the edges of the pan; it should be about ¼ inch thick. Remove the parchment paper.
4. Bake for 20 minutes, or until lightly browned.
5. Spread the marinara or Alfredo sauce over the crust, then add the toppings for the variation of your choice. Return the pan to the oven for 5 minutes, or until the cheese is melted (for the Chicken Parmesan Pizza) or the sauce is bubbling (for the Chicken Alfredo Pizza).
6. Slice and serve hot.

Make-ahead tip: Bake the crust by following Steps 1 through 4 above, then let the crust cool completely. Freeze the crust in a zip-top freezer bag for up to 1 month. When ready to use, let the crust thaw in the refrigerator overnight, then reheat in a preheated 350°F oven before adding toppings and baking as directed in Step 5.

| CRUST ONLY, WITHOUT TOPPINGS |

calories 239 | fat 14g | protein 25g | total carbs 1g | dietary fiber 0g | net carbs 1g

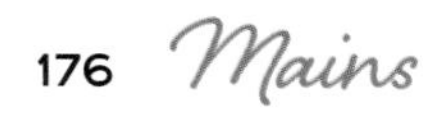

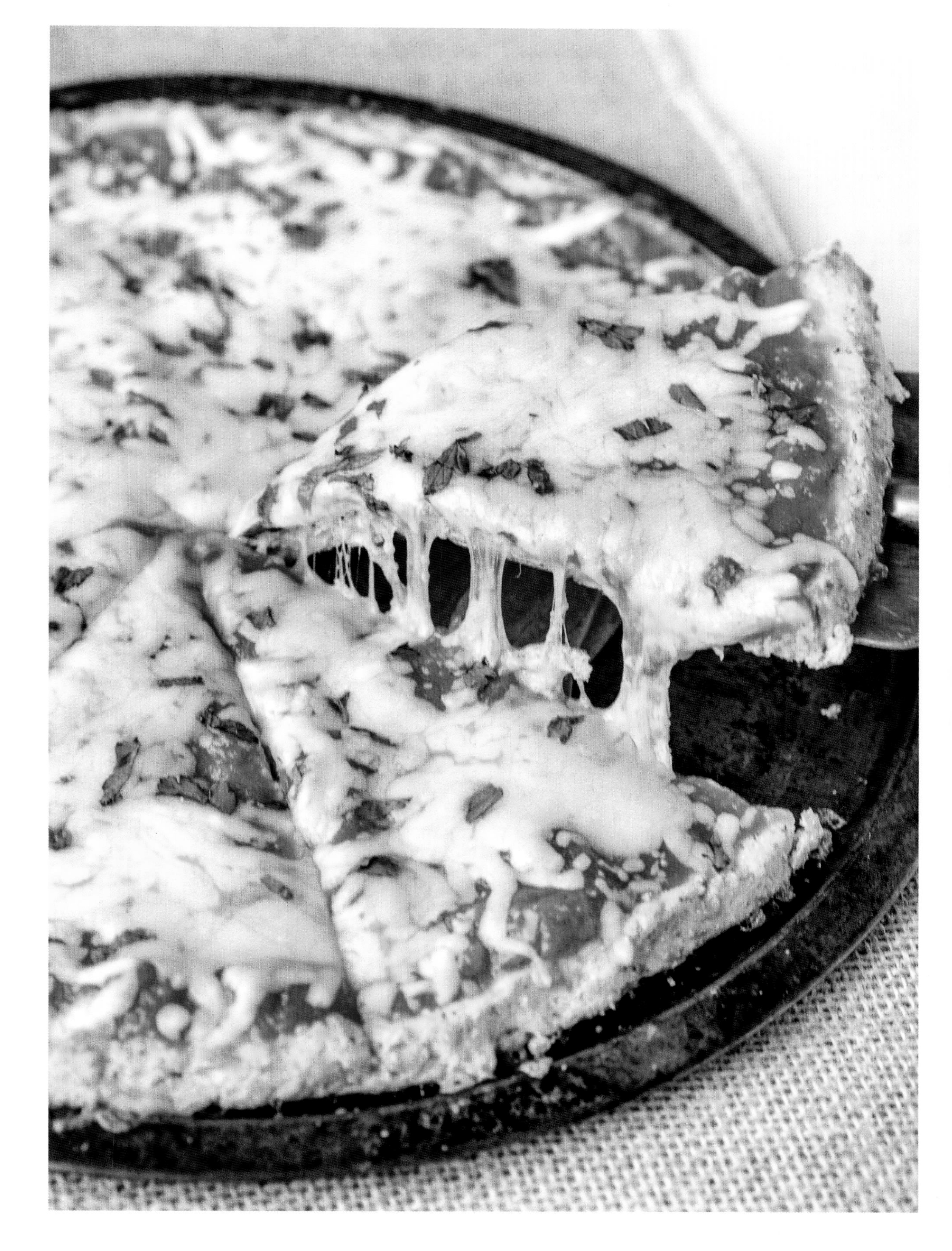

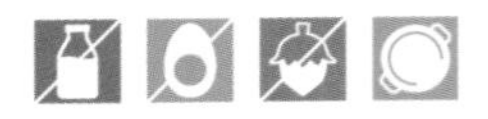

SHEET PAN ITALIAN SAUSAGE AND VEGETABLES

YIELD: 8 servings

PREP TIME: 15 minutes

COOK TIME: 45 minutes

This dish is tasty and simple, and it involves vegetables I know my kids will eat. My daughter loves roasted cauliflower, but my sons hate it; they do like Brussels sprouts, though, so I'm still winning with this recipe.

4 cups cauliflower florets (from 1 large head, about 2½ pounds)

8 ounces Brussels sprouts, ends trimmed, halved

4 ounces radishes, halved

1 small red onion, sliced

3 cloves garlic, peeled

2 tablespoons extra-virgin olive oil

½ teaspoon fine sea salt

½ teaspoon freshly ground black pepper

2 pounds mild or hot Italian sausage links

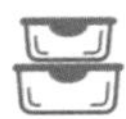

Store in an airtight container in the refrigerator for up to 3 days.

1. Preheat the oven to 400°F.

2. Arrange the vegetables and garlic on a sheet pan. Drizzle with the oil and season with the salt and pepper. Arrange the sausage links on top of the vegetables.

3. Roast for 45 minutes, or until the sausage is cooked through and the vegetables are tender. Serve hot.

calories 462 | fat 39g | protein 18g | total carbs 8g | dietary fiber 2g | net carbs 6g

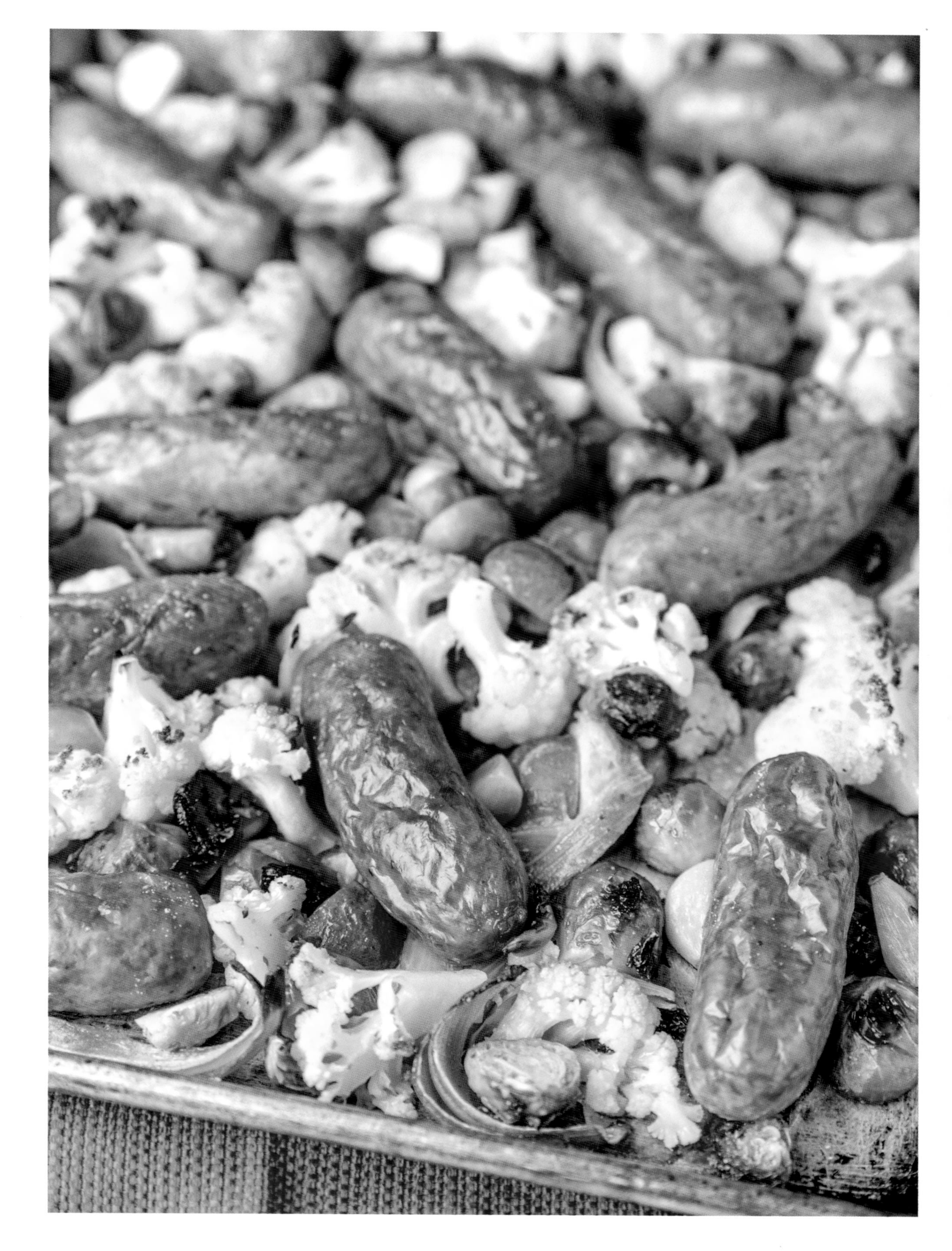

TACO CASSEROLE

YIELD: 8 servings

PREP TIME: 10 minutes (not including time to make seasoning or tortillas)

COOK TIME: 25 minutes

If you haven't already guessed it, I'll come right out and say it: I'm all about casseroles! Enjoy this Mexican-inspired dish with guacamole and Sesame Crackers (page 126), and you've got a meal your family will ask for again and again.

2 pounds grass-fed ground beef

1 cup chopped white onions

1 cup salsa

¼ cup Taco Seasoning (page 62)

3 cups shredded cheddar cheese, divided

8 "For Real" Tortillas (page 128)

SUGGESTED TOPPINGS

Sour cream

Additional salsa

Diced avocado

Chopped fresh cilantro

Store in an airtight container in the refrigerator for up to 3 days. You can also freeze the casserole after it has cooled completely. Thaw in the refrigerator overnight before reheating, covered, in a preheated 350°F oven for 30 to 40 minutes.

1. Preheat the oven to 350°F.
2. Place the ground beef and onions in a large skillet over medium-high heat. Cook, stirring often to crumble the meat, until the beef is browned and no longer pink. Stir in the salsa and taco seasoning and remove the pan from the heat.
3. Spread half of the beef mixture evenly in an 8 by 12-inch baking dish. Sprinkle 1 cup of the cheese over the meat. Arrange four of the tortillas in a single layer over the cheese. (You may need to tear some in half to completely cover the cheese without overlapping the tortillas.)
4. Spread the remaining beef mixture over the tortillas and top the meat with 1 cup of the cheese and the remaining four tortillas. Top with the remaining 1 cup of cheese.
5. Bake, uncovered, for 20 minutes. Remove from the oven and set aside to cool for 15 minutes.
6. Slice and serve with the toppings of your choice.

| WITHOUT TOPPINGS |

calories 540 | fat 38g | protein 34g | total carbs 9g | dietary fiber 4g | net carbs 5g

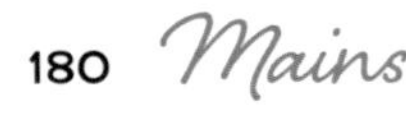

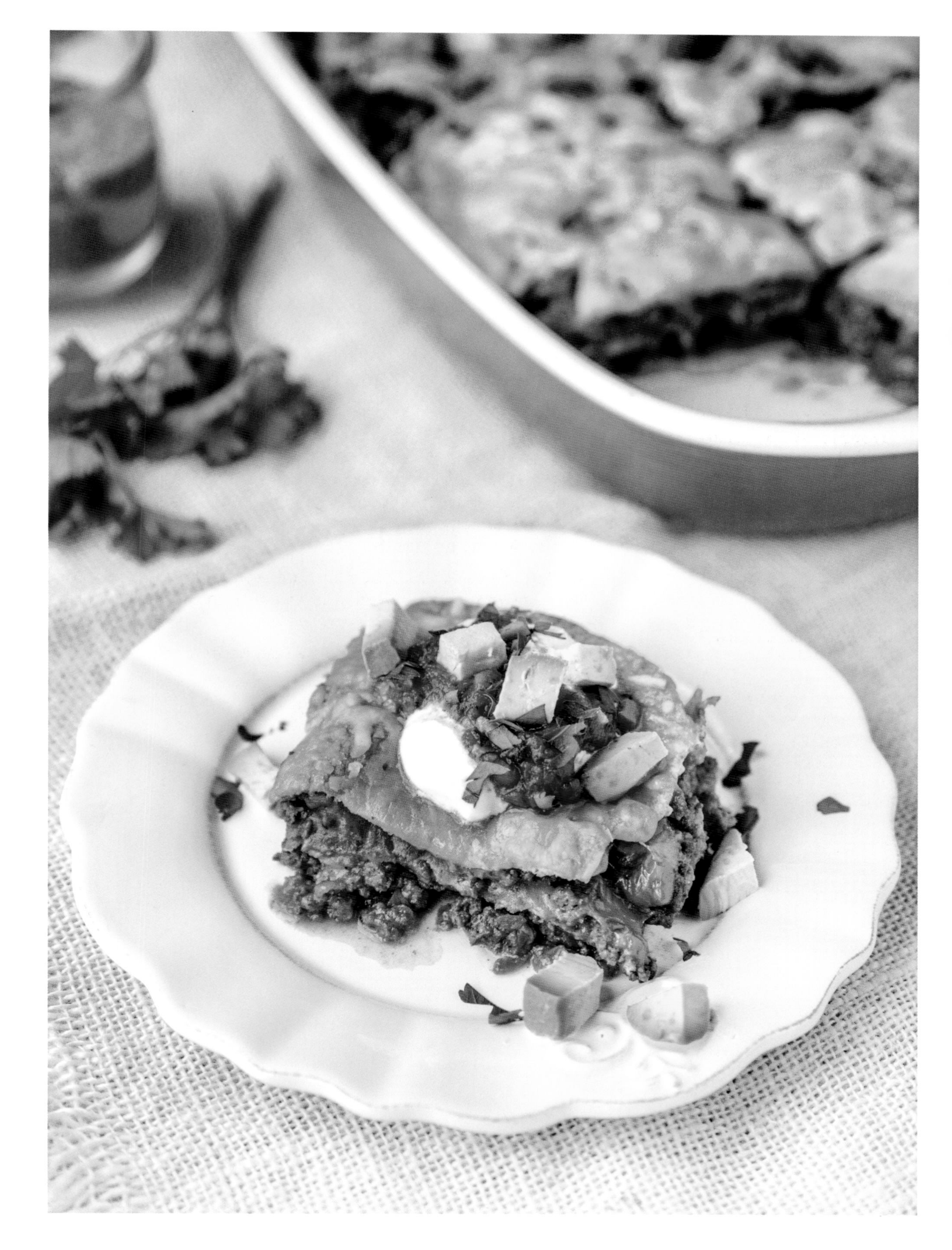

ONE-PAN PAPRIKA CHICKEN WITH CREAMY SPINACH

YIELD: 6 servings

PREP TIME: 20 minutes

COOK TIME: 40 minutes

One-pan meals are my favorite! I love it when I don't end up with a sink full of dirty pots and pans. This meal packs a flavor punch, too. If you're not a fan of spinach, substitute another green that you do like—perhaps kale.

2 pounds boneless, skinless chicken thighs

2 teaspoons smoked paprika

1 teaspoon fine sea salt

1 teaspoon freshly ground black pepper

¼ cup (½ stick) salted butter

8 ounces button mushrooms, sliced

4 cloves garlic, minced

1 cup chicken bone broth

1 cup heavy whipping cream

2 ounces cream cheese (¼ cup)

5 ounces fresh baby spinach, chopped

Chopped fresh herbs (such as thyme or parsley), for garnish (optional)

1. Preheat the oven to 400°F.
2. Season both sides of the chicken thighs with the paprika, salt, and pepper.
3. Melt the butter in a large cast-iron skillet or other ovenproof skillet over medium-high heat. Add the chicken thighs and sear for 2 to 3 minutes on each side, or until nicely browned. Remove the chicken from the pan and keep warm.
4. Add the mushrooms and garlic to the skillet and cook until the garlic is fragrant and the mushrooms are tender.
5. Add the broth, cream, and cream cheese to the skillet and stir continuously until the cream cheese is melted. Cook for 3 to 4 minutes, or until the sauce thickens. Return the chicken to the skillet and stir in the spinach.
6. Transfer the skillet to the oven and bake, uncovered, for 20 to 25 minutes, or until an instant-read thermometer inserted in the thickest part of a thigh registers 165°F.
7. Garnish with the herbs, if desired, and serve immediately.

Store in an airtight container in the refrigerator for up to 3 days.

calories 584 | fat 49g | protein 27g | total carbs 4g | dietary fiber 1g | net carbs 3g

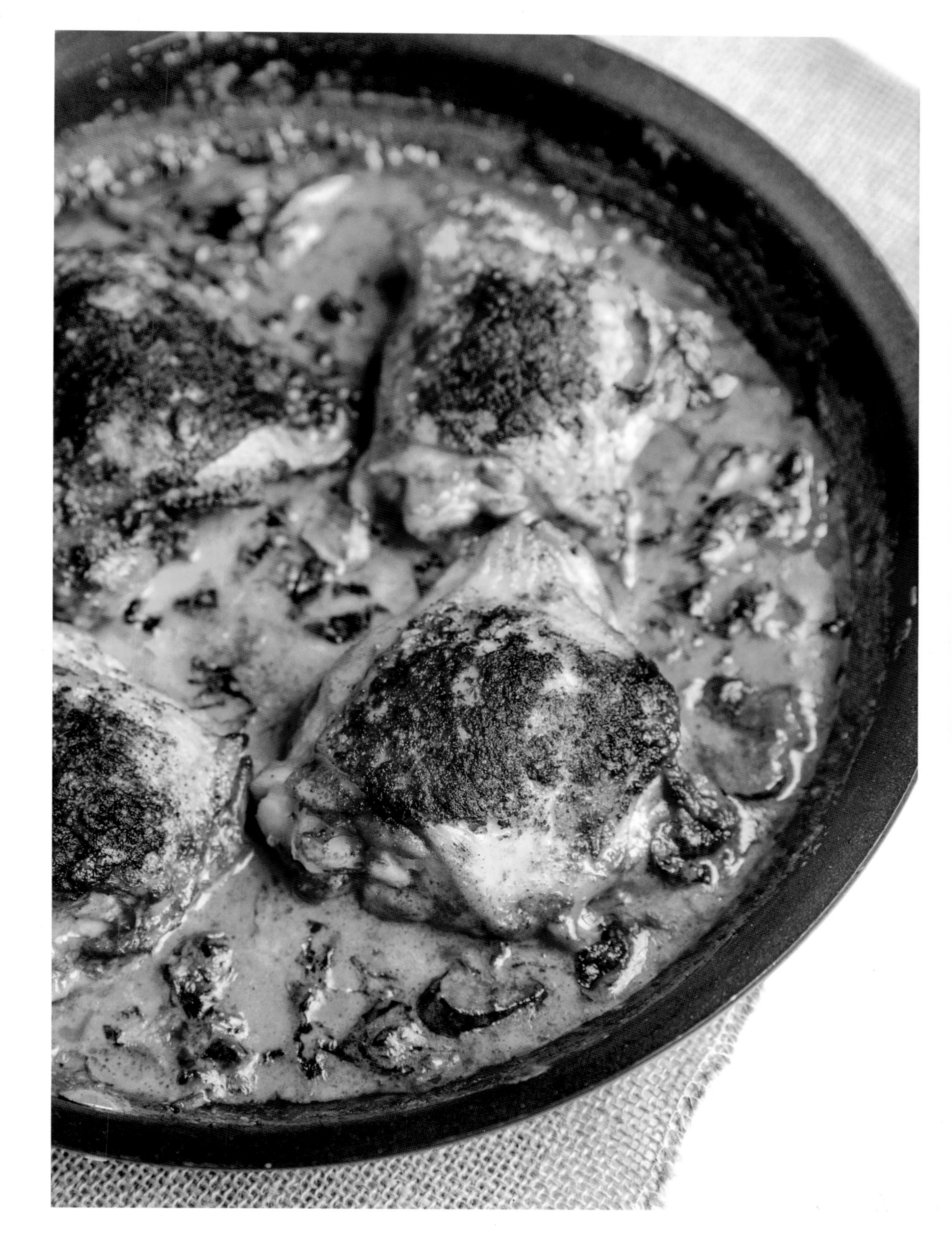

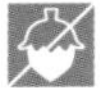

CHICKEN BROCCOLI CAESAR CASSEROLE

YIELD: 12 servings

PREP TIME: 20 minutes (not including time to make dressing)

COOK TIME: 1 hour

Here's another easy weeknight meal! Using rotisserie chicken and frozen broccoli makes this easy dish come together in about an hour.

- 6 cups shredded cooked chicken (about 2 pounds)
- 1 (8-ounce) package cream cheese, softened
- 1 cup Caesar Dressing (page 60), plus more for serving
- 2 cups cooked chopped broccoli
- 8 large eggs (see Tip, page 82)
- 2 cups shredded mozzarella cheese
- 1/2 cup heavy whipping cream
- 1/4 teaspoon fine sea salt
- 1/4 teaspoon freshly ground black pepper
- Chopped fresh flat-leaf parsley, for garnish

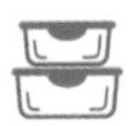

Store in an airtight container in the refrigerator for up to 3 days.

1. Preheat the oven to 350°F. Grease a 13 by 9-inch baking dish.
2. Place the chicken, cream cheese, and Caesar dressing in a mixing bowl and stir until well combined. Stir in the broccoli. Evenly spread the contents of the bowl into the prepared baking dish.
3. In the same bowl, whisk together the eggs, mozzarella, cream, salt, and pepper. Pour the egg mixture over the contents of the baking dish.
4. Bake for 45 minutes to 1 hour, or until the egg mixture is set in the center and the cheese is melted and slightly browned.
5. Serve hot, drizzled with extra dressing and garnished with parsley.

calories 396 | fat 30g | protein 26g | total carbs 2g | dietary fiber 0g | net carbs 2g

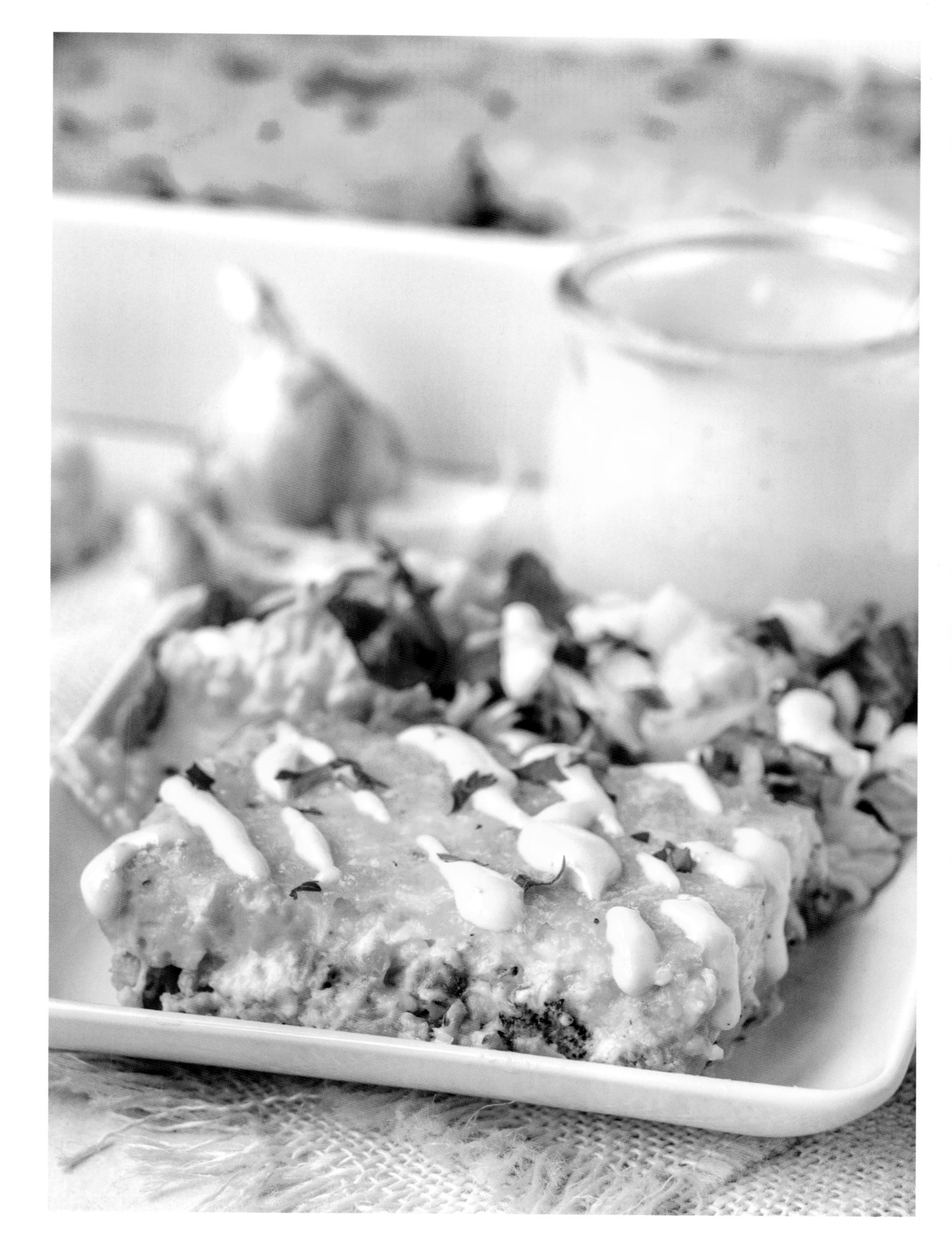

option

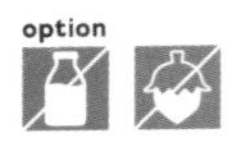

CLASSIC ITALIAN MEATBALLS

YIELD: 18 meatballs (3 per serving)

PREP TIME: 20 minutes

COOK TIME: 30 minutes

My family just loves meatballs. The addition of mayonnaise in this recipe may seem a bit weird to you, but remember: mayonnaise is really just eggs, oil, vinegar, and spices. Using it gives the meat a nice flavor and helps keep the meatballs tender.

- 1 pound grass-fed ground beef
- 1 pound pastured ground pork
- 2/3 cup grated Parmesan cheese (or nutritional yeast for dairy-free)
- 2 large eggs, beaten
- 1/3 cup avocado oil mayonnaise
- 1/4 cup chopped fresh flat-leaf parsley
- 2 teaspoons minced garlic
- 1 teaspoon crushed dried fennel seeds
- 1 teaspoon onion powder
- 1 teaspoon fine sea salt
- 1/2 teaspoon freshly ground black pepper
- Chopped fresh flat-leaf parsley, for garnish (optional)

1. Preheat the oven to 350°F. Line a sheet pan with aluminum foil or parchment paper.

2. Place all of the ingredients in a mixing bowl and use your hands to combine.

3. Form the mixture into 18 balls (2 1/4 ounces each) and arrange on the prepared sheet pan.

4. Bake for 25 to 30 minutes, or until the meatballs are nicely browned and an instant-read thermometer inserted in the thickest part of a meatball registers 165°F. Remove from the oven and set aside to rest for 5 minutes before serving.

5. Serve hot. Garnish with parsley, if desired.

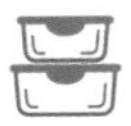

Store in an airtight container in the refrigerator for up to 3 days.

VARIATION: STOVETOP ITALIAN MEATBALLS IN MARINARA SAUCE *(pictured).* Complete Steps 2 and 3 above, but place the meatballs in a large Dutch oven or pot. To the pot, add 8 cups of marinara sauce (homemade, page 53, or store-bought) and bring to a boil over medium-high heat. Reduce the heat to low, cover, and simmer for 3 hours, or until the meatballs are cooked through. Serve hot, garnished with chopped fresh flat-leaf parsley.

calories 550 | fat 46g | protein 32g | total carbs 2g | dietary fiber 1g | net carbs 2g

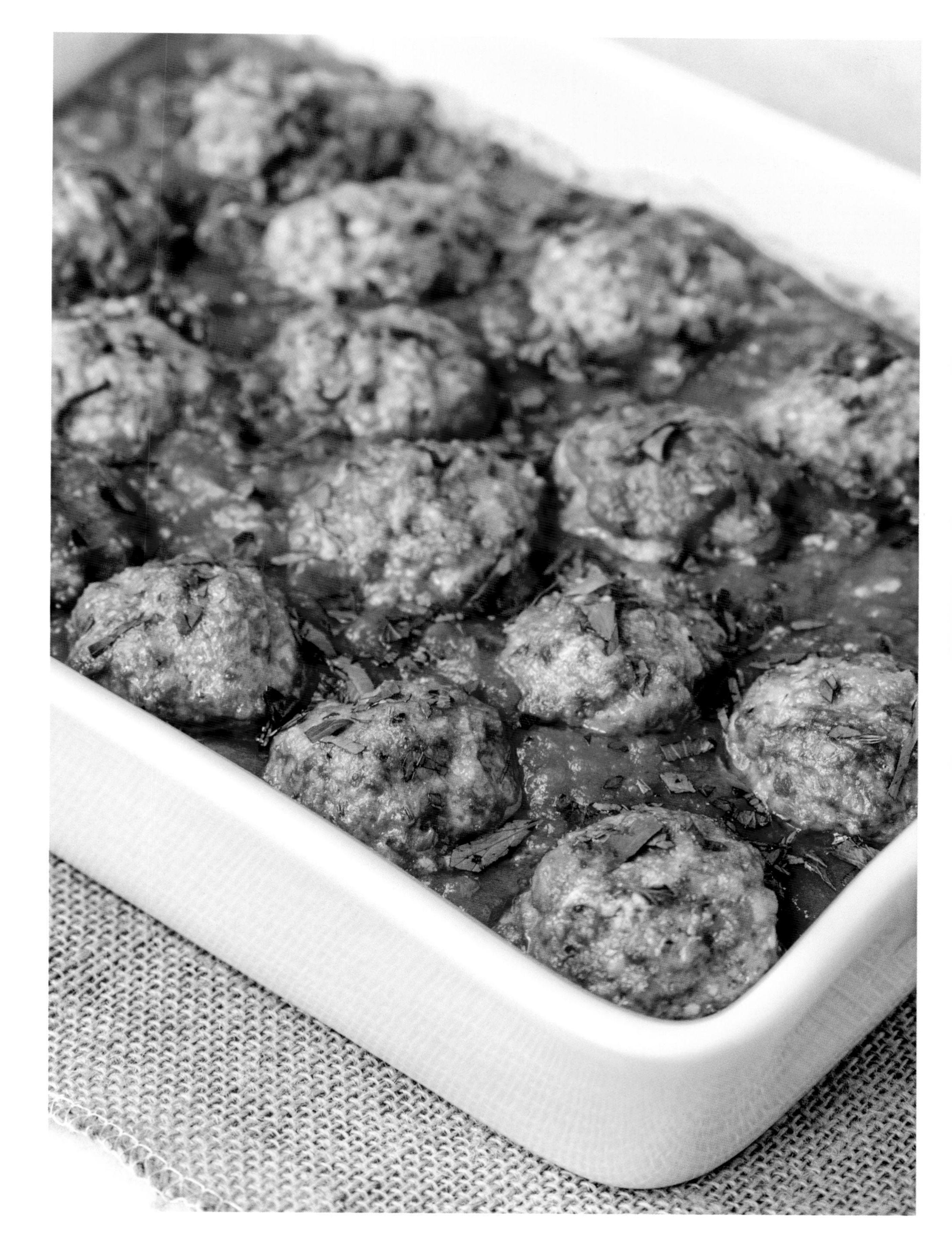

SPATCHCOCKED CHICKEN

YIELD: 12 servings

PREP TIME: 10 minutes, plus at least 1 hour to marinate

COOK TIME: 1 hour

Once you've spatchcocked a chicken, you'll never roast one any other way again. I like to serve this flavorful chicken with Jicama Fries (page 216).

1 (5-pound) whole chicken

2 tablespoons extra-virgin olive oil

2 tablespoons freshly squeezed lemon juice

2 tablespoons Chicken Spice Rub (page 47)

1. Using poultry shears, kitchen scissors, or a sharp knife, spatchcock the chicken by cutting along one side of the backbone until the body opens. Cut along the other side of the backbone to remove it completely. Open the bird and place it on a work surface, breast side up. Press down hard on the center of the breast so it lies as flat as possible.
2. In a small bowl, combine the oil, lemon juice, and spice rub.
3. Arrange the chicken, breast side up, on a sheet pan. Spread the oil mixture all over the chicken, including the underside. Refrigerate for at least 1 hour or up to 24 hours.
4. Preheat the oven to 400°F.
5. Roast the chicken, uncovered, for 45 minutes to 1 hour, or until an instant-read thermometer inserted in the thickest part of the breast registers 165°F. Remove from the oven, cover with foil, and set aside to rest for 10 minutes before carving.
6. Immediately before serving, spoon the pan juices over the chicken. Enjoy!

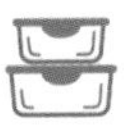

Store in an airtight container in the refrigerator for up to 3 days.

calories 218 | fat 16g | protein 16g | total carbs 0g | dietary fiber 0g | net carbs 0g

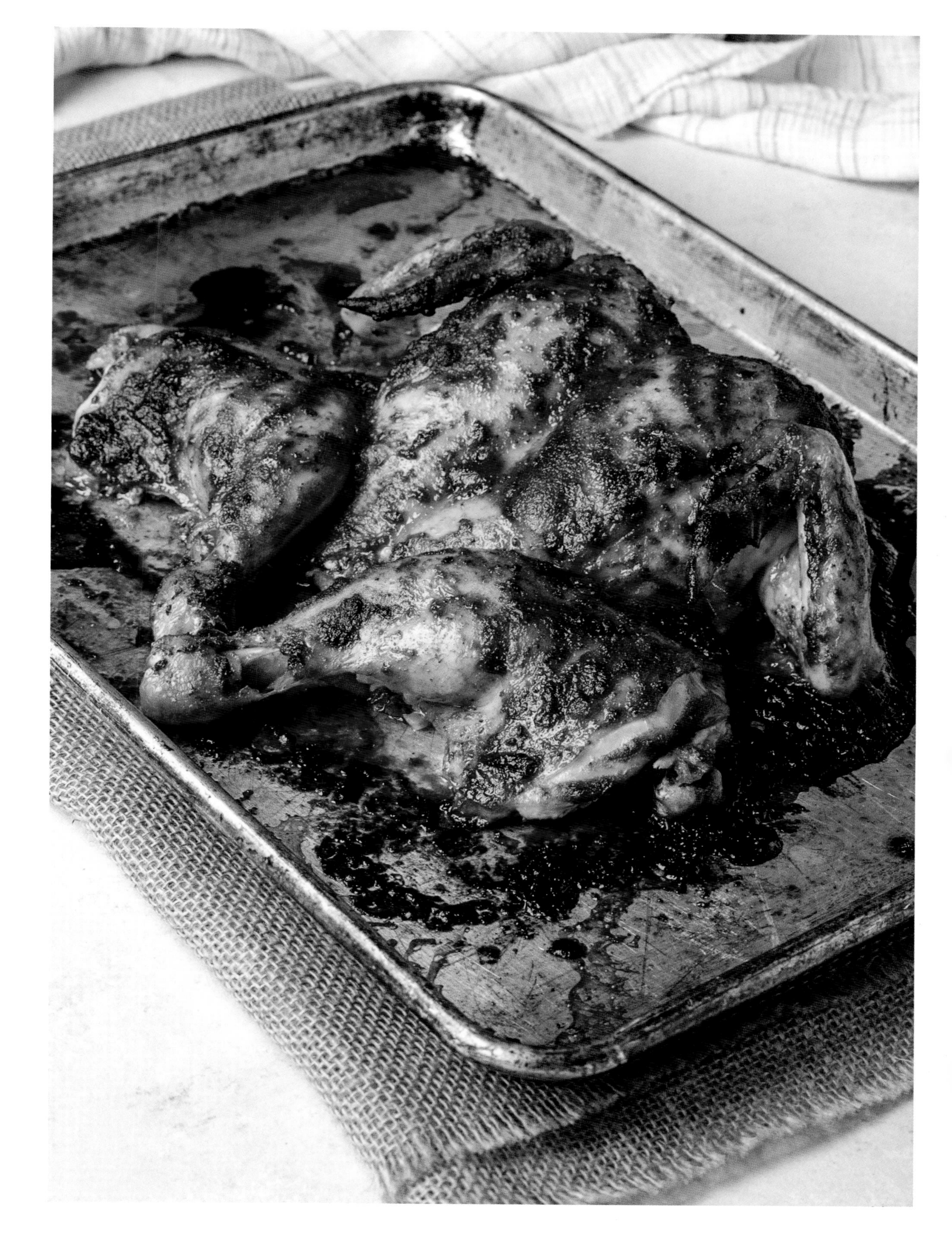

COTTAGE PIE

YIELD: 8 servings
PREP TIME: 40 minutes
COOK TIME: 1 hour 15 minutes

This cottage pie is comfort food at its best. My kids love it even though they know it is topped with mashed cauliflower. The leftovers make a great lunch, too!

FOR THE MASHED CAULIFLOWER TOPPING

Florets from 1 large head cauliflower (about 2 pounds)

2 tablespoons extra-virgin olive oil

½ teaspoon garlic powder

½ teaspoon fine sea salt

¼ teaspoon freshly ground black pepper

¼ cup (½ stick) salted butter

FOR THE BEEF FILLING

2 tablespoons extra-virgin olive oil

1 cup diced white onions

2 cloves garlic, minced

2 pounds grass-fed ground beef

2 tablespoons coconut flour

2 teaspoons Italian seasoning

2 tablespoons chopped fresh flat-leaf parsley, plus more for garnish

1½ cups beef bone broth

½ cup red wine

1 tablespoon tomato paste

½ teaspoon fine sea salt

¼ teaspoon freshly ground black pepper

1. Preheat the oven to 400°F.
2. Make the mashed cauliflower: Arrange the cauliflower florets on a sheet pan and sprinkle the oil and seasonings over them. Bake for 30 minutes.
3. Transfer the roasted cauliflower to a food processor. Add the butter and process until smooth. Set aside.
4. Make the filling: Heat the oil in a large skillet over medium-high heat. Add the onions and garlic and cook for 4 to 5 minutes, or until the onions are softened.
5. Add the ground beef to the skillet and cook, stirring often to crumble the meat, until it is browned and no longer pink. Stir in the remaining filling ingredients and simmer for 15 to 20 minutes, or until most of the liquid is absorbed. Remove from the heat.
6. Spread the contents of the skillet in a 13 by 9-inch baking dish. Spread the mashed cauliflower over the beef mixture.
7. Bake for 20 minutes, or until golden brown on top and bubbling around the edges.
8. Garnish with parsley and serve hot.

Store in an airtight container in the refrigerator for up to 3 days. You can also freeze the pie before baking. Use a freezer-safe baking dish or a metal baking pan. Follow the recipe through Step 6, then tightly cover the baking dish and freeze for up to 6 months. Thaw in the refrigerator overnight before baking; it may take an extra 10 to 15 minutes in the oven to heat through.

calories 466 | fat 36g | protein 22g | total carbs 10g | dietary fiber 3g | net carbs 7g

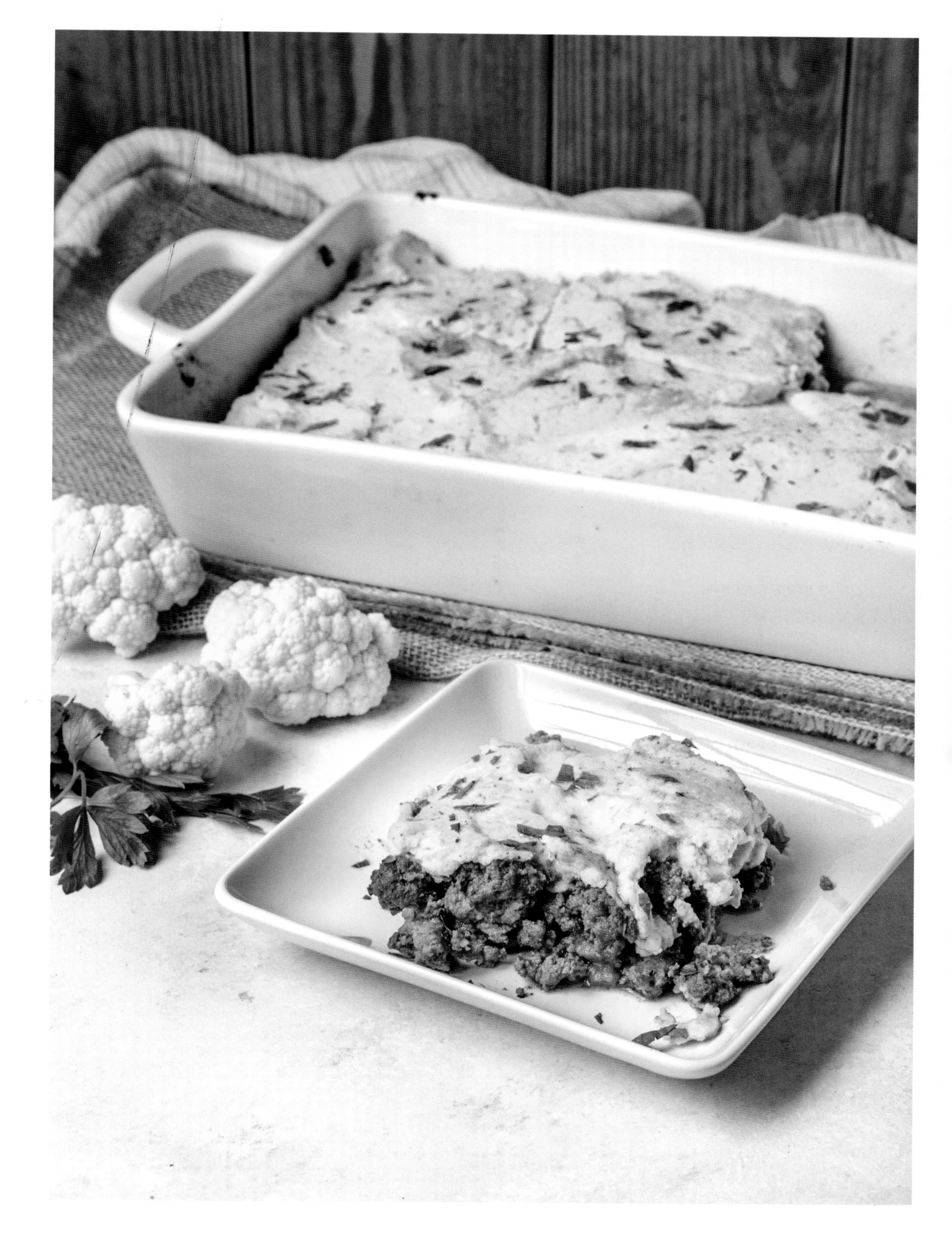

SHEET PAN LEMON GARLIC HERB SALMON AND ROASTED CAULIFLOWER

YIELD: 6 servings

PREP TIME: 15 minutes

COOK TIME: 34 minutes

Who doesn't love a meal that can be prepared on a single sheet pan? If everything cooks together, you'll have an easy meal and little to clean up. If you're sick and tired of cauliflower, substitute broccoli in this recipe.

FOR THE ROASTED CAULIFLOWER

Florets from 1 medium head cauliflower (about 1½ pounds)

2 tablespoons extra-virgin olive oil

½ teaspoon fine sea salt

¼ teaspoon freshly ground black pepper

¼ teaspoon garlic powder

FOR THE SALMON

⅓ cup chopped fresh cilantro or flat-leaf parsley

2 tablespoons extra-virgin olive oil

2 tablespoons freshly squeezed lemon juice

1 teaspoon minced garlic

6 skinless salmon fillets (about 2 pounds)

½ teaspoon fine sea salt

¼ teaspoon freshly ground black pepper

1. Preheat the oven to 400°F.
2. Make the cauliflower: Spread the cauliflower florets on a sheet pan. Drizzle the oil over the cauliflower and season with the salt, pepper, and garlic powder.
3. Roast for 20 minutes. Remove from the oven and shift the cauliflower to the edges of the pan, making room for the salmon in the center. Set aside.
4. Prepare the salmon: In a small mixing bowl, whisk together the cilantro, olive oil, lemon juice, and garlic.
5. Arrange the salmon fillets in the middle of the sheet pan and coat the fish with half of the cilantro mixture. Season with the salt and pepper, then drizzle the remaining cilantro mixture over the salmon.
6. Bake for 10 to 14 minutes, or until the salmon is opaque and flakes when prodded with a fork in the thickest part.
7. Serve hot.

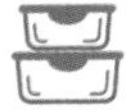
Store in an airtight container in the refrigerator for up to 2 days.

calories 329 | fat 19g | protein 32g | total carbs 6g | dietary fiber 2g | net carbs 4g

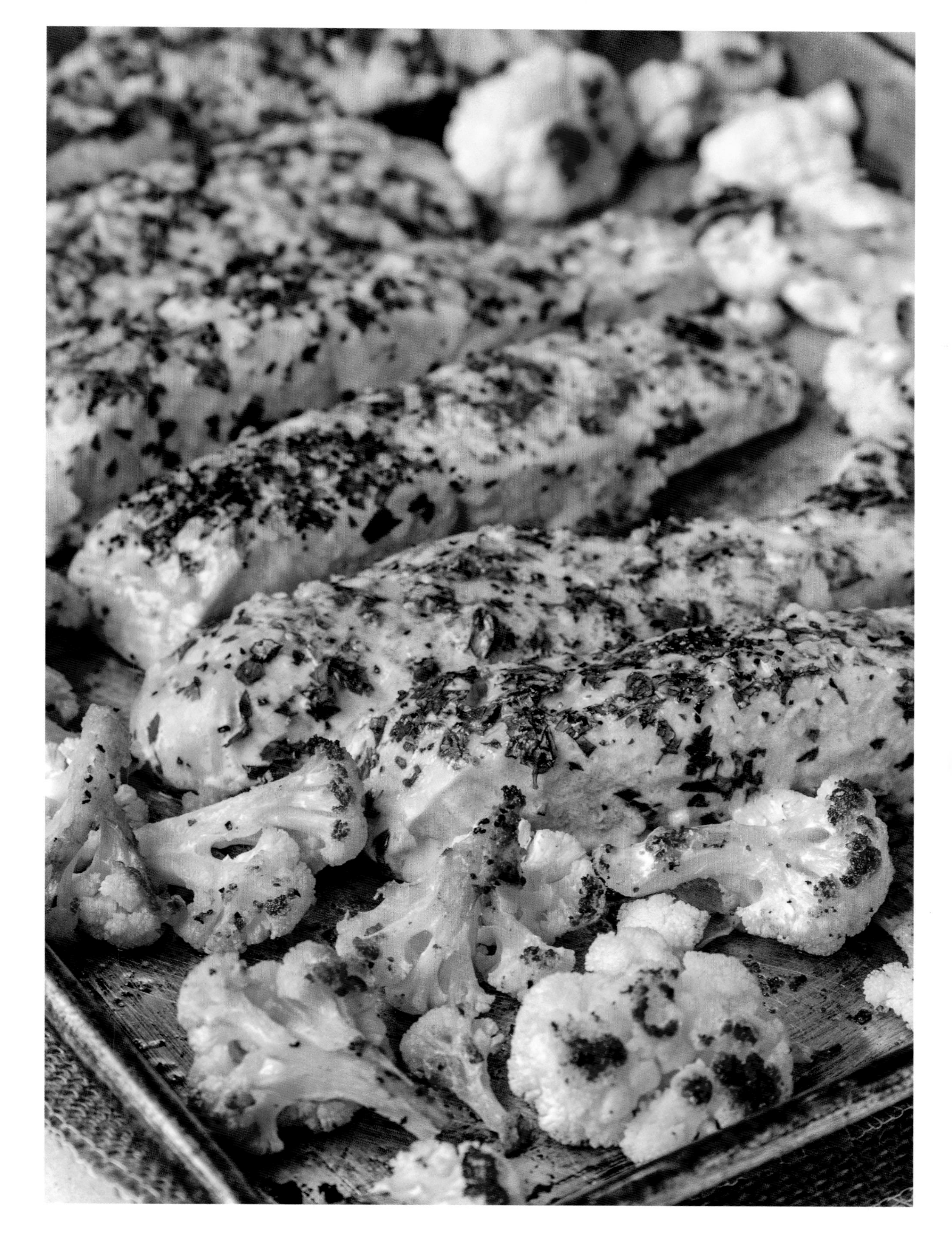

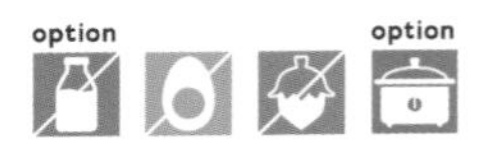

INSTANT POT (OR SLOW COOKER) BEEF SHORT RIBS

YIELD: 10 servings

PREP TIME: 10 minutes

COOK TIME: 1 hour 25 minutes or 4½ to 10½ hours, depending on method

These short ribs are pure perfection. Whether you make them quickly in an Instant Pot or choose the slow cooker method instead, the meat will fall off the bone. Your family will ask you to make this meal again and again.

5 pounds beef short ribs

1 teaspoon fine sea salt

1 teaspoon freshly ground black pepper

2 tablespoons avocado oil

1½ cups sliced white onions

3 cloves garlic, minced

1½ cups red wine

1 cup beef bone broth

2 tablespoons Worcestershire sauce

2 tablespoons tomato paste

1 batch Mashed Roasted Cauliflower (page 212), warmed, for serving (omit for dairy-free)

Chopped fresh flat-leaf parsley, for garnish

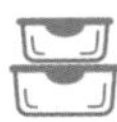

Store in an airtight container in the refrigerator for up to 3 days.

Season the ribs on both sides with the salt and pepper.

INSTANT POT DIRECTIONS:

1. Set the Instant Pot to the sauté mode and pour in the oil. Place half of the ribs in the pot and brown for 4 to 5 minutes on each side. Remove to a plate and repeat with the remaining ribs.

2. Add the onions and garlic to the pot and cook until the onions are tender and the garlic is fragrant.

3. Deglaze the pot with the wine and broth, scraping the bottom of the pot to release all of the browned bits of meat. Add the Worcestershire sauce and tomato paste and bring to a simmer. Simmer for 5 minutes.

4. Return the browned ribs to the pot, cover, and set to the stew mode on high pressure for 45 minutes. Once the cycle ends, keep in the warm mode for 15 minutes. Perform a quick release of the pressure. Remove the lid carefully, watching out for the steam.

5. Serve hot over the mashed cauliflower, garnished with parsley.

SLOW COOKER DIRECTIONS:

1. Heat the oil in a large skillet over medium-high heat. Place half the ribs in the hot skillet and cook for 5 minutes, or until the bottom side of each rib is browned. Turn over the ribs and cook for 5 minutes. Remove to a plate, add the remaining ribs, and repeat the process.

2. Place the broth and browned ribs in the slow cooker.

3. Place the onions, garlic, wine, Worcestershire sauce, and tomato paste in the skillet and stir until well combined. Bring to a boil. Boil for 5 minutes, or until the onions are tender and translucent. Pour the contents of the skillet over the ribs in the slow cooker.

4. Cover and cook on high for 4 to 6 hours or on low for 8 to 10 hours, until the meat is fall-off-the-bone tender.

5. Serve hot over the mashed cauliflower, garnished with parsley.

calories **360** | fat **19g** | protein **32g** | total carbs **4g** | dietary fiber **0g** | net carbs **4g**

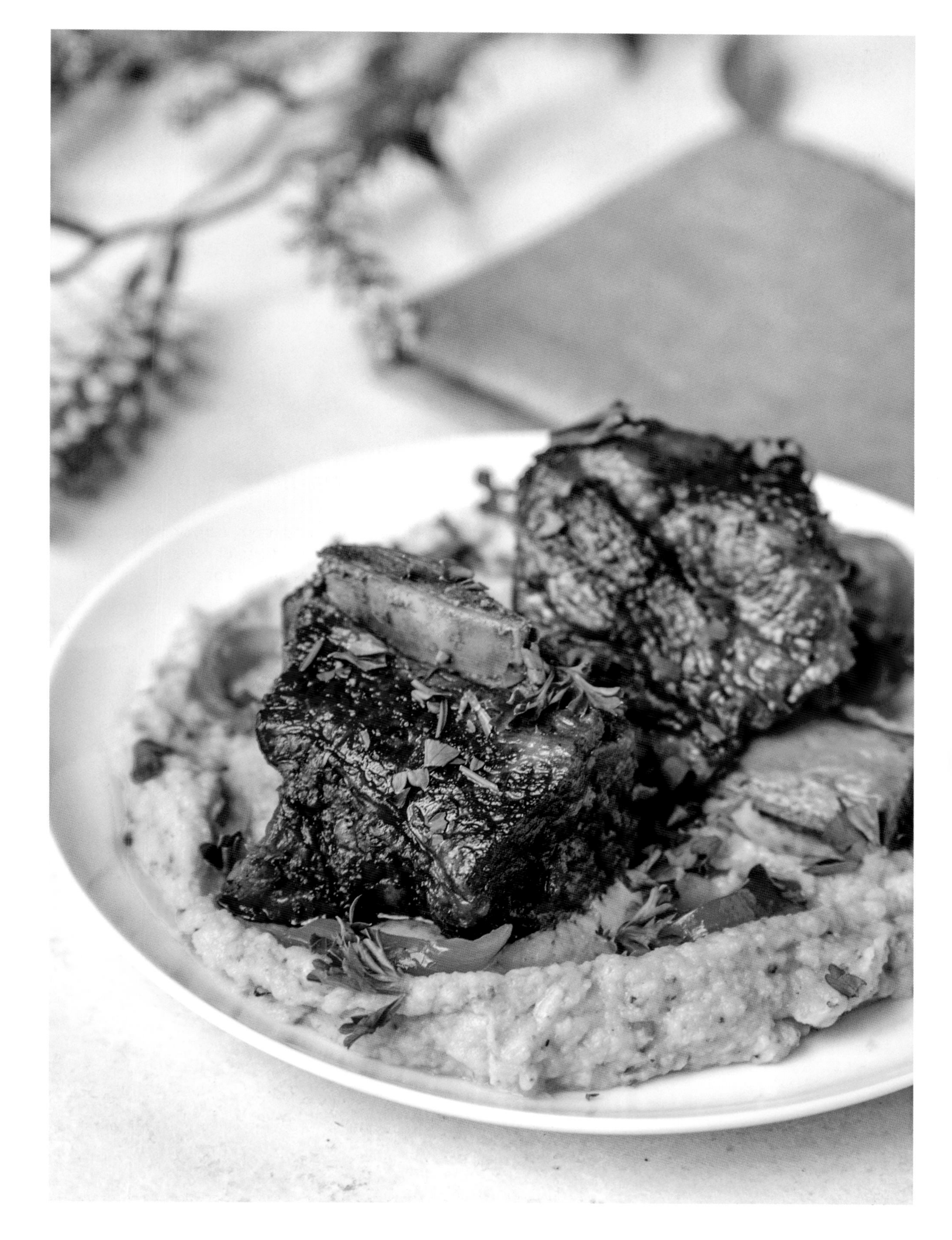

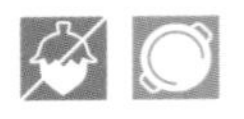

SKILLET CHICKEN PARMESAN

YIELD: 8 servings

PREP TIME: 15 minutes (not including time to make breading)

COOK TIME: 28 minutes

This is a great keto-friendly version of a traditional chicken Parmesan. At my house, it's a family favorite.

8 boneless, skinless chicken breast halves (about 2 pounds)

2 large eggs, beaten

2 tablespoons chopped fresh flat-leaf parsley, plus more for garnish

1 tablespoon minced garlic

½ teaspoon fine sea salt

¼ teaspoon freshly ground black pepper

1 cup Keto Breading (page 56)

½ cup grated Parmesan cheese

4 tablespoons avocado oil, divided

3 cups marinara sauce, store-bought or homemade (page 53)

1 cup shredded mozzarella cheese

Store in an airtight container in the refrigerator for up to 3 days or freeze for up to 6 months.

1. Place the chicken breasts between two pieces of parchment paper or plastic wrap on a level work surface. Firmly pound each breast with the smooth side of a meat mallet to a thickness of ½ inch. Set aside.

2. Place the eggs, parsley, garlic, salt, and pepper in a shallow bowl and whisk until well combined. Set aside.

3. In a second shallow bowl, combine the breading and Parmesan cheese. Set aside.

4. In a very large skillet with a lid over medium-high heat, warm 2 tablespoons of the oil.

5. One at a time, dip four of the chicken breasts in the egg mixture and then in the breading mixture. Once they are fully coated, place them in the skillet.

6. Cook the chicken for 4 to 5 minutes on each side, or until nicely browned. Remove from the skillet and set aside on a plate.

7. Warm the remaining 2 tablespoons of oil in the skillet and repeat the process with the remaining four chicken breasts. Remove the cooked chicken to the same plate.

8. Reduce the heat to low. Deglaze the skillet with the marinara sauce, stirring and scraping the bottom of the pan. Return all of the chicken to the skillet, cover, and cook for 5 to 8 minutes, or until an instant-read thermometer inserted in the thickest part of a breast registers 165°F. Remove from the heat.

9. Spoon the sauce over the chicken and sprinkle equal portions of the mozzarella cheese over each breast. Garnish with additional parsley and enjoy!

calories **423** | fat **24g** | protein **40g** | total carbs **4g** | dietary fiber **0g** | net carbs **4g**

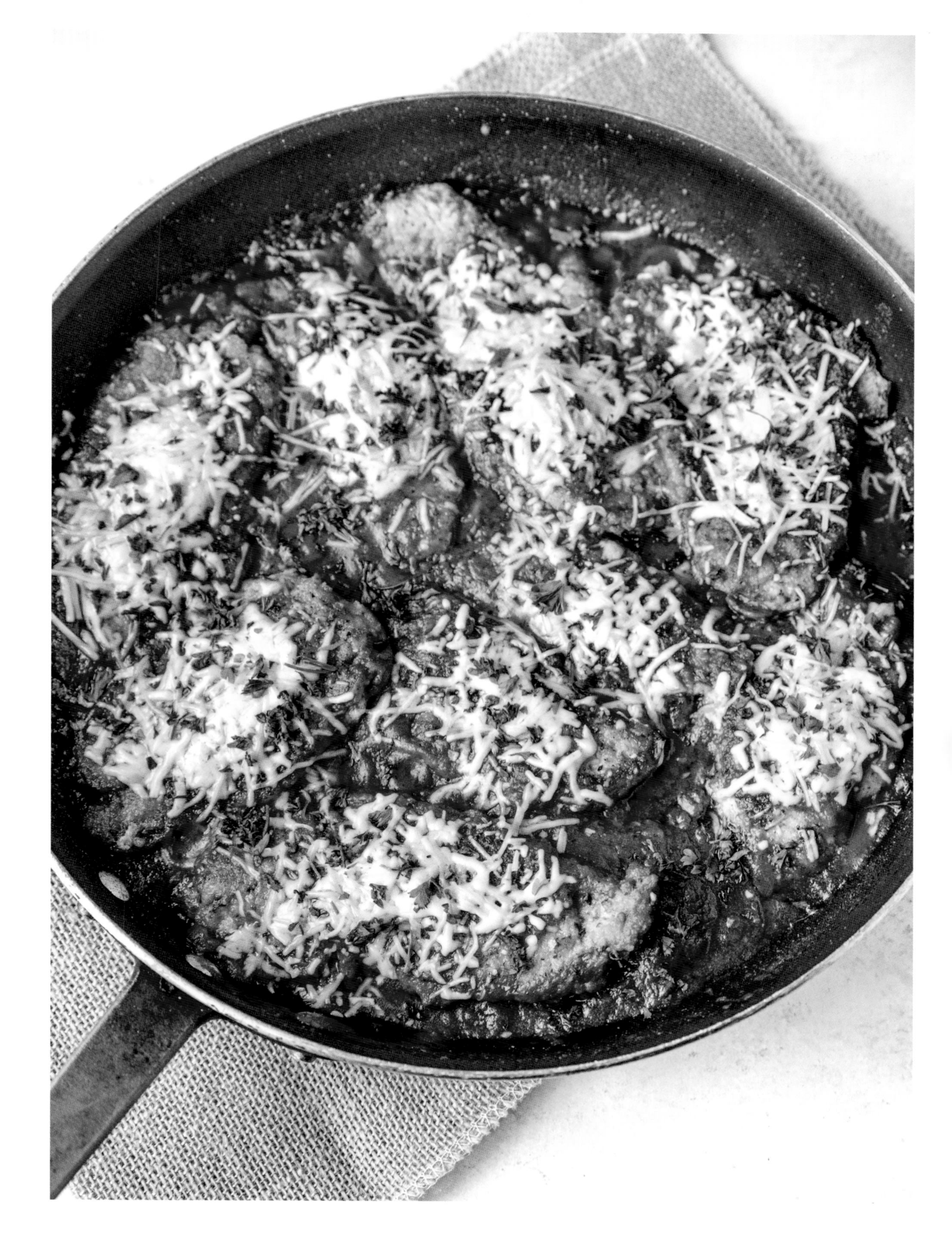

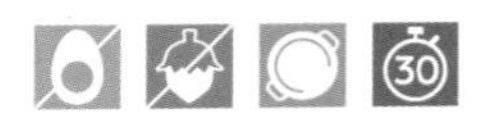

BACON CHEESEBURGER SLOPPY JOES

YIELD: 12 sandwiches (1 per serving)

PREP TIME: 10 minutes (not including time to make rolls)

COOK TIME: 20 minutes

What can I say? Bacon and cheese make everything better, so these sloppy Joes are upgraded from standard to extraordinary!

12 ounces bacon, chopped

½ cup chopped white onions

2 pounds grass-fed ground beef

2 cloves garlic, minced

1 cup beef bone broth

½ cup sugar-free ketchup, store-bought or homemade (page 50)

½ cup marinara sauce, store-bought or homemade (page 53)

¼ cup prepared yellow mustard

2 tablespoons dill pickle relish

2 cups shredded cheddar cheese

¼ teaspoon xanthan gum (optional, for thickening)

12 Hamburger Rolls (page 122), for serving

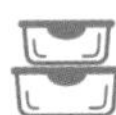

Store in an airtight container in the refrigerator for up to 3 days.

1. In a large skillet over medium-high heat, cook the bacon until crisp. Remove with a slotted spoon and set aside to cool on a plate lined with paper towels. Leave about 2 tablespoons of bacon grease in the skillet and drain the rest.

2. Add the onions to the skillet and cook over medium heat until tender and translucent. Add the ground beef and garlic and cook, stirring often to crumble the meat, until the beef is browned and no longer pink.

3. Add the broth, ketchup, marinara sauce, mustard, and relish to the skillet and bring to a simmer. Cook for about 5 minutes.

4. Add the cheese to the skillet and cook until it is melted. If the mixture is not as thick as you'd like it to be, stir in the xanthan gum until thickened. Remove from the heat.

5. Transfer the beef mixture to a serving bowl and stir in the bacon, or serve with the bacon on the side to be added as desired. Serve with the rolls and enjoy!

calories 527 | fat 43g | protein 29g | total carbs 2g | dietary fiber 0g | net carbs 2g

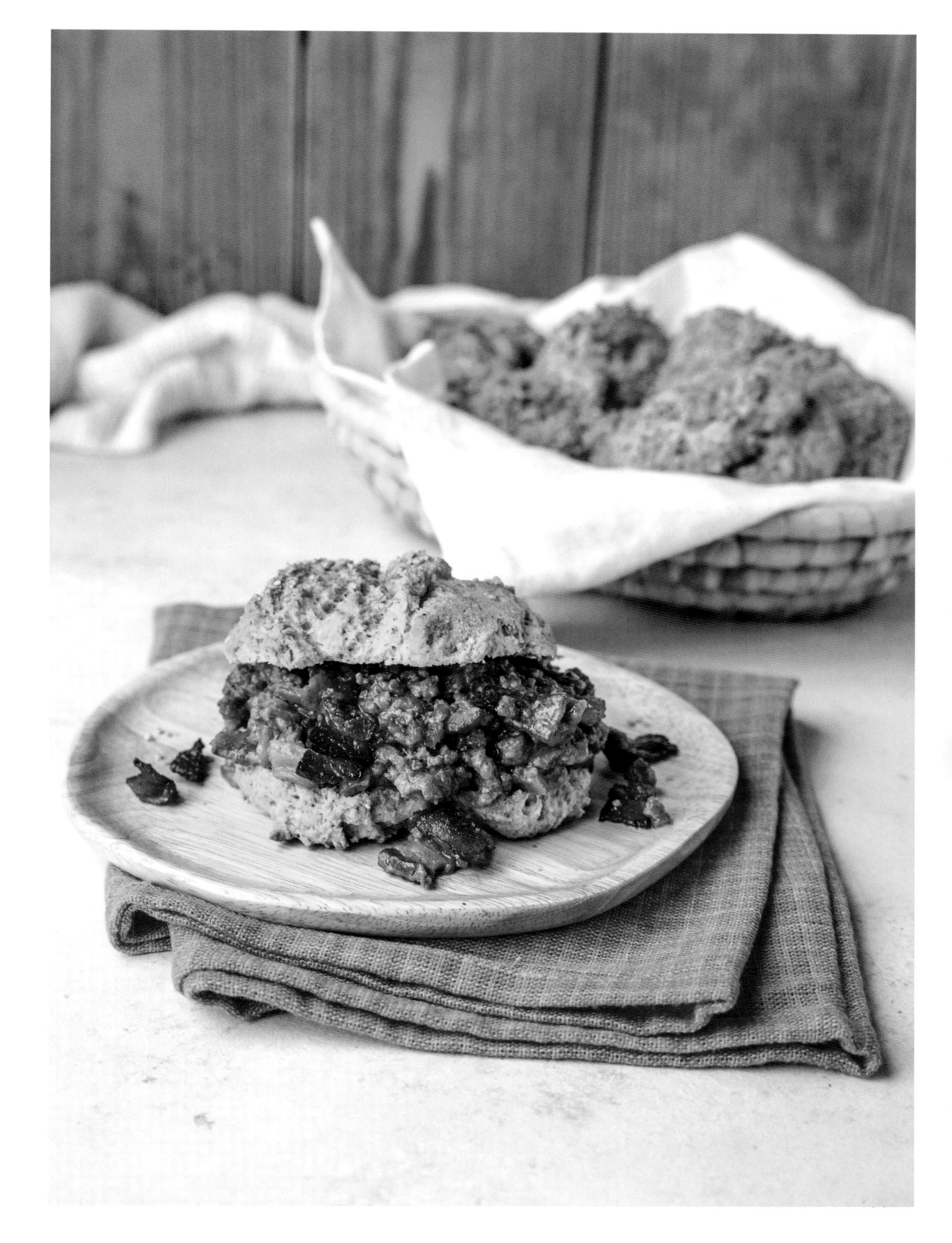

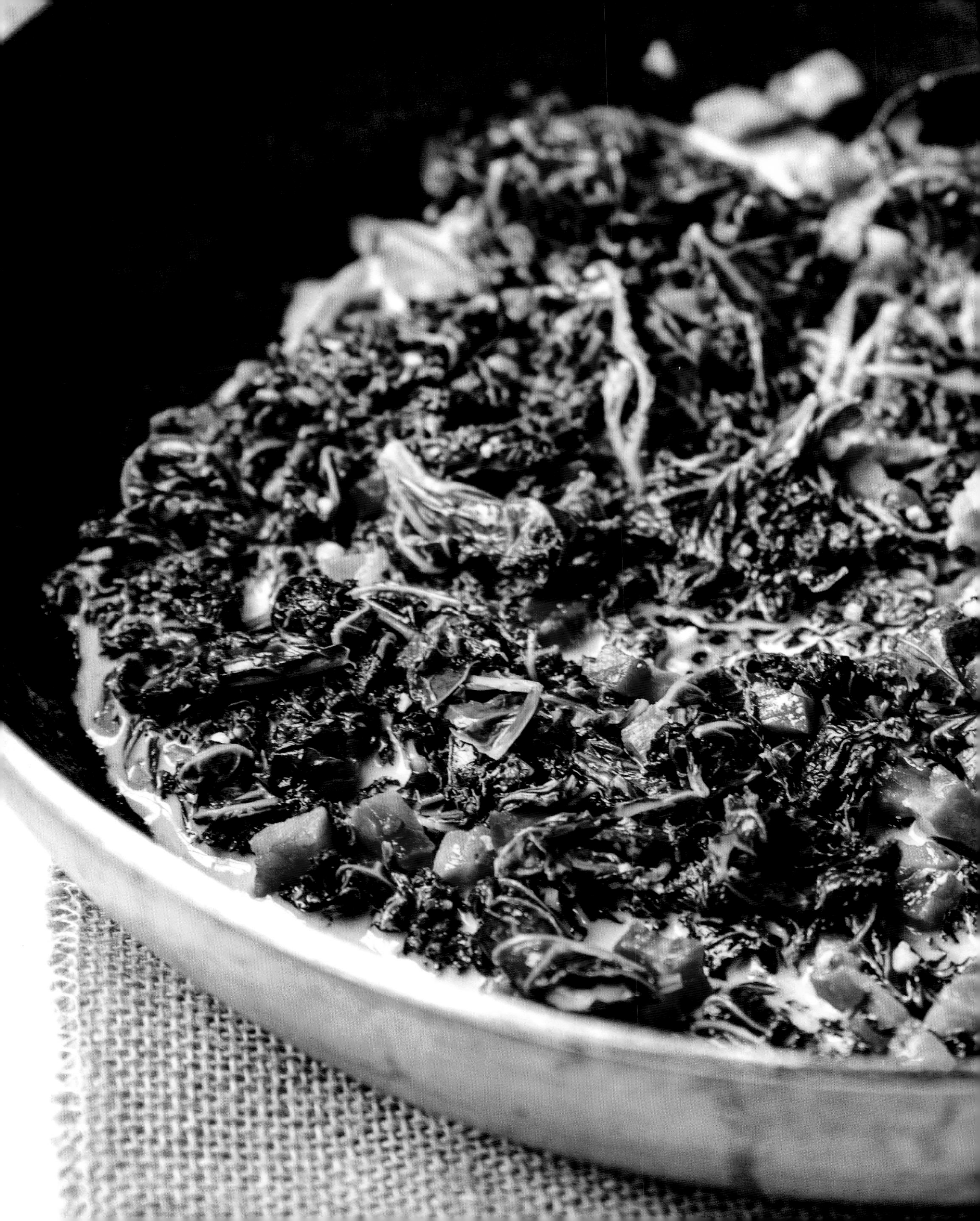

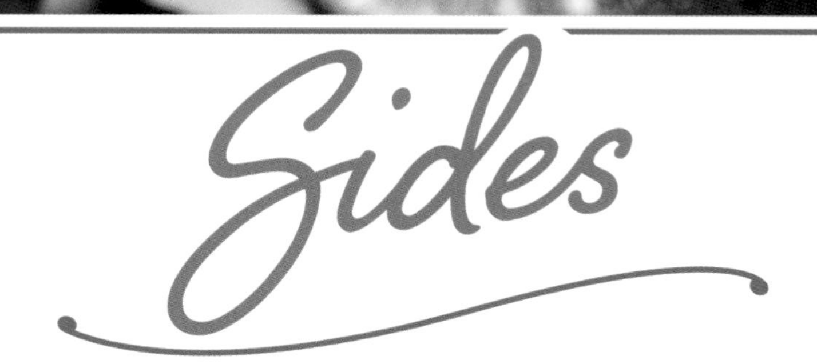
Sides

BLISTERED GARLIC GREEN BEANS

YIELD: 8 servings

PREP TIME: 5 minutes

COOK TIME: 25 minutes

I've said it many times before: I don't like standing at the stove to cook. But I'm all in for this recipe, which is super quick and doesn't require constant stirring. In case you're really stove-intolerant, I have provided oven directions as well.

1/4 cup avocado oil

2 pounds fresh green beans or haricots verts, trimmed

1/3 cup chopped fresh flat-leaf parsley

4 cloves garlic, minced

2 tablespoons freshly squeezed lemon juice

1/2 teaspoon fine sea salt

1/4 teaspoon freshly ground black pepper

Store in an airtight container in the refrigerator for up to 5 days.

STOVETOP DIRECTIONS:

1. Heat the oil in a large skillet over medium-high heat. Arrange the green beans in a single layer in the pan and cook without disturbing them for 3 to 4 minutes, or until they begin to blister.

2. Toss the beans well, cover, and cook, stirring every 5 minutes, for 10 to 20 minutes, or until all of the beans are tender and blistered. Remove from the heat.

3. Add the parsley, garlic, and lemon juice to the skillet and toss well. Season with the salt and pepper. Serve hot.

OVEN DIRECTIONS:

1. Preheat the oven to 450°F. Line a sheet pan with parchment paper.

2. Put the beans on the prepared sheet pan and toss with the oil until well coated. Arrange the beans in a single layer and roast for 10 minutes. Turn the beans over and bake for another 5 to 10 minutes, or until browned and tender.

3. Add the parsley, garlic, and lemon juice to the skillet and toss well. Season with the salt and pepper. Serve hot.

calories 98 | fat 7g | protein 32g | total carbs 8g | dietary fiber 3g | net carbs 5g

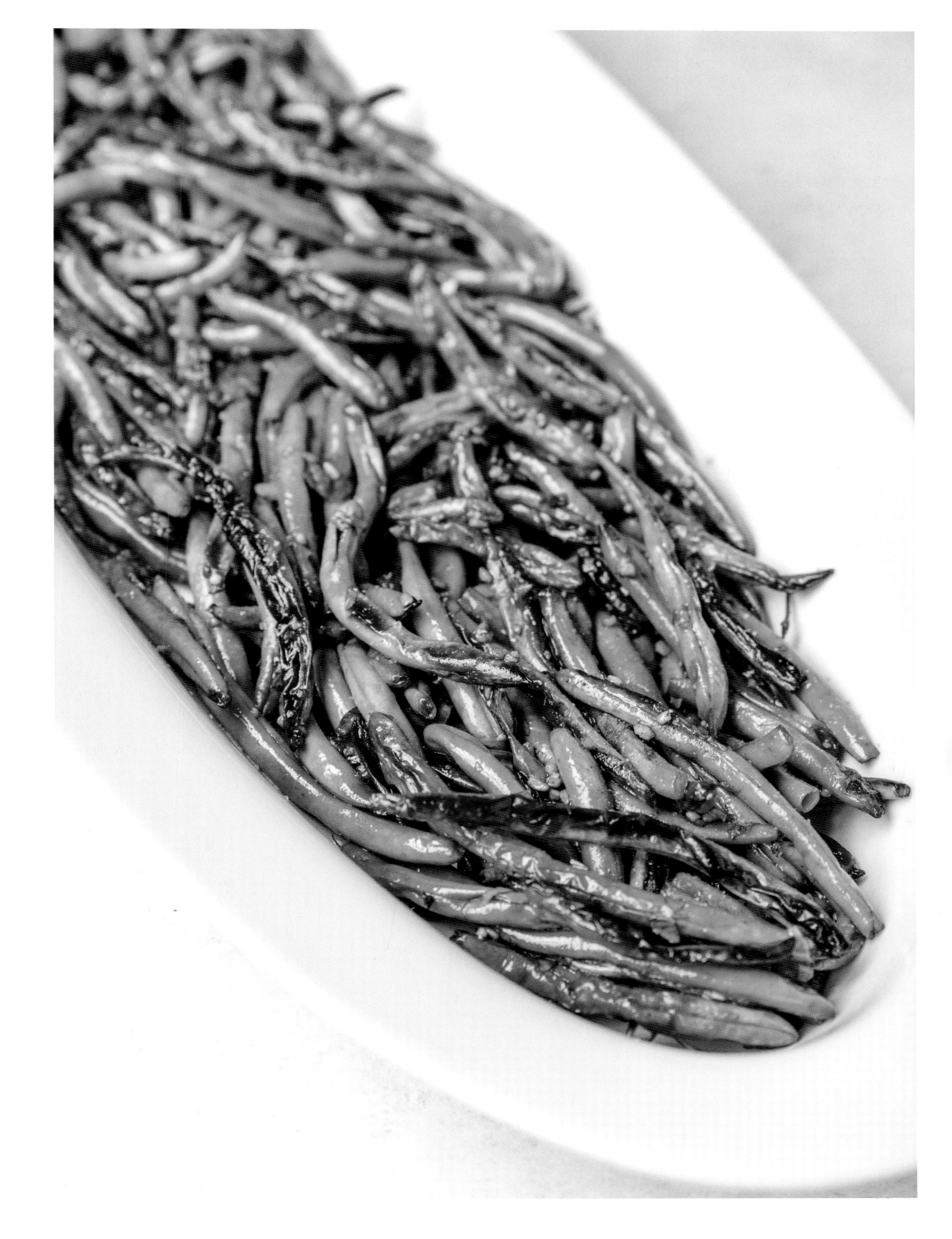

CAULIFLOWER HASH BROWNS

YIELD: 12 servings

PREP TIME: 15 minutes

COOK TIME: 32 minutes

These crispy little cauliflower hash browns are great served with eggs in the morning or with any dinner entrée.

- 1 small head cauliflower (about 1 pound), or 15 ounces fresh (not frozen) pre-riced cauliflower
- 2 large eggs, beaten
- ½ cup grated Parmesan cheese
- 3 tablespoons chopped fresh chives
- ¼ teaspoon fine sea salt
- ¼ teaspoon garlic powder
- ¼ teaspoon freshly ground black pepper

Store in an airtight container in the refrigerator for up to 5 days. Reheat in a dry skillet over medium heat until warmed through.

1. Preheat the oven to 400°F. Line a sheet pan with parchment paper.
2. If not using pre-riced cauliflower, core and then grate the cauliflower.
3. Place the riced cauliflower in a microwave-safe bowl and microwave for 5 minutes.
4. Let the cauliflower cool slightly, then wrap it in a clean towel and squeeze out as much liquid as you can. Discard the liquid.
5. Place the cauliflower in a clean bowl. Add the remaining ingredients and stir until well combined.
6. Scoop out about 2 tablespoons of the mixture and flatten it into a 3 by 2½-inch rectangle. Repeat until you have 12 rectangles.
7. Arrange the rectangles on the prepared sheet pan and bake for 25 minutes. Turn the rectangles over and broil for 1 to 2 minutes, or until crisp.
8. Serve immediately.

calories 55 | fat 2g | protein 4g | total carbs 3g | dietary fiber 1g | net carbs 2g

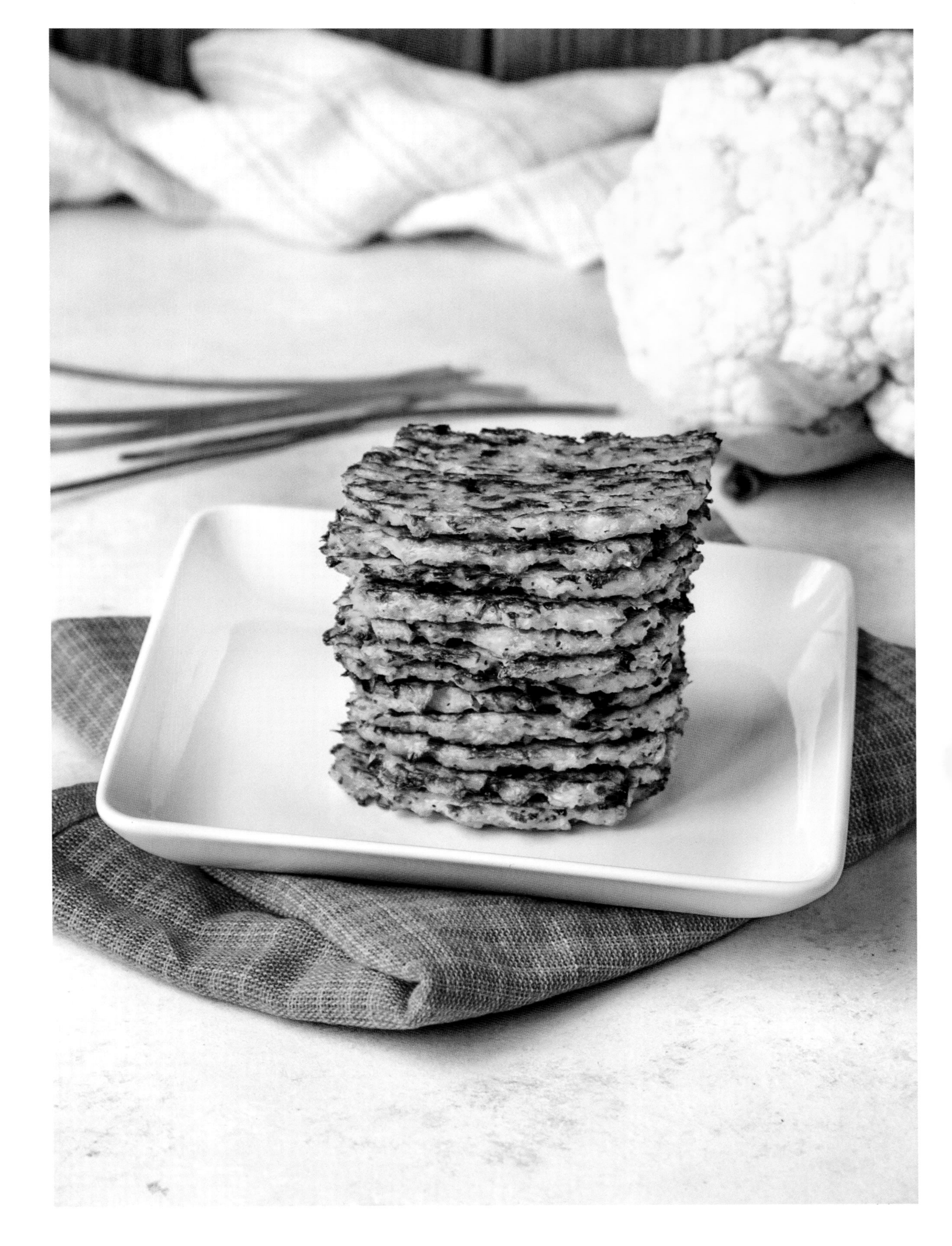

ZUCCHINI FRIES

YIELD: 4 servings

PREP TIME: 5 minutes (not including time to make breading or dressing/sauce)

COOK TIME: 10 minutes or 30 minutes, depending on method

If you've never fried breaded veggies before, you're in for a treat. These fries can also be baked, but baking won't give you the nice crispy outer coating that frying provides. Frying them takes a little time, but the end result is worth it: crispy, delicious zucchini fries!

- 1 pound zucchini (about 2 large)
- 2 large eggs, beaten
- 1 batch Keto Breading (page 56)
- ½ cup melted coconut oil, for frying
- Fry Sauce (page 52) or Ranch Dressing (page 61), for serving (optional)

Store in an airtight container in the refrigerator for up to 3 days. Reheat in the oven.

1. Line a sheet pan with parchment paper.
2. Cut off the ends of the zucchini, then slice them lengthwise into ¼-inch-wide sticks.
3. Place the eggs in one shallow bowl and the breading in a second shallow bowl.
4. One at a time, dip the zucchini sticks into the egg mixture and then into the breading mixture. Once they are fully coated, arrange them on the prepared sheet pan.

STOVETOP DIRECTIONS:

1. Pour the coconut oil into a large skillet. There should be ¼ inch of oil in the pan; add more oil if needed. Over medium-high heat, heat the oil to between 360°F and 370°F. Test the temperature by dipping the handle of a wooden spoon in the oil; if it bubbles steadily, the temperature is right. If it bubbles vigorously, it's too hot, and if there are only a few bubbles, it's not hot enough.
2. Place half of the zucchini sticks in the hot oil, being careful not to overcrowd the pan. Fry for 3 to 5 minutes, or until browned on all sides. Remove with a slotted spoon and set aside on a sheet pan lined with paper towels. Repeat with the remaining zucchini sticks.
3. Serve immediately with fry sauce or ranch dressing, if desired.

OVEN DIRECTIONS:

1. Preheat the oven to 425°F.
2. Bake the fries for 25 to 30 minutes, or until nicely browned.
3. Serve immediately with fry sauce or ranch dressing, if desired.

| FOR STOVETOP FRYING METHOD |

calories 414 | fat 32g | protein 27g | total carbs 5g | dietary fiber 1g | net carbs 4g

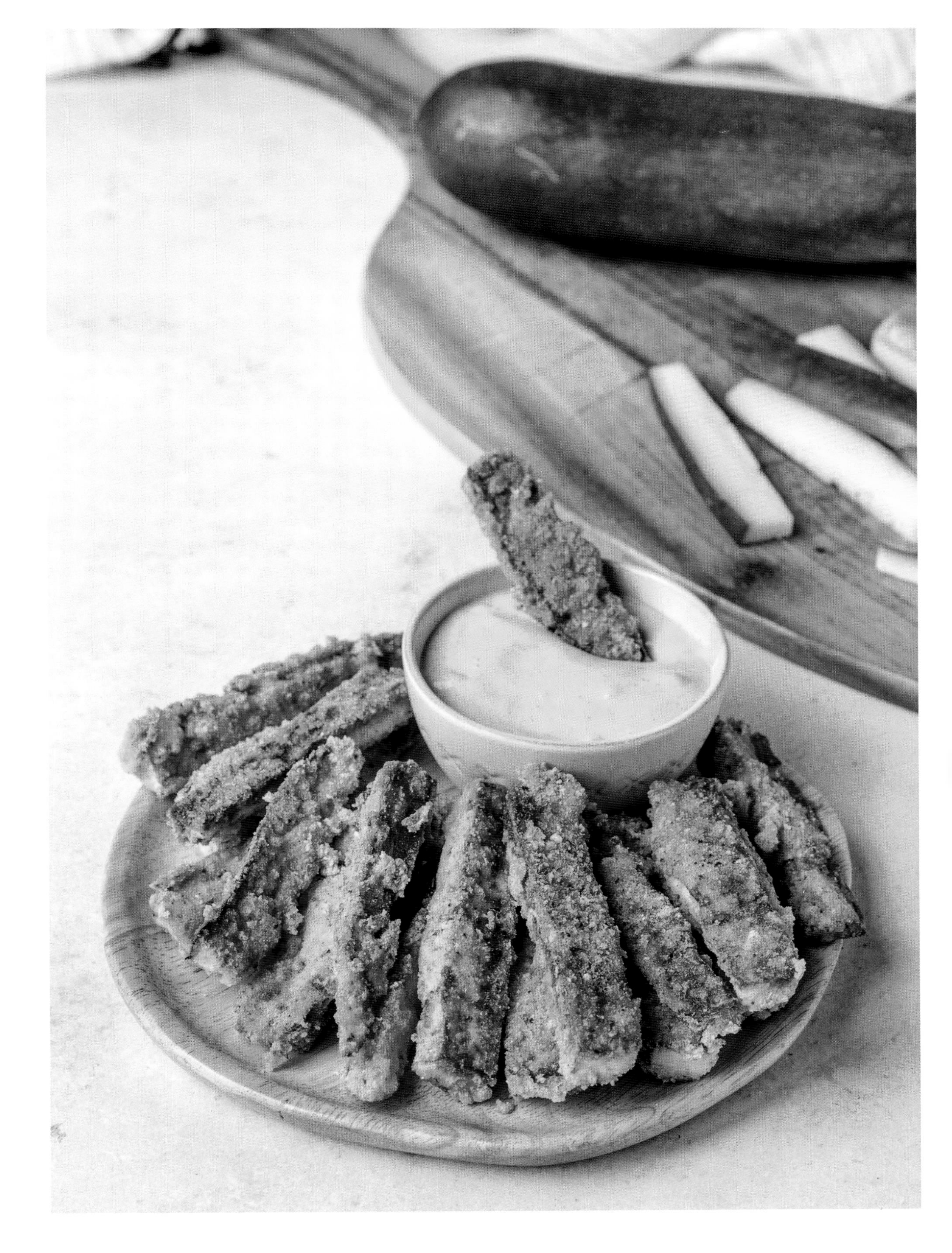

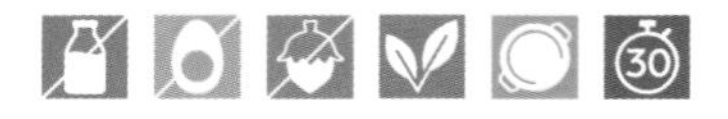

CILANTRO LIME CAULIFLOWER RICE

YIELD: 4 servings

PREP TIME: 5 minutes

COOK TIME: 8 minutes

This simple side dish is a great companion to just about any entrée. If you don't like cilantro, substitute fresh parsley.

2 tablespoons extra-virgin olive oil

1 pound fresh (not frozen) riced cauliflower

¼ cup freshly squeezed lime juice

½ cup chopped fresh cilantro

1 clove garlic, minced

½ teaspoon fine sea salt

¼ teaspoon freshly ground black pepper

1. Heat the oil in a large skillet over medium heat. Add the riced cauliflower and sauté for 2 to 3 minutes. Add the lime juice, cover, and cook for 5 minutes, or until the cauliflower is tender. Remove the pan from the heat.

2. Stir in the cilantro, garlic, salt, and pepper and serve immediately.

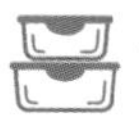

Store in an airtight container in the refrigerator for up to 5 days.

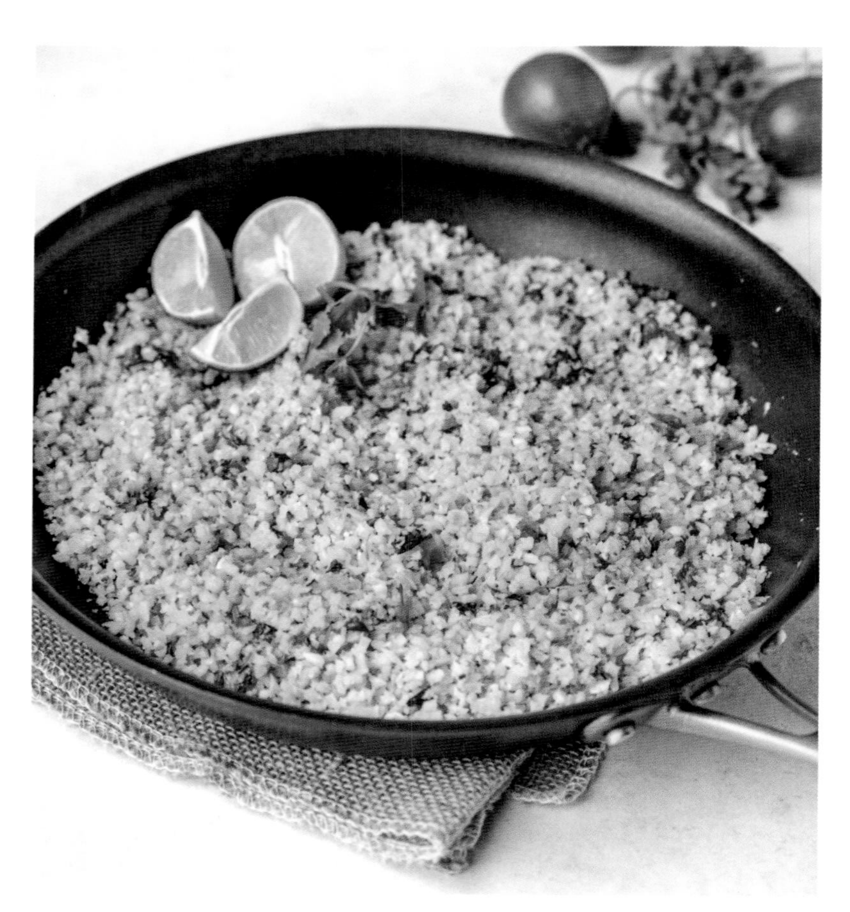

calories 95 | fat 7g | protein 2g | total carbs 7g | dietary fiber 2g | net carbs 5g

option

ROASTED CABBAGE STEAKS

YIELD: 8 servings

PREP TIME: 10 minutes

COOK TIME: 30 minutes

This is a hearty side dish—and a tasty one at that. You can skip the pancetta if you like, but if you do, be sure to add some fine sea salt to compensate.

1 large head green cabbage (about 2 pounds)

2 tablespoons extra-virgin olive oil

1 teaspoon minced garlic

¼ teaspoon onion powder

¼ teaspoon freshly ground black pepper

2 ounces pancetta or bacon, chopped

1. Preheat the oven to 400°F.
2. Slice off the bottom of the head of cabbage so it can sit upright on a cutting board. Cut the cabbage into ½-inch-thick slices.
3. Brush the oil on both sides of the cabbage slices and arrange them on a sheet pan. Sprinkle the garlic, onion powder, and pepper over the cabbage slices and top with the pancetta.
4. Roast for 25 to 30 minutes, or until the cabbage steaks are lightly browned around the edges and the pancetta is crisp.
5. Serve hot.

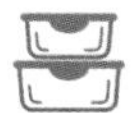
Store in an airtight container in the refrigerator for up to 3 days.

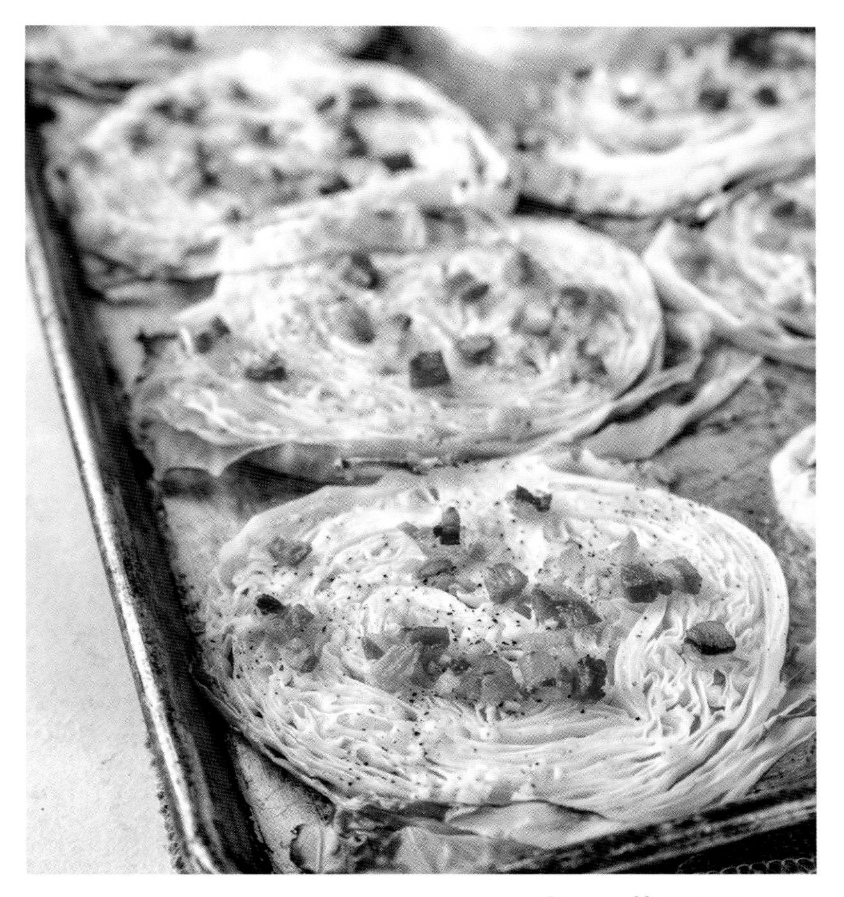

calories 89 | fat 6g | protein 2g | total carbs 6g | dietary fiber 2g | net carbs 4g

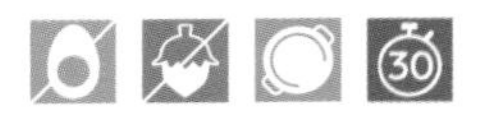

CREAMY KALE WITH PANCETTA

YIELD: 8 servings

PREP TIME: 5 minutes

COOK TIME: 10 minutes

Pancetta is the Italian version of bacon. Both meats are cut from the belly of the pig and seasoned with salt and pepper, but pancetta is curled up in a roll and remains in a casing to hold its shape. Another difference: it's not smoked, like bacon. Pancetta has its own unique taste. While you can substitute bacon in this recipe, I suggest giving pancetta a try for a nice change of pace.

4 ounces pancetta, chopped

1 teaspoon minced garlic

12 ounces curly kale, stems and stalks removed, chopped

1 cup heavy whipping cream

¼ teaspoon freshly ground black pepper

⅛ teaspoon freshly grated nutmeg

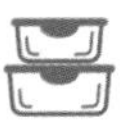

Store in an airtight container in the refrigerator for up to 3 days.

1. In a large skillet over medium heat, cook the pancetta until crisp. Remove with a slotted spoon, leaving the drippings in the pan, and set aside to cool on a plate lined with paper towels.

2. Reduce the heat to low, add the garlic, and cook until fragrant. Add the kale and cream and cook for about 5 minutes, until the kale is wilted. Remove from the heat.

3. Sprinkle the pepper and nutmeg over the kale, top with the pancetta, and serve immediately.

calories 180 | fat 16g | protein 3g | total carbs 4g | dietary fiber 0g | net carbs 4g

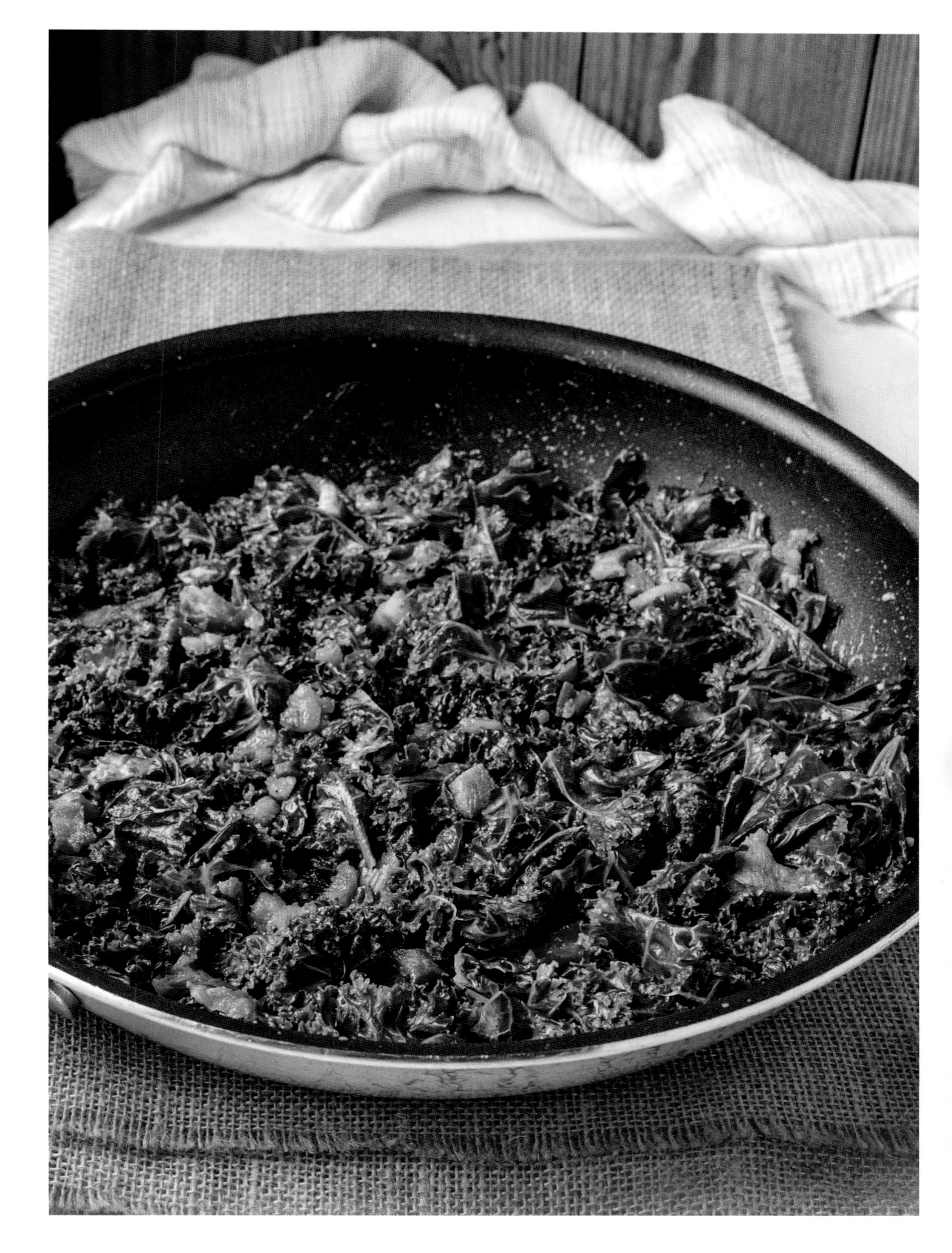

MASHED ROASTED CAULIFLOWER

YIELD: 8 servings

PREP TIME: 5 minutes

COOK TIME: 30 minutes

This is the keto side dish that goes with everything. It's wonderful with my Instant Pot (or Slow Cooker) Beef Short Ribs (page 194) or any other entrée you love. Roasting the cauliflower imparts a lot of flavor, but if you're short on time, you can use thawed frozen cauliflower florets and skip the roasting step. If you do, simply add the olive oil and seasonings to the food processor in Step 4.

Florets from 1 large head cauliflower (about 2 pounds)

2 tablespoons extra-virgin olive oil

½ teaspoon garlic powder

½ teaspoon fine sea salt

¼ teaspoon freshly ground black pepper

¼ cup (½ stick) salted butter, sliced

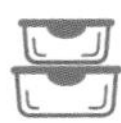

Store in an airtight container in the refrigerator for up to 5 days.

1. Preheat the oven to 400°F.
2. Arrange the cauliflower florets on a sheet pan. Drizzle the oil over the cauliflower and stir until well coated. Sprinkle the garlic powder, salt, and pepper over the cauliflower.
3. Roast for 30 minutes, or until tender.
4. Transfer the roasted cauliflower to a food processor, add the butter, and process until the mixture has a smooth, mashed potato-like texture.
5. Enjoy immediately!

calories 110 | fat 9g | protein 2g | total carbs 5g | dietary fiber 2g | net carbs 3g

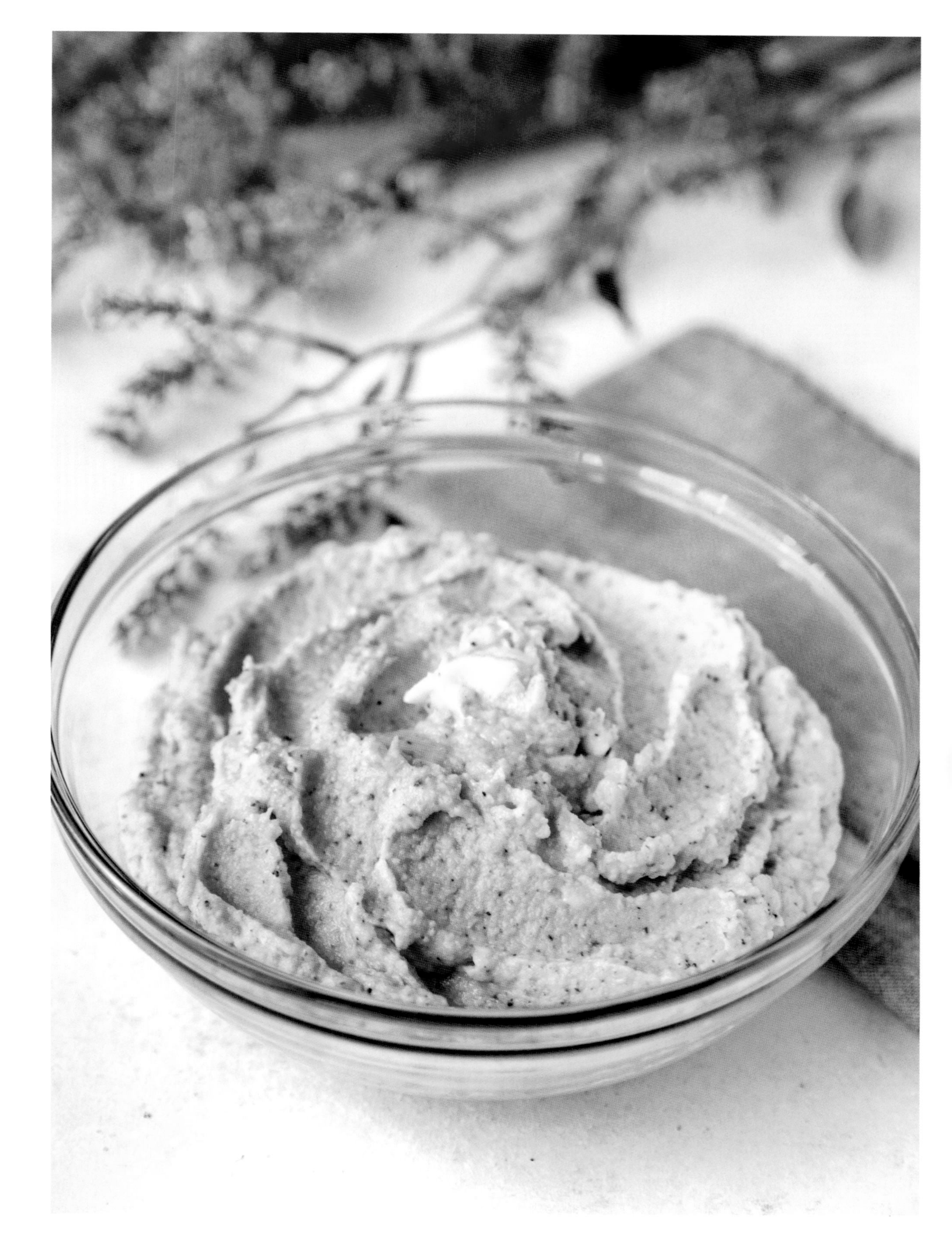

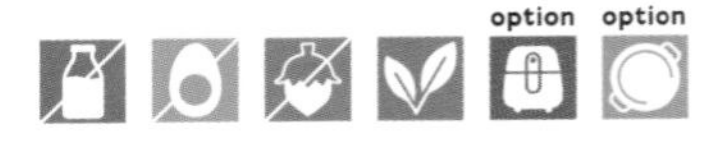

CRISPY BRUSSELS SPROUTS

YIELD: 10 servings

PREP TIME: 15 minutes

COOK TIME: 45 minutes or 20 minutes, depending on method

I've got three kids, and they all like different vegetables. My daughter despises Brussels sprouts, but my boys love them—but only if they are nice and crispy, like they are in this dish.

2 pounds Brussels sprouts

4 cloves garlic, minced

¼ cup avocado oil

½ teaspoon fine sea salt

½ teaspoon freshly ground black pepper

These Brussels are best eaten immediately, but leftovers can be stored in an airtight container in the refrigerator for up to 3 days.

1. Trim the ends of the Brussels sprouts. Cut the sprouts into quarters if they are large or in half if they are small. Arrange them on a sheet pan.

2. Sprinkle the garlic over the Brussels sprouts, then pour the oil over them. Toss the Brussels sprouts in the garlic and oil until they are nicely coated. Season with the salt and pepper and toss again.

OVEN DIRECTIONS:

1. Preheat the oven to 400°F.

2. Roast the Brussels sprouts for 30 minutes. Remove from the oven and toss well.

3. Raise the oven temperature to 450°F and roast for 10 to 15 minutes, or until the outer edges of the leaves are browned.

4. Serve hot.

AIR FRYER DIRECTIONS:

1. Set the air fryer to 400°F.

2. If you have a large air fryer, put all of the Brussels sprouts in the basket; if you have a smaller air fryer, you will need to cook them in two batches. Set the air fryer to cook for 15 minutes. Remove the basket and toss well.

3. Raise the temperature to 425°F and cook for 5 minutes.

4. Serve hot.

calories 93 | fat 5g | protein 3g | total carbs 8g | dietary fiber 3g | net carbs 5g

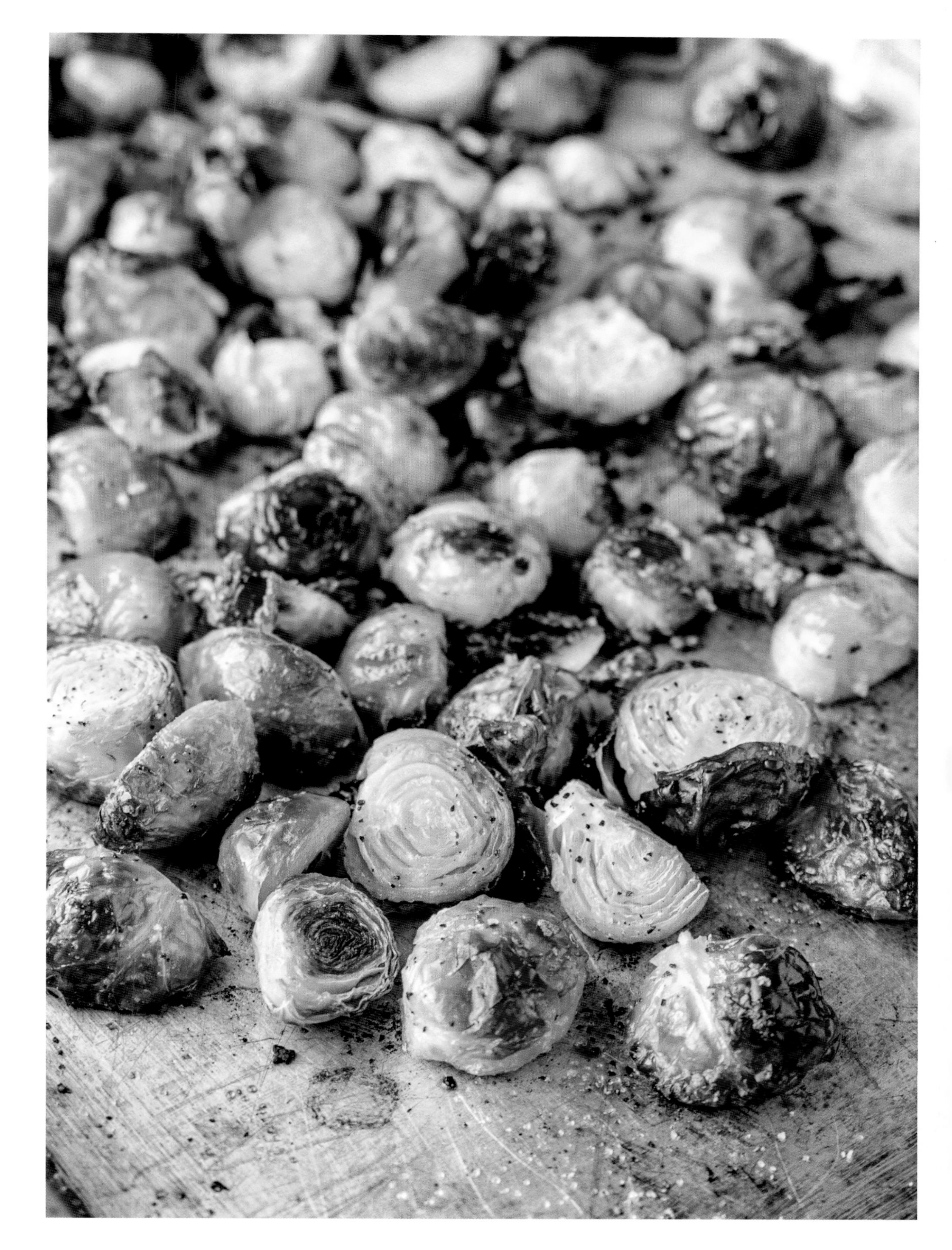

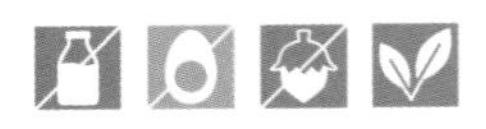

JICAMA FRIES

YIELD: 8 servings

PREP TIME: 15 minutes

COOK TIME: 50 minutes

Jicama, a Mexican root vegetable, looks a lot like a white potato. It doesn't taste like a white potato, but it's got a great texture for making fries. You can find pre-sliced jicama at Whole Foods or Trader Joe's.

2 pounds fresh jicama

1½ teaspoons fine sea salt, divided

2 tablespoons extra-virgin olive oil

1 teaspoon smoked paprika

½ teaspoon ground cumin

½ teaspoon onion powder

¼ teaspoon freshly ground black pepper

Sugar-free ketchup, store-bought or homemade (page 50), or Egg-Free Mayo (page 48), for serving

1. Peel the jicama and slice it lengthwise into ¼-inch-wide sticks.
2. Bring a medium pot of water to a boil. Add the jicama and 1 teaspoon of the salt and boil for 10 minutes. Drain and pat dry.
3. Preheat the oven to 425°F.
4. Place the jicama on a sheet pan and toss with the oil.
5. In a small bowl, combine the remaining ½ teaspoon of salt with the paprika, cumin, onion powder, and pepper. Season the jicama sticks with half of the spice mixture. Turn the fries over and season the other side with the remaining spice mixture.
6. Bake the fries for 20 minutes. Remove from the oven, turn the jicama over, and bake for 15 minutes, or until tender.
7. Broil for 3 to 4 minutes, or until browned and crisp.
8. Enjoy immediately with ketchup or mayo for dipping.

Store in an airtight container in the refrigerator for up to 5 days.

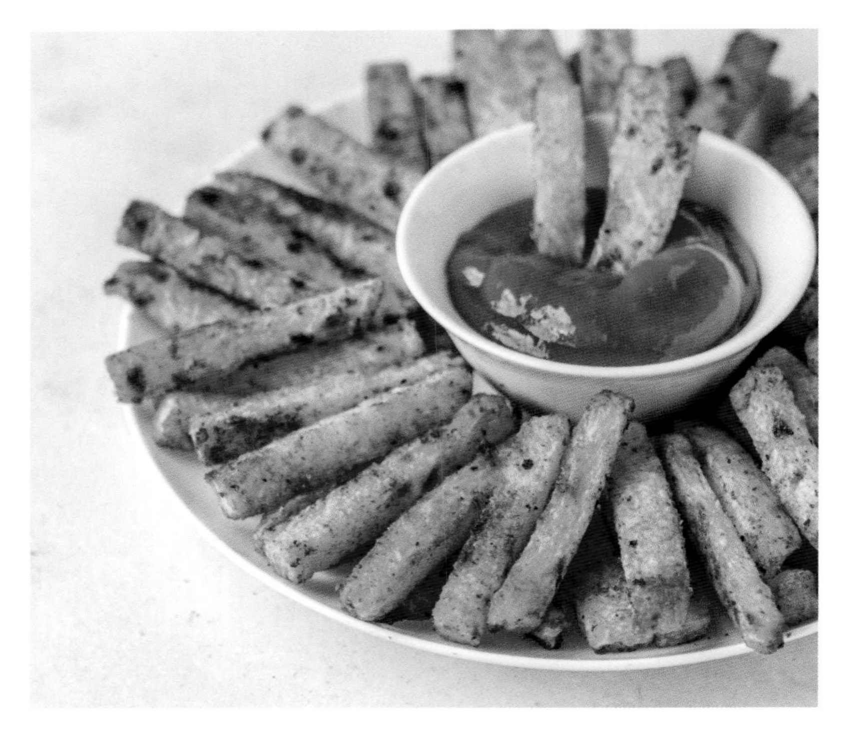

calories 75 | fat 3g | protein 0g | total carbs 10g | dietary fiber 5g | net carbs 5g

ZUCCHINI NOODLES WITHOUT A SPIRALIZER

YIELD: 8 servings

PREP TIME: 10 minutes

COOK TIME: 5 minutes

Even if you don't own a spiralizer gadget, you can still make your own zucchini noodles using a serrated vegetable peeler. Serve with Classic Italian Meatballs (page 186) and Alfredo Sauce (page 44) or Quick Marinara Sauce (page 53).

1½ pounds zucchini (about 3 large), ends removed

2 tablespoons extra-virgin olive oil

2 teaspoons minced garlic

½ teaspoon fine sea salt

1. If desired, peel the zucchini. Hold one end of a zucchini at an angle and, using a serrated vegetable peeler, apply light pressure as you glide the tool down the side of the zucchini, letting the noodles fall onto a clean surface. Continue to peel until you get to the center with the seeds; discard the center. Repeat with the other zucchini.

2. Heat the oil in a large skillet over medium heat. Add the garlic and cook until fragrant. Add the zucchini noodles and sauté, tossing constantly with tongs, for 3 to 4 minutes, or until al dente.

3. Remove from the heat, season with the salt, and serve hot.

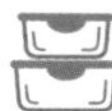 *Store in an airtight container in the refrigerator for up to 5 days.*

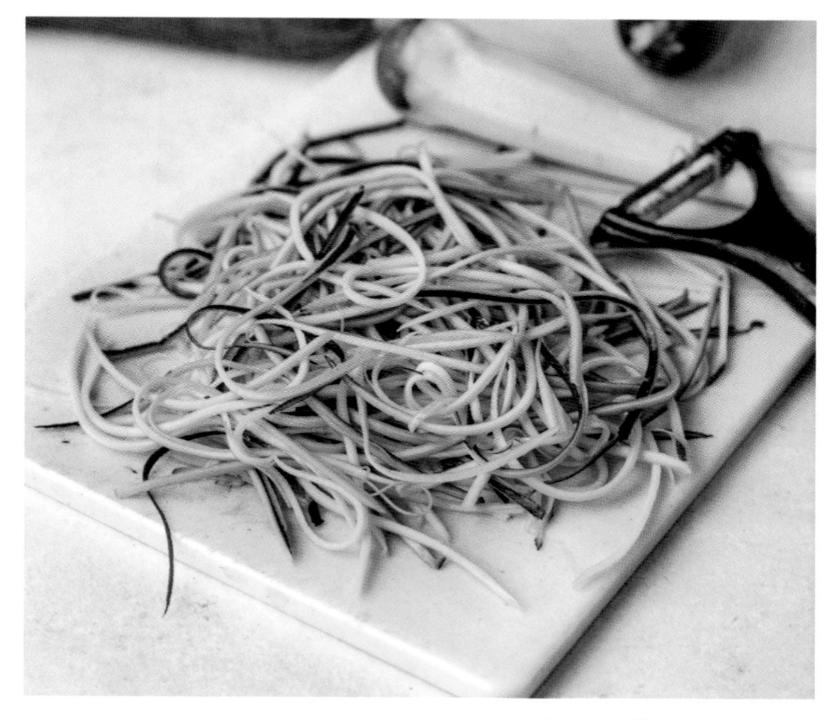

calories 46 | fat 3g | protein 1g | total carbs 2g | dietary fiber 0g | net carbs 2g

ZUCCHINI TOTS

YIELD: 21 tots (3 per serving)

PREP TIME: 15 minutes, plus 10 minutes for zucchini to drain

COOK TIME: 25 minutes

If I slice up zucchini, my kids won't touch it, but when I add cheese and turn it into tots, they'll eat them up. This recipe is a little time-consuming, but it's worth the effort to change up the usual veggie sides. I like to dip these tots in my homemade egg-free mayo (page 48).

- 4 cups shredded zucchini (about 4 medium)
- 1 teaspoon fine sea salt, divided
- 1/2 cup shredded part-skim mozzarella cheese
- 2 large eggs, beaten
- 1/4 cup coconut flour
- 1/4 cup grated Parmesan cheese
- 2 tablespoons chopped fresh flat-leaf parsley
- 2 tablespoons chopped green onions
- 1/2 teaspoon freshly ground black pepper

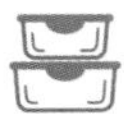
Store in an airtight container in the refrigerator for up to 1 week.

1. Preheat the oven to 400°F. Line a sheet pan with parchment paper.
2. Place the zucchini in a bowl and sprinkle it with 1/2 teaspoon of the salt. Set aside for 10 minutes.
3. After 10 minutes, wrap the zucchini in a clean towel and squeeze out as much liquid as you can. Discard the liquid.
4. Place the zucchini, the remaining 1/2 teaspoon of salt, and the remaining ingredients in the bowl of a stand mixer (or a large bowl if using an electric hand mixer) and mix until well combined.
5. Using a 1 1/2-tablespoon cookie scoop, form the mixture into 21 tots. Arrange the tots on the prepared sheet pan.
6. Bake for 15 minutes. Remove from the oven, turn the tots over, and bake for another 5 to 10 minutes, or until nicely browned.
7. Serve hot.

calories 87 | fat 4g | protein 6g | total carbs 5g | dietary fiber 2g | net carbs 3g

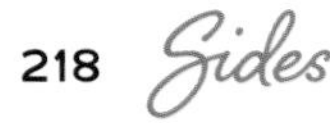

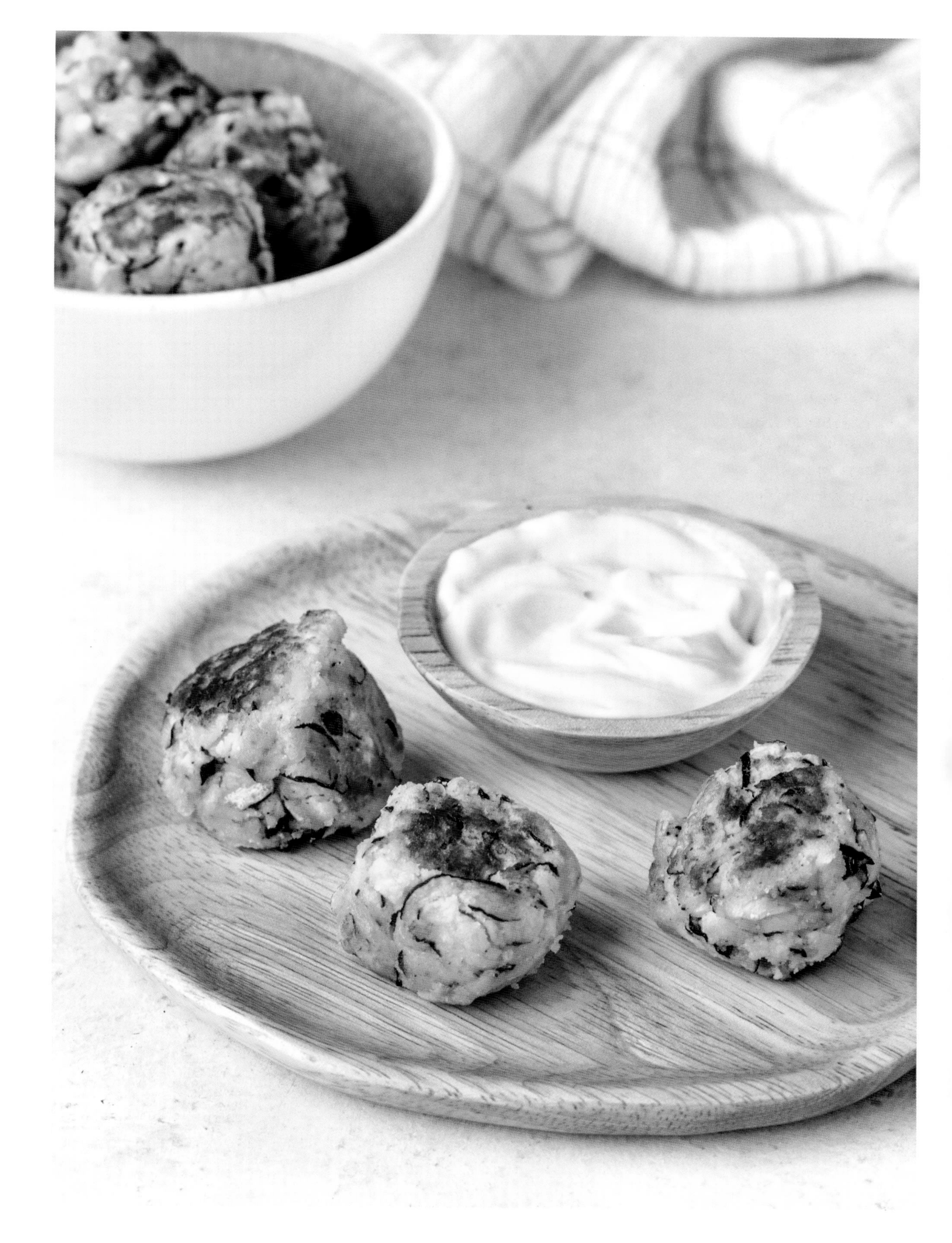

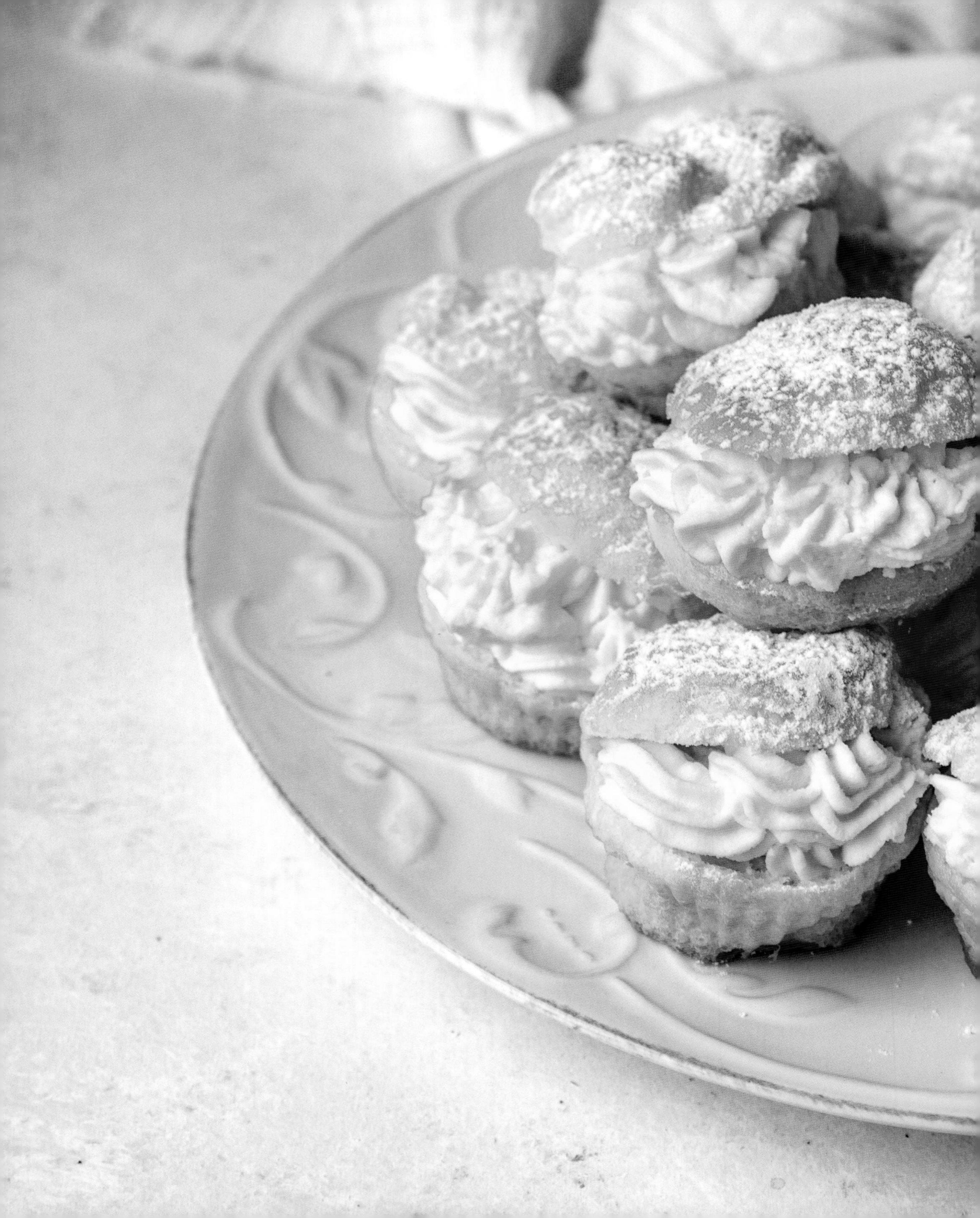

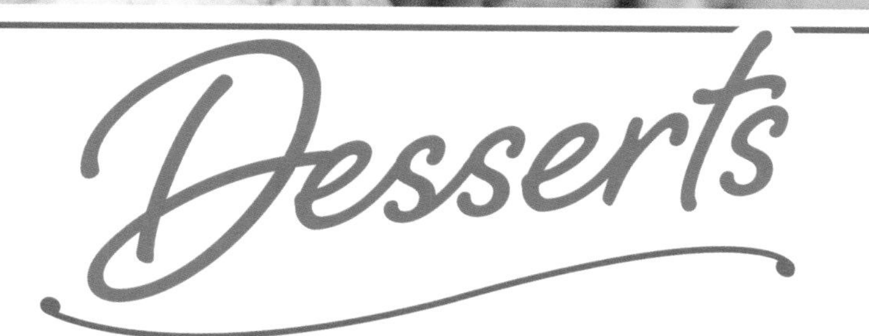

Desserts

APPLE CRISP

YIELD: 6 servings

PREP TIME: 30 minutes

COOK TIME: 35 minutes

I have not told my kids or my husband that I make this recipe with zucchini. They will find out when they read this book, but until then, I will make it again and again and never say a word. The texture of zucchini works perfectly to replace apple, but you must purchase the apple extract to truly pull it off.

4 cups peeled and sliced zucchini (about 3 medium)

3 tablespoons salted butter or coconut oil

1/3 cup freshly squeezed lemon juice

1/2 cup (112g) Swerve granular sweetener

1 1/2 teaspoons apple extract

1 teaspoon apple pie spice

1/4 teaspoon fine sea salt

1/4 teaspoon xanthan gum

FOR THE CRUMB TOPPING

1/2 cup (1 stick) salted butter or coconut oil, softened

1/2 cup (60g) coconut flour

1/2 cup (95g) packed Swerve brown sugar sweetener

Pinch of fine sea salt

Vanilla Gelato (page 254) or store-bought keto vanilla ice cream, for serving (optional)

SPECIAL EQUIPMENT:

6 (4-inch) tart pans or 5-inch ramekins

1. Preheat the oven to 350°F.

2. Place the zucchini and butter in a large skillet. Cover and cook over medium heat until the zucchini is tender, about 15 minutes. Add the lemon juice, granular sweetener, apple extract, apple pie spice, salt, and xanthan gum and stir until well combined.

3. Evenly distribute the zucchini mixture among six 4-inch tart pans or 5-ounce ramekins.

4. Make the crumb topping: Place the topping ingredients in a small bowl and stir until crumbs form. Sprinkle the topping over the zucchini mixture in each pan.

5. Bake for 20 minutes, or until golden brown and bubbling. Serve with keto vanilla gelato or ice cream, if desired, and enjoy!

Cover each tart pan or ramekin with plastic wrap and store in the refrigerator for up to 3 days.

calories 245 | fat 22g | protein 2g | total carbs 9g | dietary fiber 4g | net carbs 5g

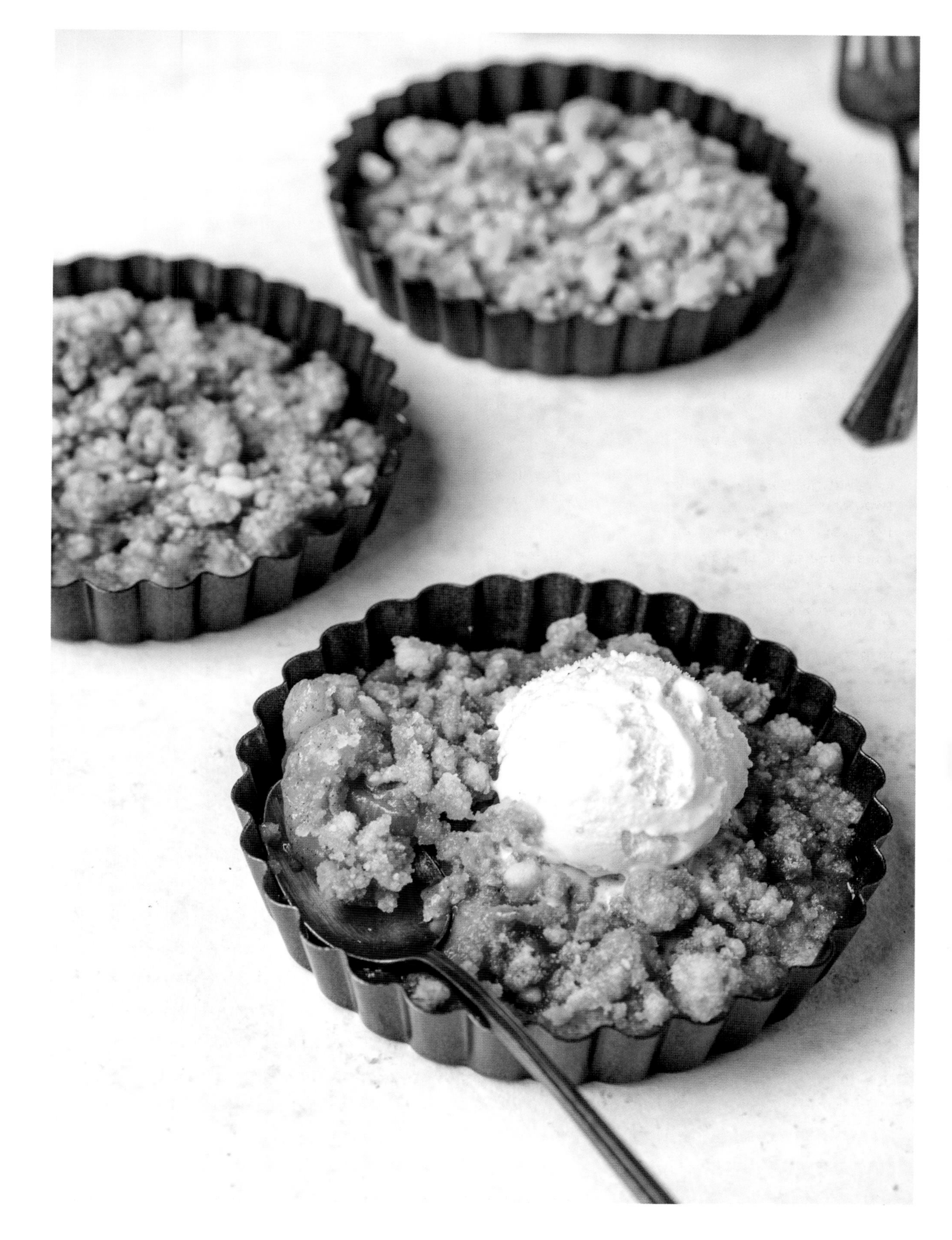

BOSTON CREAM CUPCAKES

YIELD: 12 cupcakes (1 per serving)

PREP TIME: 30 minutes, plus at least 2½ hours to cool and chill filling

COOK TIME: 55 minutes

A cupcake that honors my New England roots! Boston cream donuts were a favorite of mine growing up. Now I make these cupcakes instead, and my kids absolutely love them!

FOR THE CREAM FILLING

- 1½ cups heavy whipping cream
- 4 large egg yolks
- ½ cup Swerve confectioners'-style sweetener
- ¼ teaspoon fine sea salt
- 2 teaspoons vanilla extract
- ½ teaspoon vanilla-flavored liquid stevia
- 1 teaspoon xanthan gum

FOR THE CUPCAKES

- 2 large eggs
- ½ cup (1 stick) unsalted butter, softened
- ⅓ cup unsweetened almond milk
- 1 teaspoon vanilla extract
- 1 teaspoon vanilla-flavored liquid stevia
- 1¼ cups (130g) blanched almond flour
- ½ cup (65g) Swerve confectioners'-style sweetener
- ¼ cup (25g) unflavored whey protein powder
- 1 teaspoon baking powder
- 1 teaspoon baking soda
- ½ teaspoon xanthan gum
- ¼ teaspoon fine sea salt

FOR THE GANACHE

- ⅔ cup heavy whipping cream
- 4 ounces sugar-free chocolate or dark chocolate (85% cacao)

MAKE THE FILLING:

1. Warm the cream in a medium saucepan over medium-low heat. While the cream is heating, whisk the egg yolks in a small bowl until they are light in color.
2. Once the cream is hot but not boiling, pour a small amount of the cream into the whisked egg yolks to temper them. Whisk to combine, then add a bit more cream to the yolks. Pour the tempered yolk mixture into the saucepan and reduce the heat to low while continuing to whisk the mixture.
3. Add the confectioners'-style sweetener and salt and continue to whisk until the mixture is boiling. Remove from the heat and whisk in the vanilla extract and stevia.
4. Sprinkle the xanthan gum over the filling and whisk until all of it is absorbed. Allow to cool on the stovetop for about 30 minutes, then refrigerate for 2 to 3 hours before filling the cupcakes.

MAKE THE CUPCAKES:

1. Preheat the oven to 325°F. Grease a 12-well silicone muffin pan and place it on a sheet pan for support in the oven. Use paper liners in a metal muffin pan if you don't have a silicone one.
2. Place the eggs, butter, almond milk, vanilla extract, and stevia in the bowl of a stand mixer (or a medium bowl if using an electric hand mixer) and mix until combined.
3. In a separate bowl, whisk together the dry ingredients. Add half of the dry ingredients to the wet ingredients and mix until incorporated. Repeat with the remaining dry ingredients.
4. Evenly fill the prepared muffin wells with the batter. Bake for 20 minutes, or until the cupcakes bounce back to the touch. Allow to cool completely before adding the filling.
5. When ready to fill the cupcakes, slice them in half horizontally and evenly pipe or spread the filling on the bottom half of each cupcake. Place the tops back on and set aside while you make the ganache.

calories 353 | fat 33g | protein 0g | total carbs 5g | dietary fiber 1g | net carbs 4g

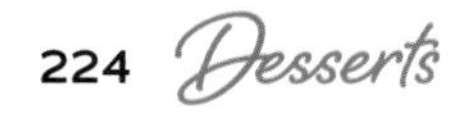

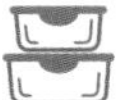 *Store in an airtight container in the refrigerator for up to 3 days.*

MAKE THE GANACHE:

1. Bring the cream to a boil in a small saucepan over medium-low heat. Meanwhile, chop the chocolate into small pieces and place in a small bowl.

2. Once the cream is boiling, sprinkle the chopped chocolate over the cream and turn off the heat. Let stand for 5 minutes before stirring. After 5 minutes, stir until the ganache is completely smooth and there are no lumps.

3. Pour the ganache over the tops of the cupcakes. Keep in mind that the longer the ganache sits, the thicker it becomes. You may need to spread it on the cupcakes rather than pour it.

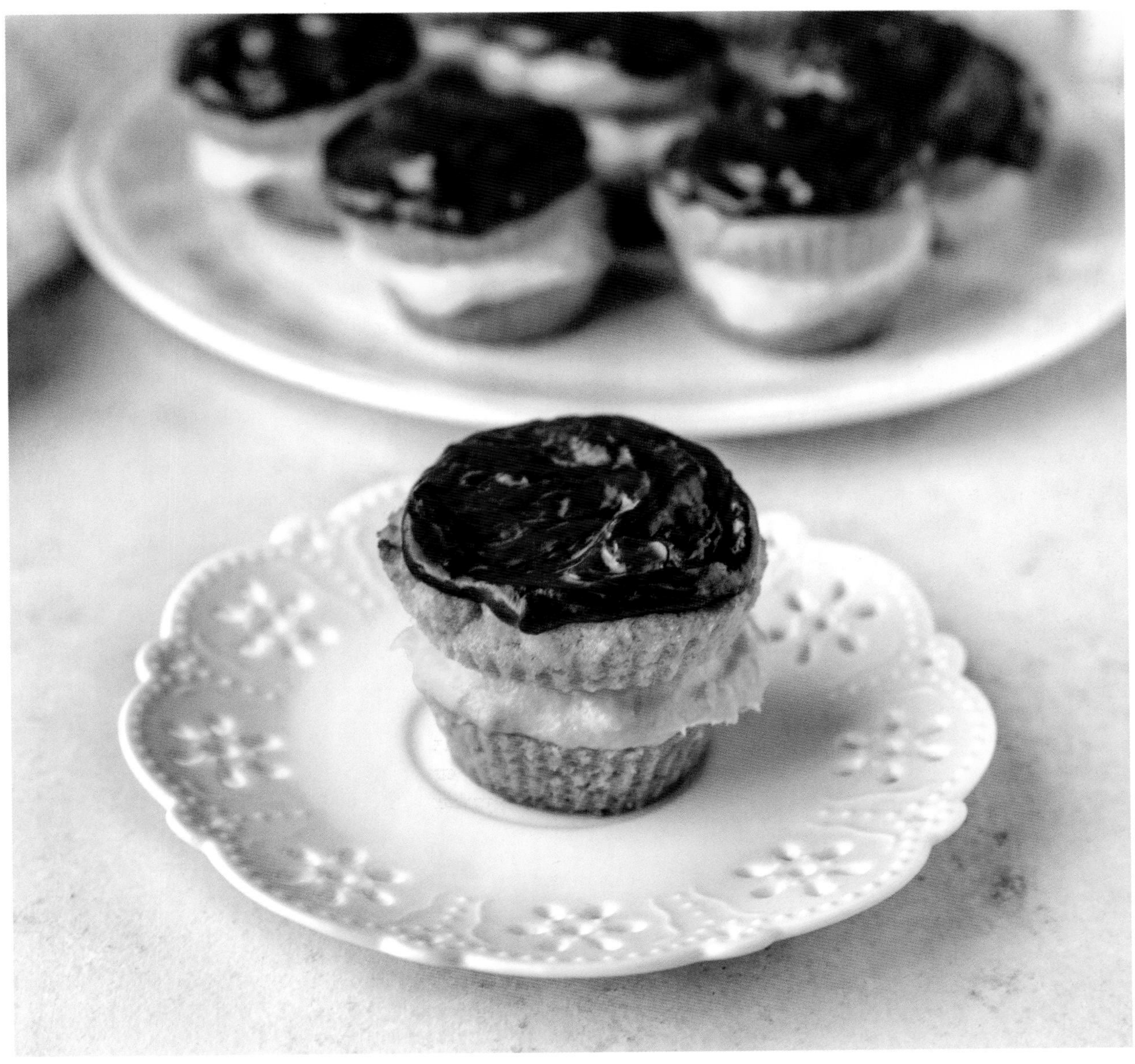

BUCKEYE FAT BOMB BARS

YIELD: 16 bars (1 per serving)

PREP TIME: 5 minutes, plus 30 minutes to chill

COOK TIME: 10 minutes

The ultimate fat bomb! When you need something decadent to curb a craving, having these bars in the fridge or freezer is a lifesaver. Nothing satisfies me more than the combination of creamy peanut butter and chocolate. Your non-keto friends will be shocked when they try these!

1¼ cups unsweetened smooth peanut butter

½ cup (1 stick) unsalted butter

½ cup blanched almond flour

1 teaspoon unflavored or vanilla-flavored liquid stevia

1 teaspoon vanilla extract

6 ounces sugar-free chocolate chips, store-bought or homemade (page 230)

⅛ teaspoon fine sea salt

¾ cup heavy whipping cream

Store in an airtight container in the refrigerator for up to 2 weeks or in the freezer for up to 2 months.

1. Line an 8-inch square baking dish with parchment paper, allowing enough paper to hang over the sides for easy removal.

2. Place the peanut butter and butter in a small saucepan over low heat or in a microwave-safe bowl. Heat on the stovetop or microwave for 1 minute, until the butter is melted. Stir until combined and smooth.

3. Stir in the almond flour, stevia, and vanilla extract. Spread the mixture in the prepared baking dish.

4. Place the chocolate chips and salt in a medium heatproof bowl. Heat the cream in a small saucepan over medium heat until bubbles start to form around the edges. Pour the hot cream over the chocolate and let sit for 5 minutes; do not stir. After 5 minutes, whisk until smooth. Pour the chocolate mixture over the peanut butter mixture in the baking dish.

5. Refrigerate until set, about 30 minutes. Once set, cut into 16 bars and serve.

calories **271** | fat **24g** | protein **6g** | total carbs **6g** | dietary fiber **1g** | net carbs **5g**

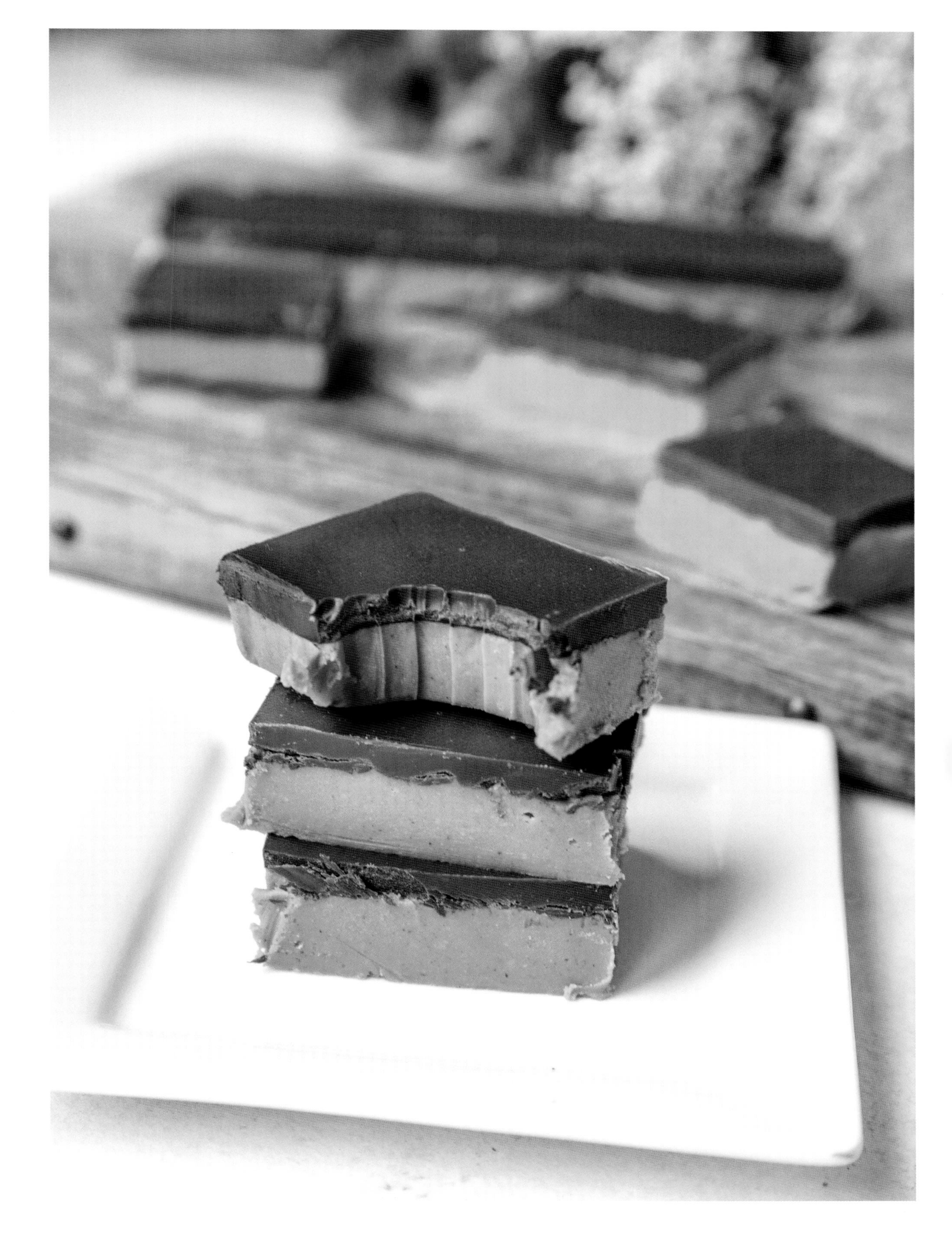

CANNOLI

YIELD: 12 cannoli (1 per serving)

PREP TIME: 20 minutes (not including time to make shells)

Cannoli are an Italian staple at Christmastime and even on Easter. Although they are time-consuming to make, they are a favorite for special occasions and are sure to win over the non-keto crowd!

FOR THE FILLING

8 ounces ricotta cheese (1 cup)

8 ounces mascarpone cheese (1 cup)

1/3 cup Swerve confectioners'-style sweetener, plus more for dusting

Pinch of fine sea salt

1/2 cup heavy whipping cream

1 teaspoon vanilla extract

1/2 teaspoon grated lemon zest

Dark chocolate (85% cacao) shavings or chips, for sprinkling (optional)

12 Cannoli Shells (page 256)

SPECIAL EQUIPMENT:

Pastry bag with piping tip

1. Place the ricotta and mascarpone in the bowl of a stand mixer (or a medium bowl if using an electric hand mixer) and mix on high until smooth.

2. Scrape down the bowl and add the sweetener and salt. Mix again until smooth, then taste and add more sweetener, if desired.

3. Add the cream, vanilla extract, and lemon zest and mix until it holds soft peaks; this could take up to 5 minutes.

4. Transfer the filling to a pastry bag. Insert the bag tip into one end of a cannoli shell and pipe the cream filling halfway into the shell and outward, then turn the shell around and pipe the cream into the other end to fill the shell. Repeat with the remaining shells and filling.

5. Sprinkle the filling on each end with chocolate shavings, if desired, and dust the shells with more confectioners'-style sweetener. The cannoli are best served immediately. Otherwise, refrigerate until ready to serve.

calories 240 | fat 22g | protein 5g | total carbs 2g | dietary fiber 1g | net carbs 1g

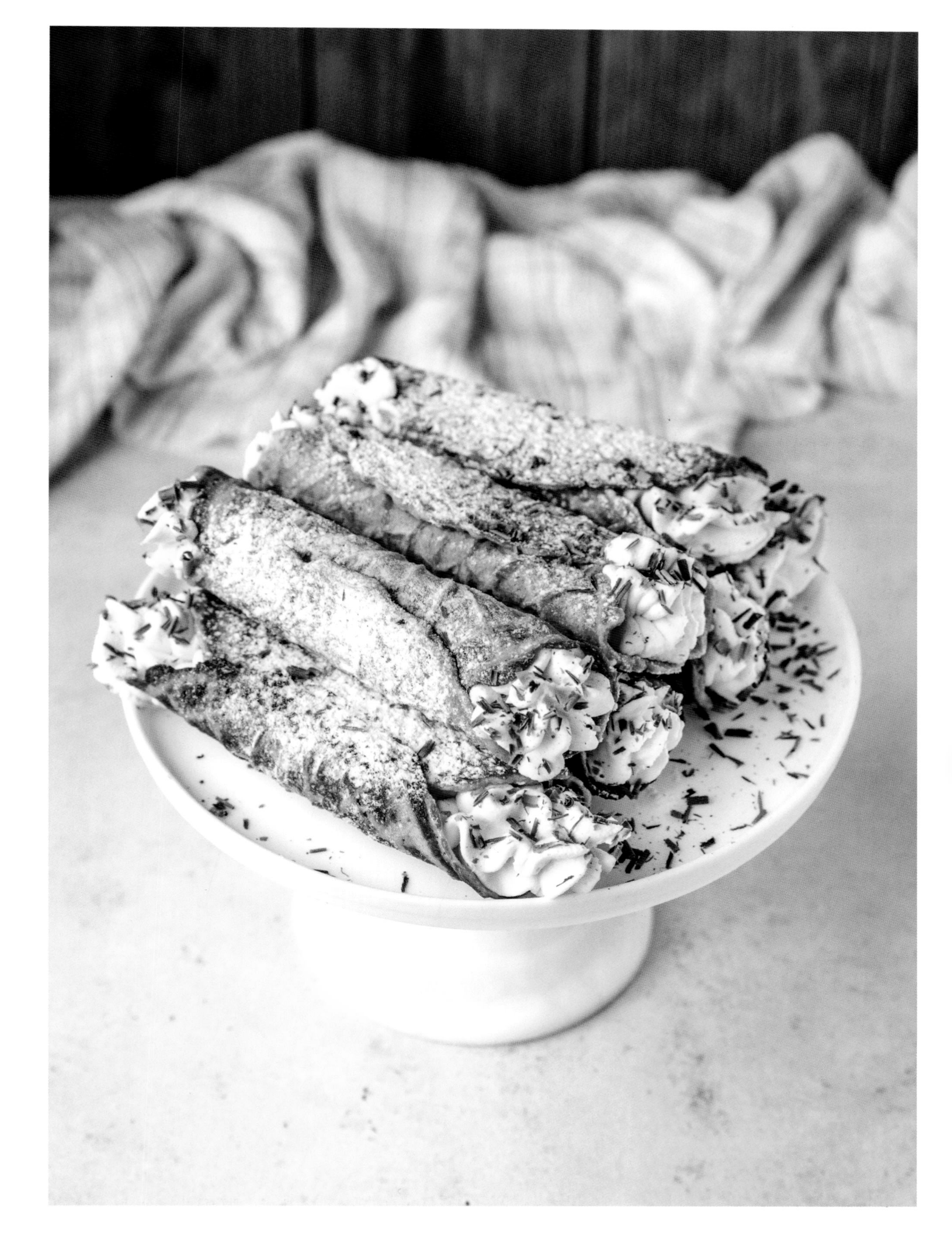

CHOCOLATE BARS OR CHOCOLATE CHIPS

YIELD: 8 ounces (1 ounce per serving)

PREP TIME: 5 minutes, plus 1 hour to chill

COOK TIME: 3 minutes

A truly natural sugar-free candy bar or chocolate chips! This keto chocolate won't cause the digestive side effects that typical sugar-free chocolate made with maltitol would. This recipe yields 8 ounces of chocolate. If you make bars, use two 4-ounce silicone bar molds, yielding two bars. If you make chips, you will need 8 silicone chocolate chip molds, since one mold holds 1 ounce of chocolate.

4 ounces cacao butter

3 ounces unsweetened chocolate, chopped

¼ cup Swerve confectioners'-style sweetener

1 tablespoon unsweetened cocoa powder

1 tablespoon heavy whipping cream

1 teaspoon coffee extract

1 teaspoon vanilla extract

1 teaspoon vanilla-flavored liquid stevia

¼ teaspoon fine sea salt

SPECIAL EQUIPMENT:

2 (4-ounce) silicone chocolate bar molds or 8 silicone chocolate chip molds

Store in an airtight container in the refrigerator for up to 1 month or in the freezer for up to 3 months.

1. Place the cacao butter and chocolate in a small saucepan over medium-low heat and stir until melted. Whisk in the confectioners'-style sweetener and cocoa powder. Turn off the heat and whisk in the remaining ingredients until smooth. Taste and add more confectioners'-style sweetener, if desired.
2. Pour the chocolate into the molds and refrigerate for 1 hour.

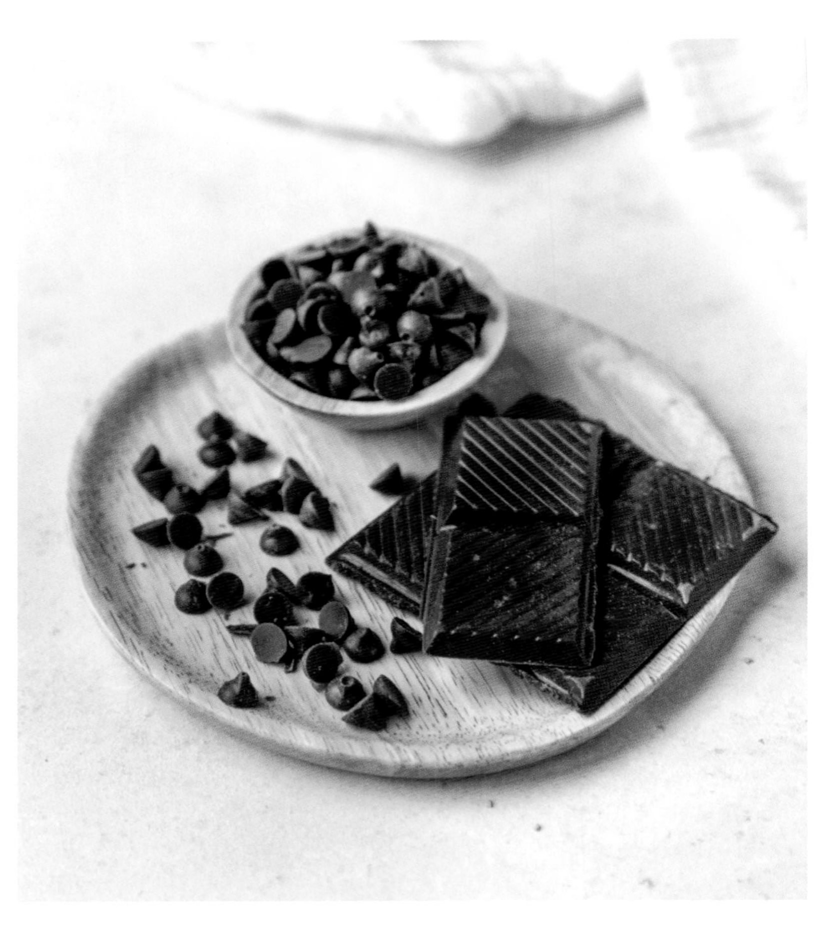

calories 182 | fat 20g | protein 1g | total carbs 3g | dietary fiber 1g | net carbs 2g

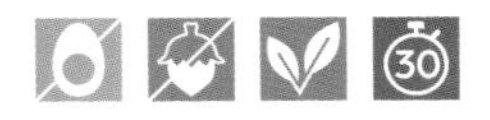

VANILLA BUTTERCREAM FROSTING

YIELD: 1¼ cups (2 tablespoons per serving)

PREP TIME: 5 minutes

A classic buttercream frosting to enjoy on cupcakes, cakes, or cookies. You can swap out the coconut milk for unsweetened almond milk if you prefer.

- ½ cup (1 stick) salted butter, softened
- 1 cup Swerve confectioners'-style sweetener
- 2 to 3 tablespoons coconut milk
- 1 teaspoon vanilla extract

Place the butter, sweetener, 2 tablespoons of coconut milk, and the vanilla in the bowl of a stand mixer (or a medium bowl if using an electric hand mixer) and mix on high until smooth. If the frosting seems too thick to spread, add another tablespoon of coconut milk and mix again.

Store in an airtight container in the pantry for up to 2 weeks. The frosting does not need to be refrigerated but can be frozen for up to 3 months. To use frozen frosting, let it thaw in the refrigerator overnight, then beat it with a mixer to get it creamy and smooth again.

Tip: For colored frosting, simply add a few drops of natural food coloring in the color(s) of your choice. I buy mine at Whole Foods.

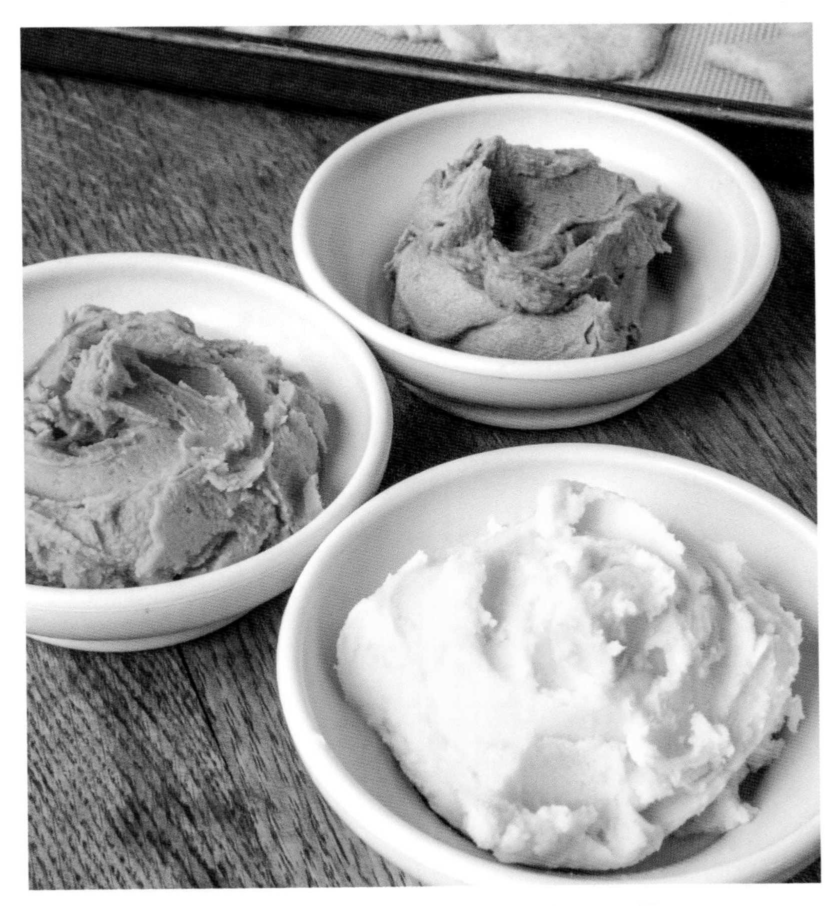

calories 87 | fat 9g | protein 0g | total carbs 0g | dietary fiber 0g | net carbs 0g

CHOCOLATE BUTTERCREAM FROSTING

YIELD: 1½ cups (2 tablespoons per serving)

PREP TIME: 15 minutes

COOK TIME: 10 minutes

Chocolate heaven right here! Be careful with this one, or you might just enjoy one too many spoonfuls.

½ cup (1 stick) unsalted butter, softened

1 cup Swerve confectioners'-style sweetener

4 ounces dark chocolate (85% cacao) or sugar-free chocolate, chopped

1 teaspoon instant espresso powder or instant coffee granules

2 to 3 tablespoons heavy whipping cream

1 teaspoon vanilla extract

⅛ teaspoon fine sea salt

Store in an airtight container in the refrigerator for up to 1 week or in the freezer for up to 3 months. To use frozen frosting, let it thaw in the refrigerator overnight, then beat it with a mixer to get it creamy and smooth again.

1. Place the butter and sweetener in the bowl of a stand mixer (or a medium bowl if using an electric hand mixer) and mix until smooth.

2. Place the chocolate in a small saucepan over low heat and stir, or place in a microwave-safe bowl and microwave for 1 to 2 minutes, until melted. Stir in the espresso powder, remove from the heat, and allow to cool for about 15 minutes.

3. Carefully pour the melted chocolate mixture into the bowl with the butter mixture. Mix on low to incorporate.

4. Add 2 tablespoons of cream, the vanilla extract, and salt. Scrape down the sides of the bowl and mix again until smooth. If the frosting seems too thick to spread, add another tablespoon of cream and mix again.

calories 90 | fat 8g | protein 0g | total carbs 2g | dietary fiber 1g | net carbs 1g

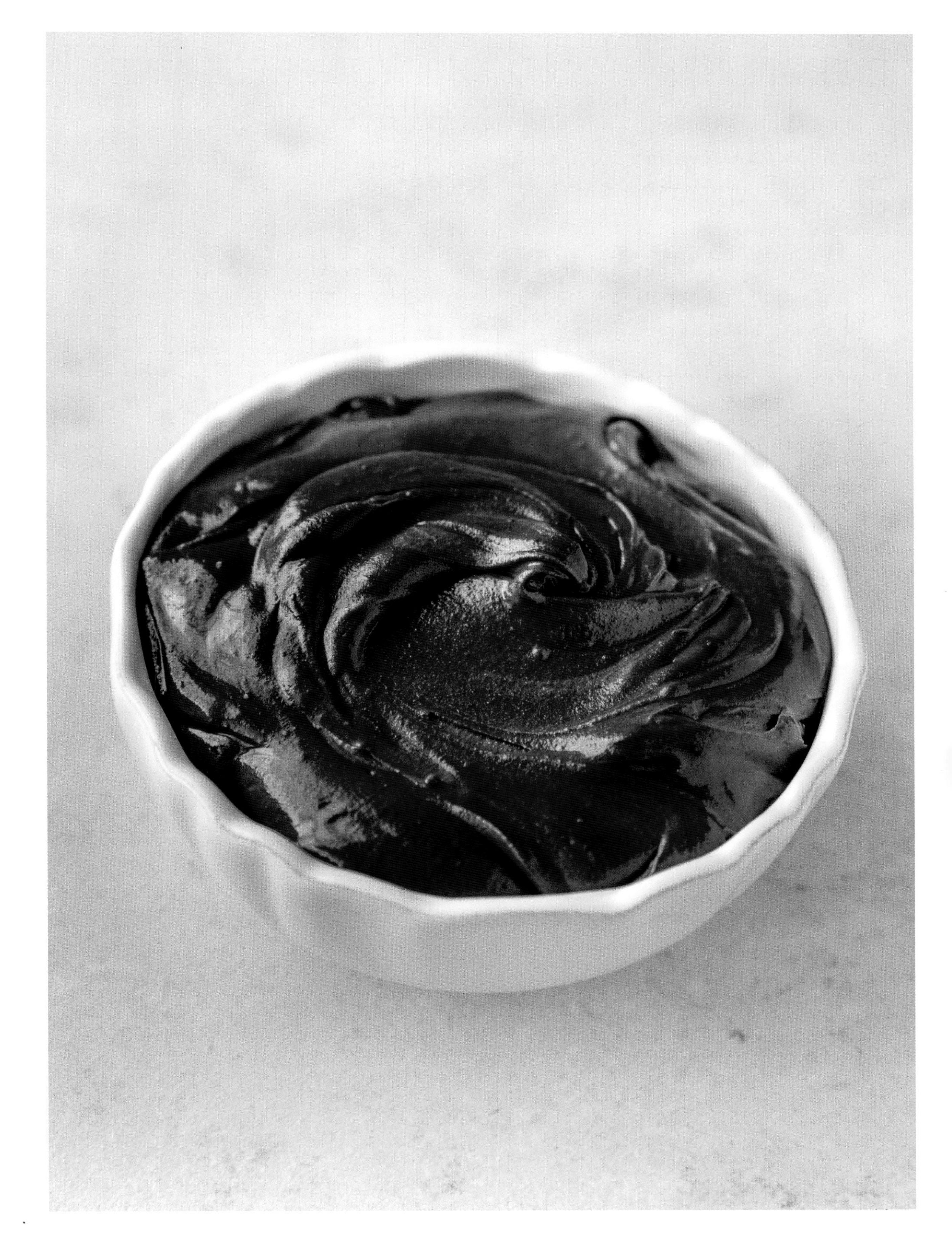

option

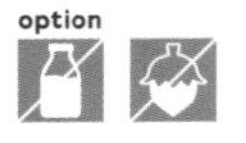

CHOCOLATE CHIP COOKIES

YIELD: 24 cookies (2 per serving)

PREP TIME: 15 minutes, plus at least 2 hours to chill dough

COOK TIME: 20 minutes

These cookies are made with an ingredient that might surprise you: tahini! I've made them without the tahini and used an additional ½ cup of sesame flour instead. My hubby said they were more cakelike that way and loved them. I prefer them with the tahini; it creates more of a chewy bite. If you don't have a nut allergy to accommodate, feel free to use almond flour in place of the sesame flour and the nut butter of your choice in place of the tahini. I've also made these cookies without the cream cheese, and again I thought they were good, but more cakelike. The cream cheese adds fat and gives them more of a traditional cookie texture.

4 ounces cream cheese (½ cup), softened (use dairy-free cream cheese or coconut cream for dairy-free)

½ cup (1 stick) unsalted butter, softened

½ cup tahini

½ teaspoon vanilla extract

½ teaspoon vanilla-flavored liquid stevia

2 large eggs

2 large egg yolks

1½ cups (180g) sesame flour

1 cup (130g) Swerve confectioners'-style sweetener

1 teaspoon baking powder

1 teaspoon unflavored gelatin

½ teaspoon fine sea salt

1 cup sugar-free chocolate chips, store-bought or homemade (page 230)

1. Place the cream cheese, butter, tahini, vanilla extract, stevia, whole eggs, and egg yolks in the bowl of a stand mixer (or a medium bowl if using an electric hand mixer) and mix on high until well combined.

2. Add the sesame flour, confectioners'-style sweetener, baking powder, gelatin, and salt and mix until well incorporated. Stir in the chocolate chips by hand.

3. Form the dough into a ball and wrap in plastic wrap. Refrigerate for 2 to 3 hours.

4. When you're ready to bake the cookies, preheat the oven to 350°F and line two cookie sheets with parchment paper.

5. Using a 1¼-tablespoon cookie scoop, make 24 balls of dough, place 12 balls on one prepared cookie sheet and 12 on the other cookie sheet, spacing them 1 inch apart. Flatten the balls with your palm.

6. Bake for 18 to 20 minutes, or until the cookies are golden brown. Serve warm or remove to a cooling rack to cool before storing.

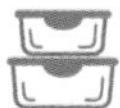

Store in an airtight container in the pantry for up to 5 days or in the refrigerator for up to 10 days.

Tip: You can bake only half of the cookies and freeze the remaining balls of dough between sheets of parchment paper in an airtight container to bake later.

calories 127 | fat 11g | protein 5g | total carbs 3g | dietary fiber 1g | net carbs 2g

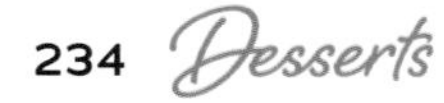

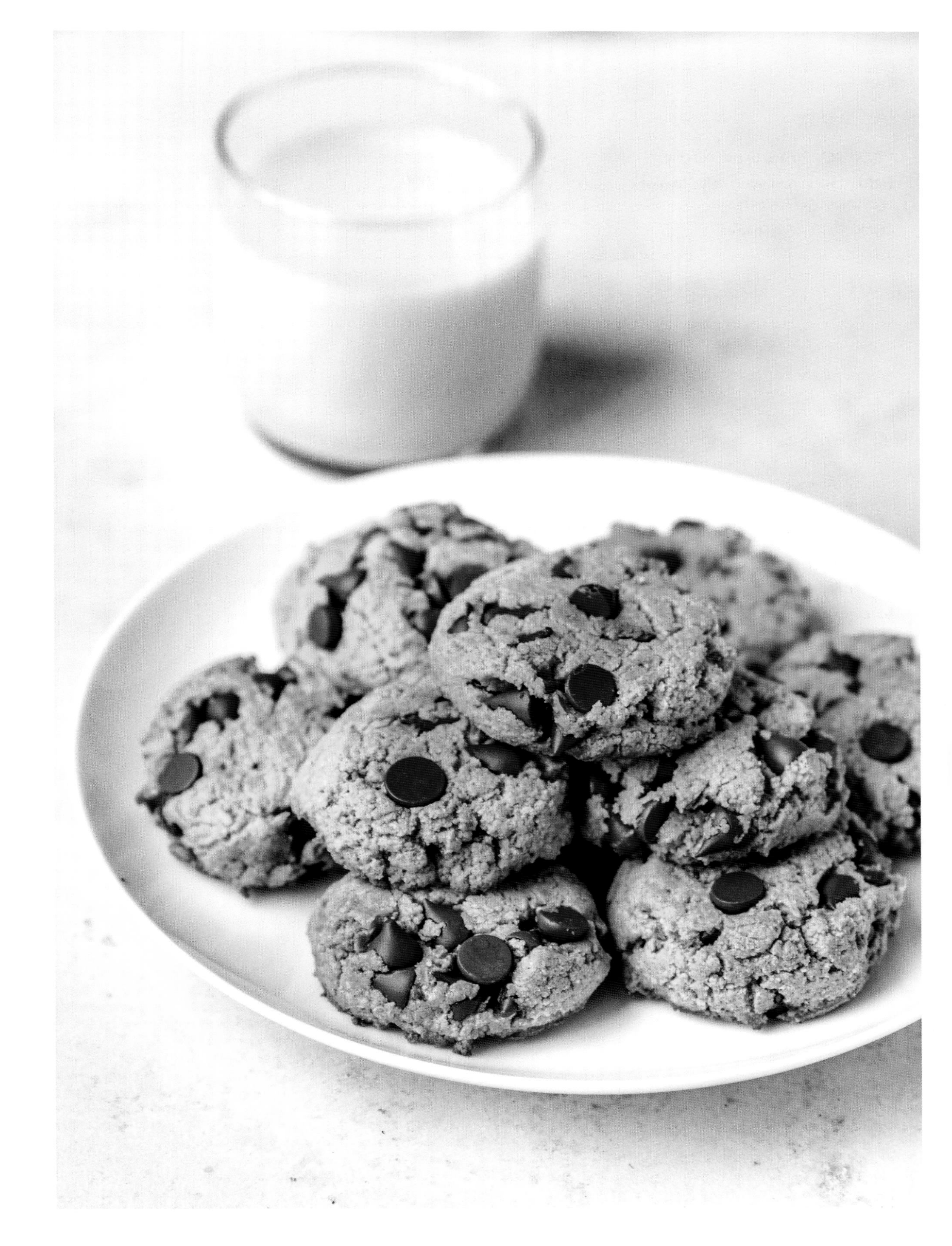

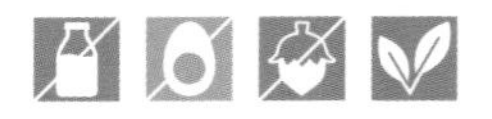

DAIRY-FREE FUDGE

YIELD: 18 pieces (1 per serving)

PREP TIME: 5 minutes, plus 3 hours to chill

COOK TIME: 15 minutes

Finally, a creamy dairy-free fudge! My daughter, who avoids dairy, requested a fudge that she could enjoy, so I worked on this recipe for a long time to get that creamy texture—and it is perfect.

8 ounces dark chocolate (85% cacao)

4 ounces cacao butter

1 cup unsweetened coconut milk (preferably not canned)

1/2 cup coconut oil

1 teaspoon vanilla extract

1/2 teaspoon fine sea salt

1/4 cup Swerve confectioners'-style sweetener, or 1/2 teaspoon chocolate-flavored liquid stevia (optional)

Store in an airtight container in the refrigerator for up to 5 days or in the freezer for up to 3 months.

1. Line a 9 by 5-inch loaf pan with parchment paper, allowing enough paper to hang over the sides for easier removal.
2. Chop the chocolate and cacao butter into small pieces, then place in a medium saucepan with the coconut milk and coconut oil. Melt over low heat, stirring continually, until there are no lumps. Remove the pan from the heat.
3. Add the vanilla extract and salt and stir to combine. Allow the fudge to cool slightly, then taste it. Add the sweetener, if desired.
4. Pour the fudge into the prepared loaf pan and refrigerate for 3 hours.
5. Cut the fudge into 18 equal-sized pieces and enjoy.

calories 189 | fat 19g | protein 1g | total carbs 4g | dietary fiber 1g | net carbs 3g

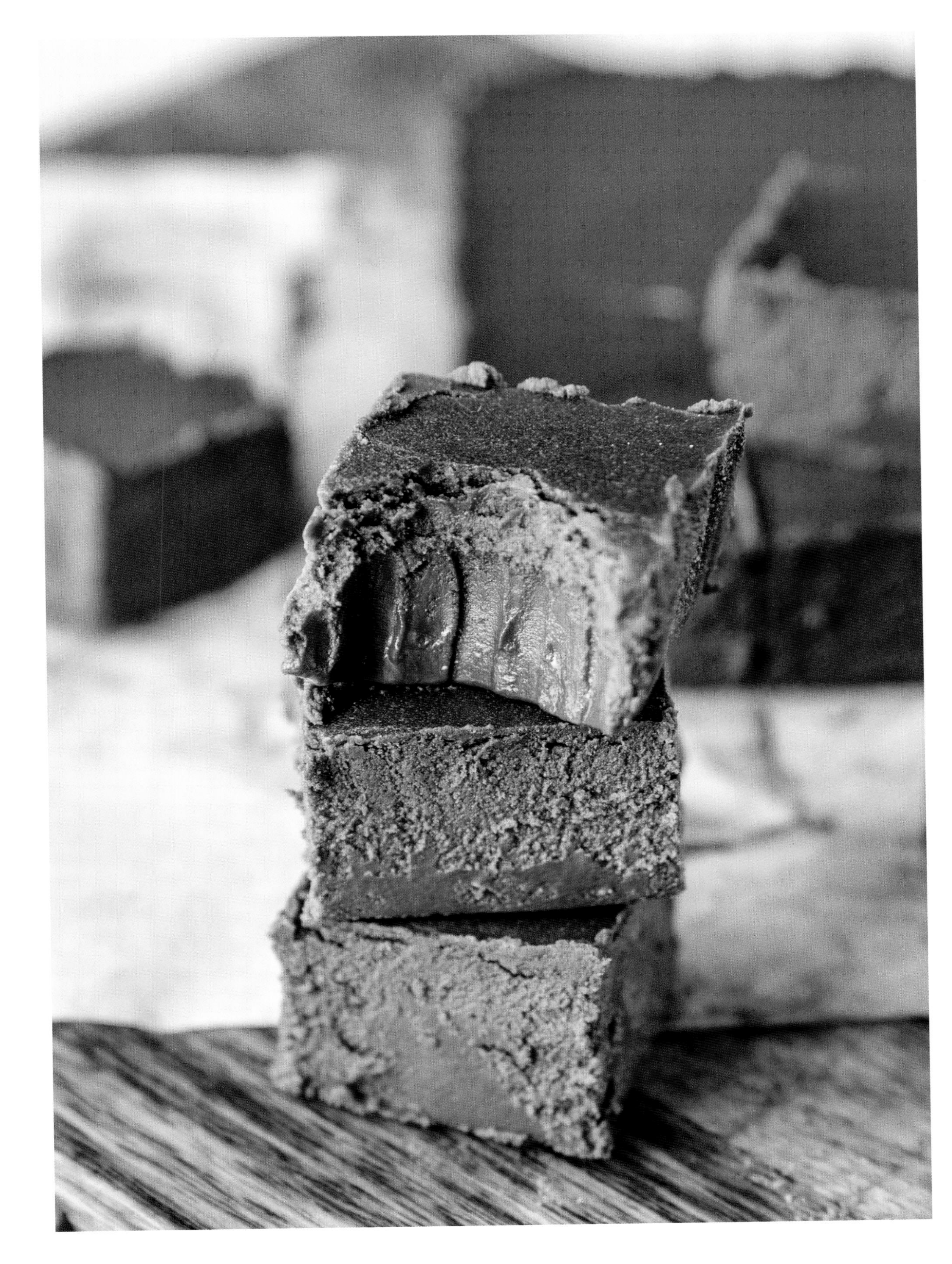

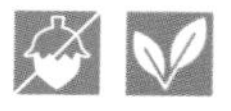

ITALIAN CREAM PUFFS

YIELD: 24 cream puffs (1 per serving)

PREP TIME: 30 minutes

COOK TIME: 20 minutes

While they may be a bit time-consuming to prepare, these cream puffs are well worth the effort. The traditional cream puffs that I grew up enjoying were always filled with custard cream, but you could also use whipped cream or even ice cream. A simple dusting of confectioners'-style sweetener is all you need to serve these cream puffs to company.

FOR THE PUFFS

- 4 large eggs, separated
- ½ teaspoon cream of tartar
- 4 ounces cream cheese (½ cup), softened
- ½ teaspoon vanilla extract
- ⅓ cup (28g) unflavored egg white protein powder
- 1 teaspoon baking powder
- ½ teaspoon baking soda
- ¼ teaspoon vanilla-flavored liquid stevia
- Pinch of fine sea salt

FOR THE CUSTARD FILLING

- 8 ounces mascarpone cheese (1 cup)
- 1 teaspoon vanilla extract
- ½ cup Swerve confectioners'-style sweetener
- Pinch of fine sea salt
- ½ cup heavy whipping cream

- 2 tablespoons Swerve confectioners'-style sweetener, for sprinkling (optional)

SPECIAL EQUIPMENT:

Pastry bag with piping tip

Store in an airtight container in the refrigerator for up to 3 days.

MAKE THE PUFFS:

1. Preheat the oven to 300°F. Line two sheet pans with parchment paper or grease a 24-well mini muffin pan. (Using a mini muffin pan will give you more formed puffs that have some height.)

2. Place the egg whites and cream of tartar in the bowl of a stand mixer (or a medium bowl if using an electric hand mixer) and whip until stiff peaks form. Set aside.

3. Place the egg yolks in a small bowl and set aside. Whisk the remaining ingredients for the puffs in a large bowl, then add the yolks. Stir until combined. Fold in the whipped egg whites.

4. Using a 1½-tablespoon cookie scoop, make 24 mounds of dough, placing 12 on each prepared sheet pan or one in each well of the prepared mini muffin pan. Bake for 20 minutes, or until lightly browned. Allow to cool completely before filling.

MAKE THE CUSTARD FILLING:

1. While the puffs are baking, place the mascarpone, vanilla extract, confectioners'-style sweetener, and salt in the bowl of the stand mixer (or a medium bowl if using the hand mixer) and mix on high until well combined.

2. Pour in the cream, change to the whisk attachment, and whisk on high until the mixture has thickened. Refrigerate until ready to fill the puffs.

ASSEMBLE THE CREAM PUFFS:

1. Slice the cooled puffs in half.

2. Transfer the custard filling to a pastry bag and pipe it evenly onto the bottom half of each puff.

3. Place the tops of the puffs on the filling and sprinkle with the confectioners'-style sweetener, if desired.

calories 91 | fat 8g | protein 2g | total carbs 0g | dietary fiber 0g | net carbs 0g

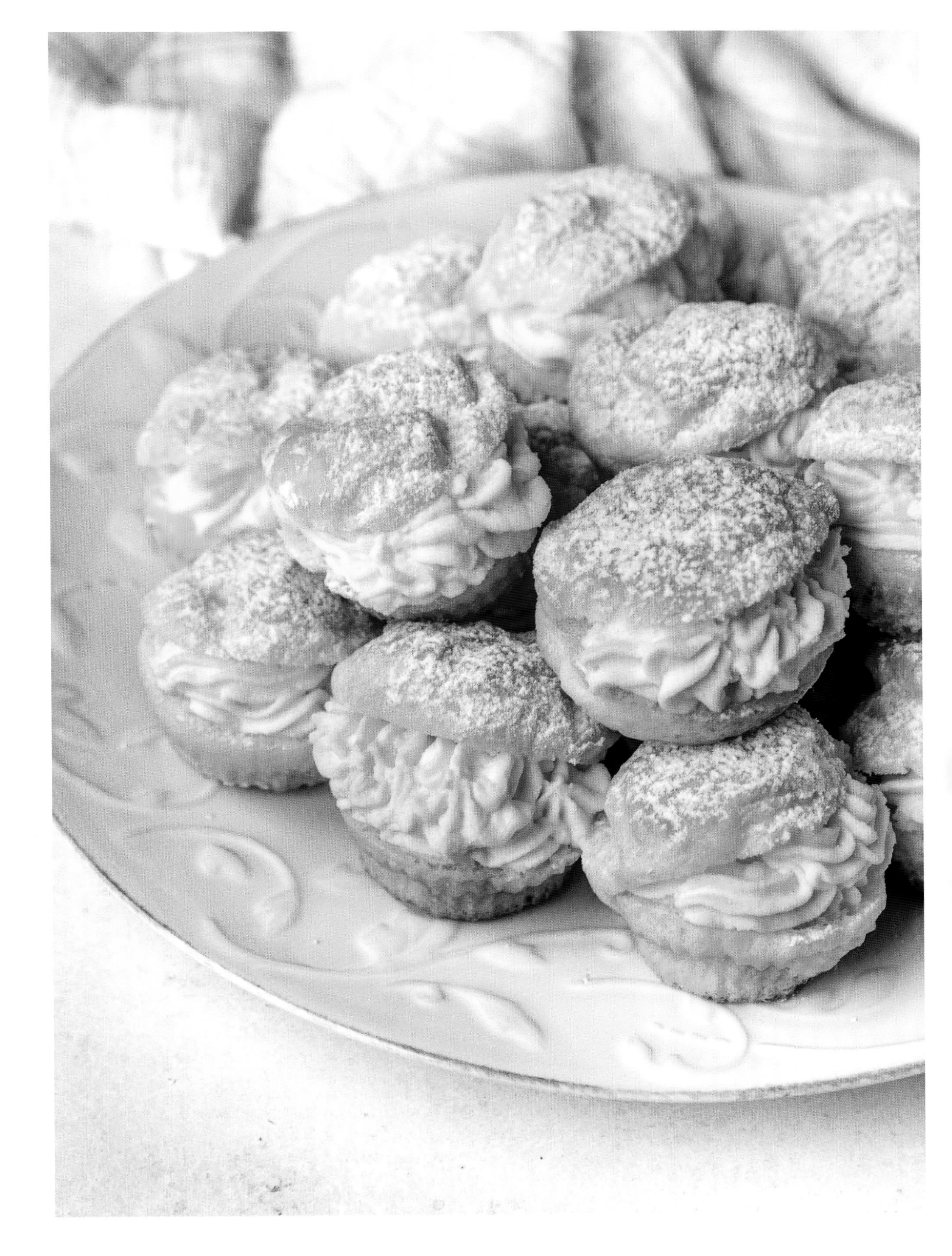

option

FUDGY BROWNIES

YIELD: 16 brownies (1 per serving)

PREP TIME: 15 minutes

COOK TIME: 27 minutes

This is my go-to brownie recipe. Whenever we want a fudgy chocolate something, I make these treats to satisfy us all! When we want double-chocolate brownies, I mix in more chocolate chips by hand at the end.

1 cup sugar-free chocolate chips, store-bought or homemade (page 230), plus an additional cup if desired

½ cup (1 stick) unsalted butter or coconut oil

½ cup avocado oil

¼ cup heavy whipping cream or coconut cream

2 large eggs

1 large egg yolk

2 teaspoons vanilla extract

1 teaspoon chocolate-flavored liquid stevia

¾ cup (143g) packed Swerve brown sugar sweetener

⅓ cup (30g) chocolate-flavored protein powder

¼ cup (33g) coconut flour

¼ cup (25g) unsweetened cocoa powder

2 teaspoons instant espresso powder or instant coffee granules

½ teaspoon baking powder

¼ teaspoon fine sea salt

1. Melt the chocolate chips and butter in a small saucepan over low heat or in a microwave-safe bowl in the microwave for 1 to 2 minutes. Stir until completely smooth. Set aside.

2. Preheat the oven to 350°F. Line an 8-inch square baking dish with parchment paper or grease the dish.

3. Place the avocado oil, cream, whole eggs, egg yolk, vanilla extract, and stevia in the bowl of a stand mixer (or a medium bowl if using an electric hand mixer) and mix on medium until combined.

4. Turn the mixer to low and slowly pour in the melted chocolate mixture.

5. Add the remaining ingredients and mix until well combined. Stir in the additional cup of chocolate chips by hand, if using.

6. Pour the batter into the prepared baking dish and bake for 25 minutes. The brownies might look underbaked after 25 minutes, but it's best to take the dish out of the oven before the brownies look done to achieve that gooey texture.

7. Allow to cool in the pan for 15 minutes before slicing into 16 squares. The brownies are best enjoyed the same day, but you can store them in an airtight container in the fridge to eat the next day.

calories **155** | fat **13g** | protein **5g** | total carbs **4g** | dietary fiber **1g** | net carbs **3g**

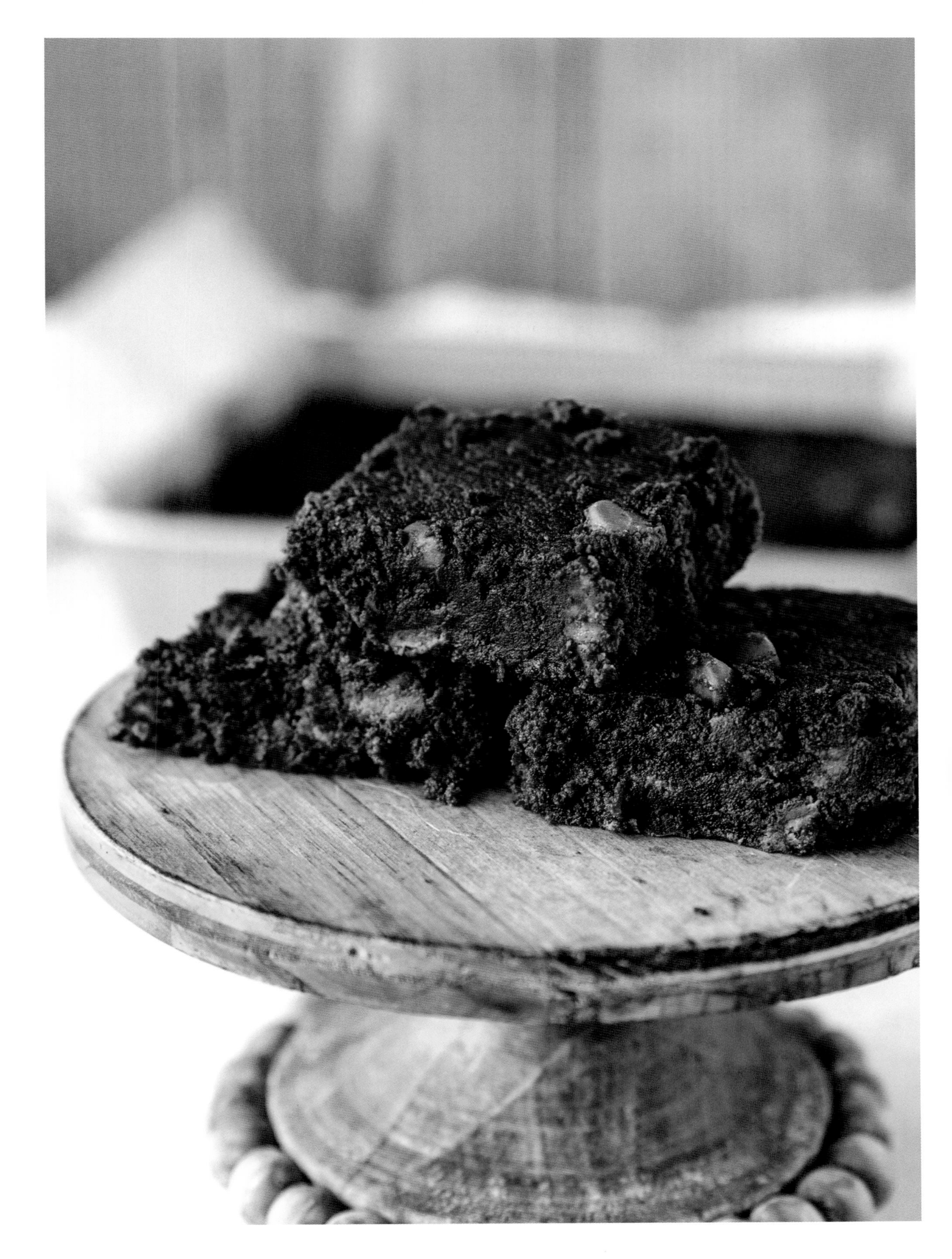

MINI CRUSTLESS BLUEBERRY LEMON CHEESECAKES

YIELD: 12 mini cheesecakes (1 per serving)

PREP TIME: 20 minutes, plus at least 2 hours to chill

COOK TIME: 25 minutes (not including time to make syrup)

These mini cheesecakes can be made into one large cheesecake if you prefer. Just use an 8-inch springform pan instead of a muffin pan. You may need to add an extra 10 to 15 minutes of baking time to get the center to set. If you're not a fan of blueberries, simply omit the blueberry syrup and enjoy the cheesecakes unfilled.

2 (8-ounce) packages cream cheese, softened

2 large eggs

1 large egg yolk

½ cup sour cream

1 tablespoon freshly squeezed lemon juice

½ teaspoon lemon-flavored liquid stevia

1 teaspoon vanilla extract

⅓ cup Swerve confectioners'-style sweetener

½ teaspoon baking powder

¼ teaspoon fine sea salt

1½ batches Blueberry Syrup (page 64)

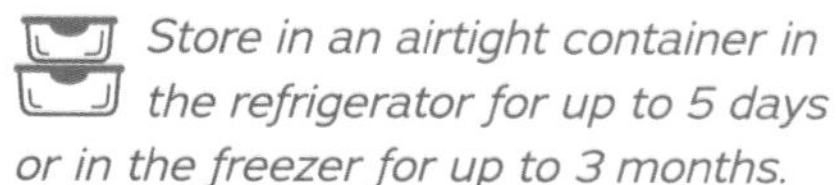

Store in an airtight container in the refrigerator for up to 5 days or in the freezer for up to 3 months.

1. Preheat the oven to 325°F. Grease a 12-well muffin pan or use silicone or paper cupcake liners.
2. Place the cream cheese in the bowl of a stand mixer (or a medium bowl if using an electric hand mixer) and mix on high until smooth, with no lumps.
3. Add the remaining ingredients and mix until well incorporated.
4. Pour the batter evenly into the wells of the prepared pan. Bake for 20 to 25 minutes, or until the edges are set and the centers are slightly jiggly.
5. Allow to cool completely, then refrigerate for 2 to 3 hours or overnight.
6. Before serving, top each cheesecake with 2 tablespoons of blueberry syrup.

| WITHOUT BLUEBERRY SYRUP |

calories 245 | fat 12g | protein 28g | total carbs 3g | dietary fiber 0g | net carbs 3g

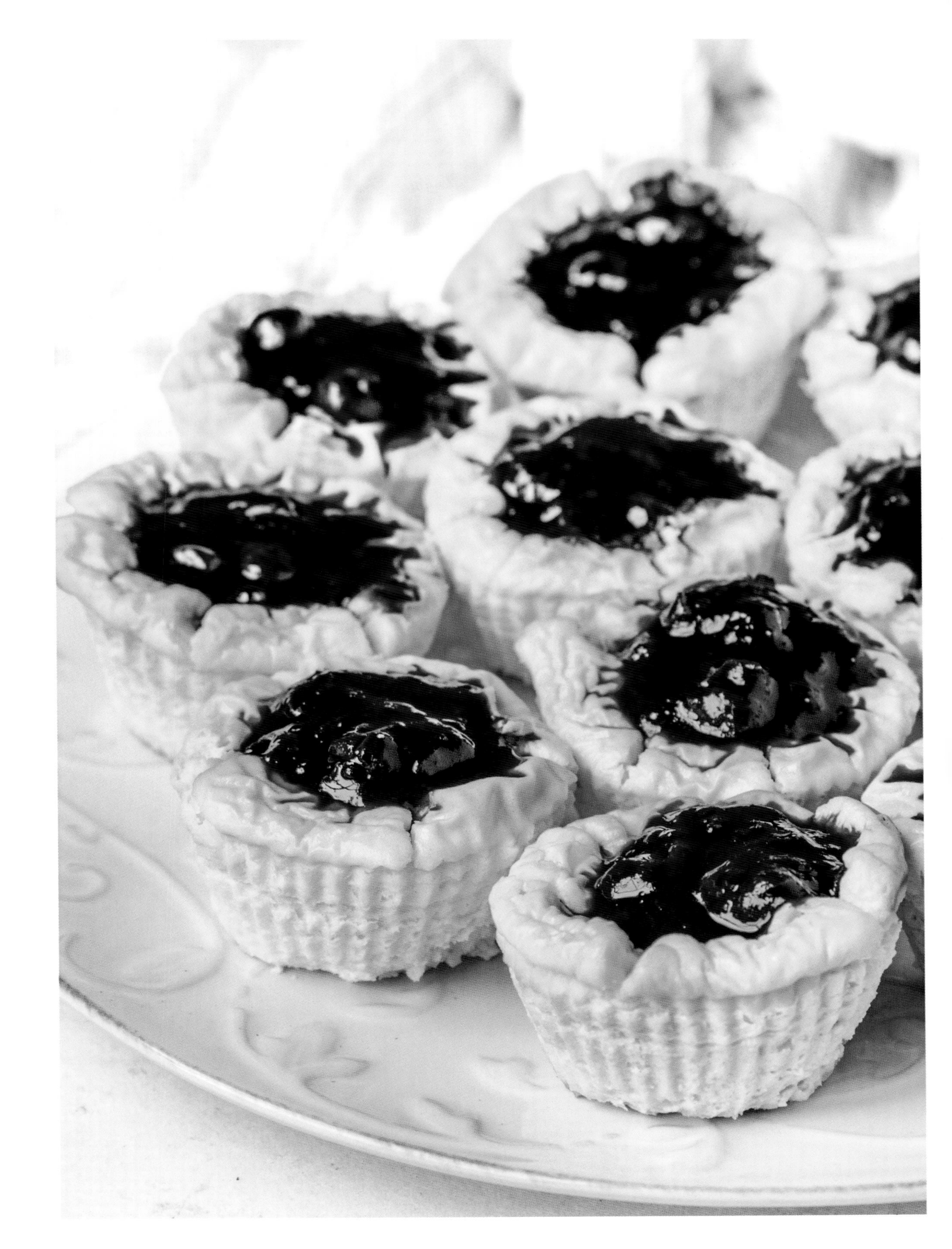

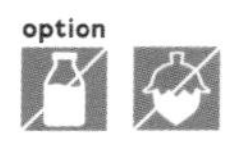

GINGERBREAD BISCOTTI

YIELD: 12 biscotti (1 per serving)

PREP TIME: 20 minutes, plus at least 40 minutes to cool and chill

COOK TIME: 55 minutes

Biscotti are one of my dad's favorite treats. Who doesn't love a delicious biscotto with coffee? I adapted this recipe from my popular chocolate biscotti recipe on my website, and I think the gingerbread flavor is spectacular for the holiday season.

2 cups (240g) sesame flour

1/2 cup (95g) packed Swerve brown sugar sweetener

2 tablespoons unflavored gelatin

2 teaspoons baking powder

1 teaspoon xanthan gum

1 teaspoon ground cinnamon

1 teaspoon ginger powder

1/2 teaspoon ground cloves

1/2 teaspoon baking soda

1/4 teaspoon fine sea salt

1/2 cup (1 stick) unsalted butter or coconut oil, melted but not hot

1 teaspoon maple extract

2 large eggs, beaten

1 teaspoon vanilla-flavored liquid stevia

FOR THE CHOCOLATE COATING (OPTIONAL)

2 1/2 ounces sugar-free chocolate chips, store-bought or homemade (page 230)

1 tablespoon salted butter

1/4 teaspoon ground cinnamon

Wrap in aluminum foil and store on the counter to keep crisp for up to 5 days.

1. Preheat the oven to 325°F. Line a cookie sheet with parchment paper.

2. Place the sesame flour, brown sugar sweetener, gelatin, baking powder, xanthan gum, cinnamon, ginger, cloves, baking soda, and salt in the bowl of a stand mixer fitted with the whisk attachment (or a large bowl if using an electric hand mixer) and whisk to combine.

3. Add the melted butter and maple extract and stir until incorporated. Stir in the eggs and stevia.

4. Transfer the dough to the prepared cookie sheet and use your hands to form it into a 10 by 4-inch rectangle.

5. Bake for 25 minutes. Remove from the oven and allow to cool for 30 minutes.

6. Using a sharp knife, very gently cut the rectangle down the longer length into 12 slices. Lay the slices cut side down on the cookie sheet. Bake for 15 minutes, then gently flip over and bake for another 10 minutes. Let cool completely before adding the chocolate coating, if desired.

7. While the biscotti are cooling, make the chocolate coating (if using): Melt the chocolate and butter in a small saucepan over low heat, then stir until completely smooth. Add the cinnamon and stir until fully incorporated.

8. Lay a sheet of parchment paper on a sheet pan. Dip one end of each biscotto into the chocolate, then lay the cookies on the parchment. Drizzle the remaining chocolate over the cookies, then place the sheet pan in the refrigerator for 10 to 15 minutes, or until the chocolate is set.

calories 161 | fat 11g | protein 10g | total carbs 8g | dietary fiber 3g | net carbs 5g

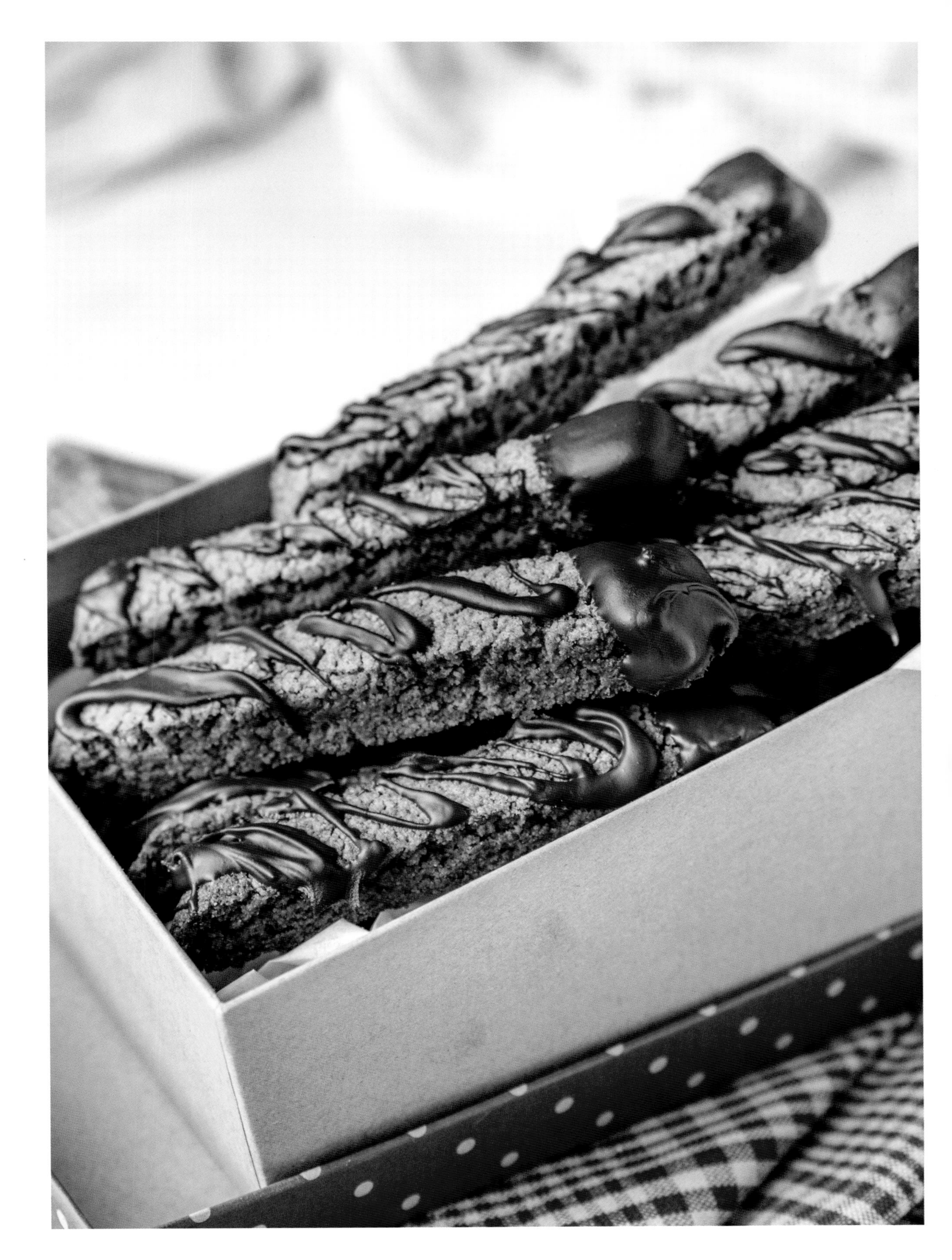

ITALIAN AMARETTI

YIELD: 24 cookies (1 per serving)

PREP TIME: 15 minutes

COOK TIME: 24 minutes

Italian amaretti are almond-flavored macaroons. They were my dad's favorite cookie growing up in Italy. He likes them chewy, so I opt to underbake mine at just 20 minutes, but you can bake them for up to 26 minutes if you prefer crispier cookies.

3 cups (312g) blanched almond flour

1 cup (225g) Swerve granular sweetener

1 teaspoon vanilla-flavored liquid stevia

1 teaspoon almond extract

1 teaspoon vanilla extract

Pinch of fine sea salt

3 large egg whites

¼ cup sliced almonds, for topping (optional)

2 tablespoons Swerve confectioners'-style sweetener, for sprinkling (optional)

Store in an airtight container on the counter for up to 3 days.

1. Preheat the oven to 300°F. Line a cookie sheet with parchment paper.

2. Place the almond flour, sweeteners, extracts, and salt in the bowl of a stand mixer (or in a medium bowl) and mix or stir to combine.

3. Add the egg whites one at a time and mix or stir until combined.

4. Use a tablespoon-sized cookie scoop to make 24 balls of dough. Place the balls on the prepared cookie sheet, spaced about an inch apart. Top with the almonds, if using.

5. Bake for 22 to 24 minutes, or until lightly golden brown.

6. Remove from the oven and sprinkle the cookies with the confectioners'-style sweetener, if desired. Allow to cool completely before serving.

calories 82 | fat 16g | protein 3g | total carbs 3g | dietary fiber 1g | net carbs 2g

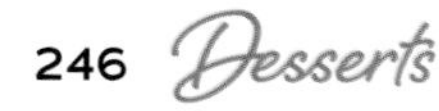

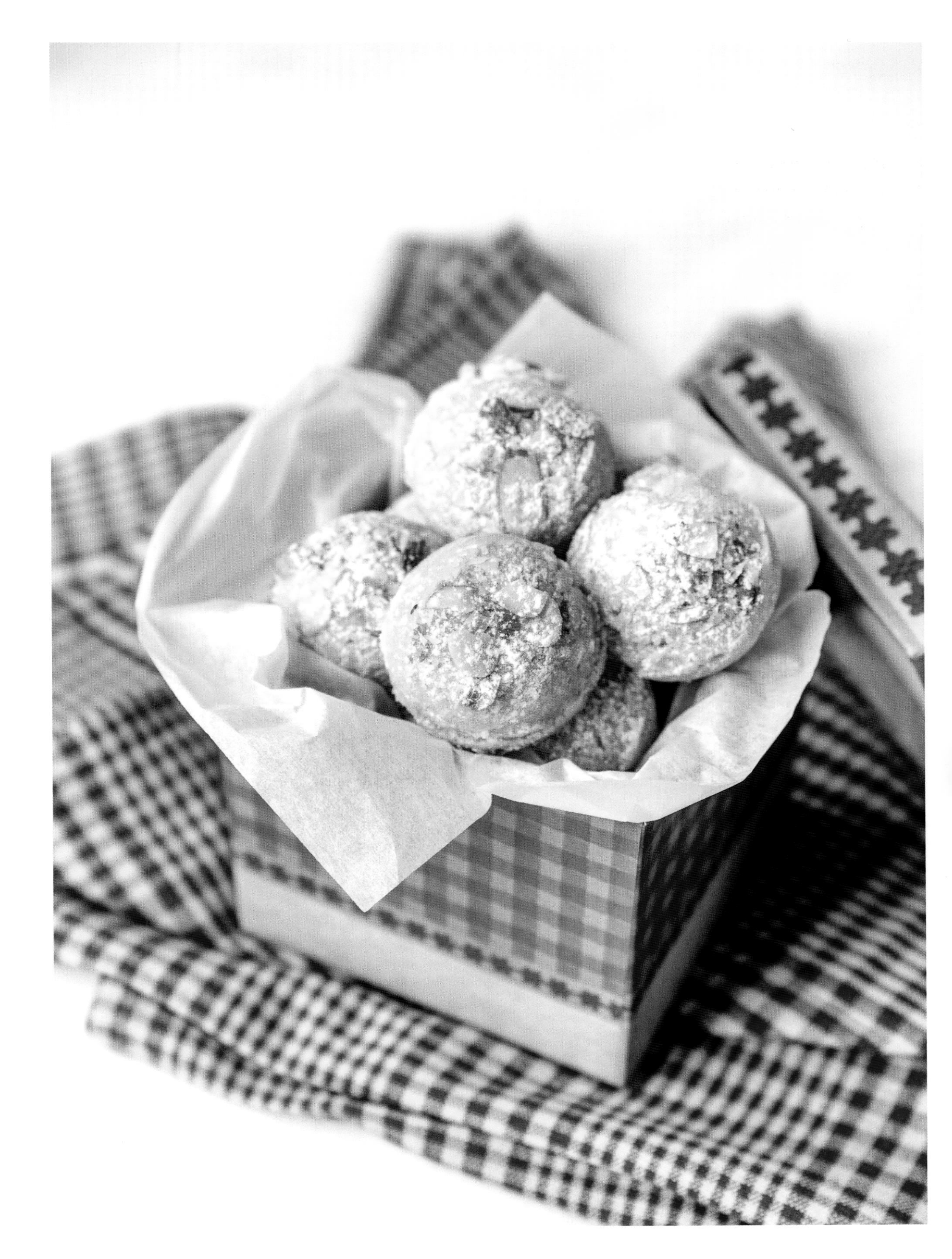

option

QUICK STRAWBERRY SHORTCAKES

YIELD: 4 servings

PREP TIME: 20 minutes

COOK TIME: 10 minutes

This lemony mug cake topped with fresh strawberries and homemade whipped cream is a sweet little treat for any day of the week.

FOR THE SHORTCAKES

¼ cup heavy whipping cream or coconut cream

2 large eggs

2 tablespoons freshly squeezed lemon juice

1 teaspoon lemon-flavored liquid stevia

3 tablespoons coconut flour

½ teaspoon baking powder

⅛ teaspoon fine sea salt

FOR THE STRAWBERRY TOPPING

1 cup sliced fresh strawberries

2 teaspoons freshly squeezed lemon juice

1 tablespoon Swerve confectioners'-style sweetener

Pinch of fine sea salt

FOR THE WHIPPED TOPPING

½ cup heavy whipping cream or coconut cream

2 tablespoons Swerve confectioners'-style sweetener, or ½ teaspoon vanilla-flavored liquid stevia

SPECIAL EQUIPMENT:

4 (7-ounce) ramekins

1. Preheat the oven to 350°F and grease four 7-ounce ramekins.
2. Make the shortcakes: In a large bowl, whisk together all of the shortcake ingredients. Pour the batter evenly into the prepared ramekins.
3. Bake for 10 minutes, or until a toothpick inserted in the center of a cake comes out clean. Allow to cool completely.
4. Make the strawberry topping: Place all of the ingredients in a medium bowl and stir to combine.
5. Make the whipped topping: Place the cream and sweetener in the bowl of a stand mixer fitted with the whisk attachment (or in a medium bowl if using an electric hand mixer). Mix on high until stiff peaks form. Taste and add more sweetener, if desired.
6. Assemble the strawberry shortcakes: Place each shortcake on a serving plate. Top each shortcake with ¼ cup of the strawberries and a dollop of the whipped topping. Enjoy!

Store the cakes, without toppings, in an airtight container in the refrigerator for up to 5 days.

calories 221 | fat 18g | protein 4g | total carbs 7g | dietary fiber 2g | net carbs 5g

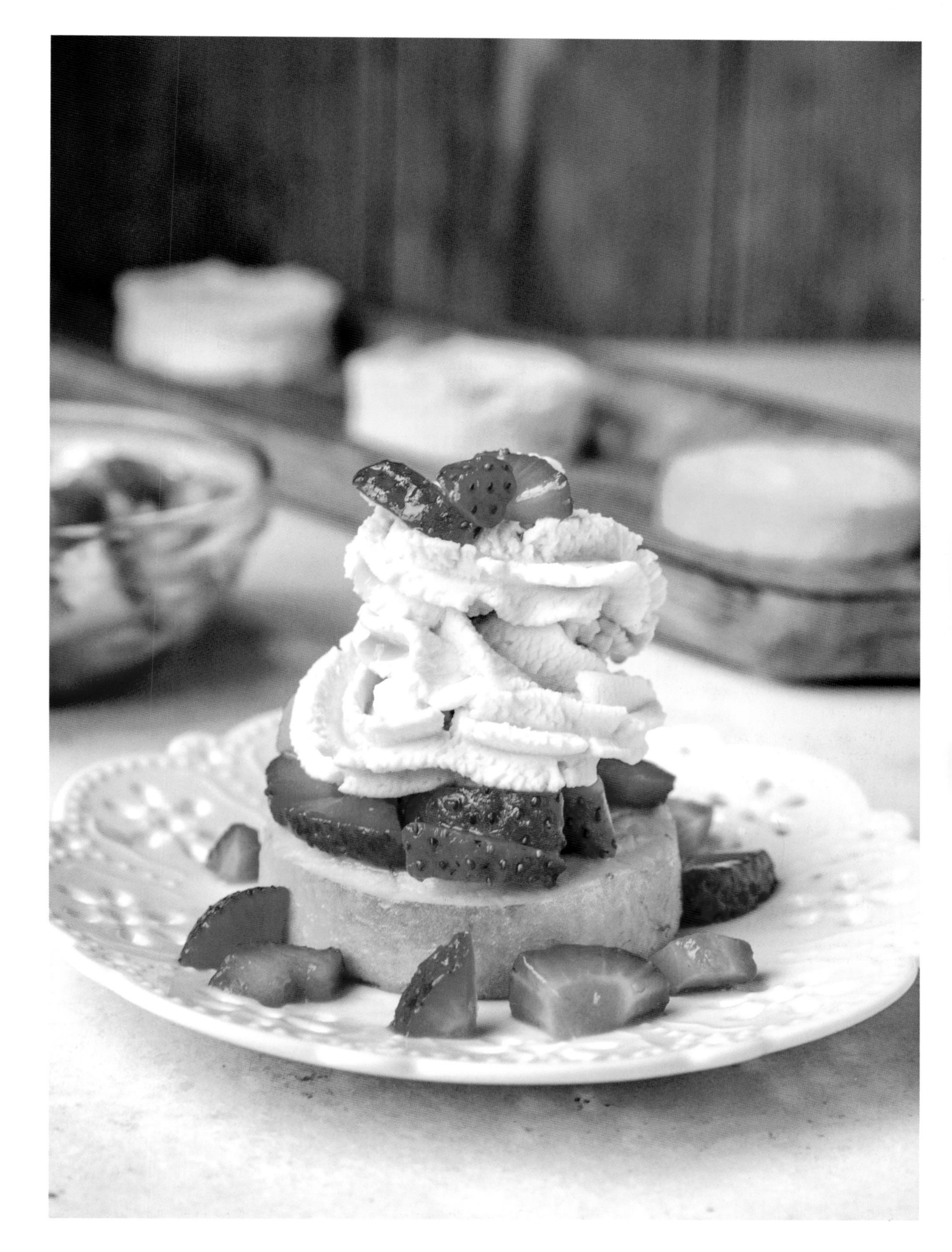

TRIPLE-LAYER CHOCOLATE CAKE

YIELD: one 9-inch three-layer cake (16 servings)

PREP TIME: 20 minutes (not including time to make frosting)

COOK TIME: 25 minutes

I'm not a fan of making a dessert like this on a weekly basis, but we all need a cake for birthdays and other special occasions. Why is mayo added to this cake, you ask? Mayo is essentially oil, eggs, and vinegar. Vinegar reacts with baking soda to aerate the cake, making this one of the moistest cakes you'll ever eat. The espresso powder elevates the flavor of the chocolate.

Don't want to make a three-layer cake? Use two eggs and divide the rest of the ingredients by three to make a single round cake. This recipe yields sixteen servings because it is very rich; you need only a small piece to satisfy. For a lighter dessert, skip the frosting and top the cake with Whipped Cream (page 73) or Coconut Whipped Cream (page 66).

1½ cups (180g) sesame flour

1½ cups (335g) Swerve granular sweetener

1 cup (95g) unsweetened cocoa powder

¾ cup (85g) ground flaxseed

1 tablespoon baking powder

2½ teaspoons baking soda

2 teaspoons instant espresso powder or instant coffee granules

1½ teaspoons xanthan gum

1½ cups avocado oil mayonnaise

4 large eggs

2 teaspoons vanilla extract

1½ cups water

3 batches Chocolate Buttercream Frosting (page 232)

Store covered on the counter for up to 3 days or in the refrigerator for up to a week. You can also wrap individual slices in plastic wrap, then seal in a zip-top freezer bag and freeze for up to 4 months.

1. Preheat the oven to 350°F. Grease three 9-inch round cake pans.
2. In a large bowl, whisk together the sesame flour, sweetener, cocoa powder, ground flaxseed, baking powder, baking soda, espresso powder, and xanthan gum.
3. Place the mayonnaise, eggs, and vanilla extract in the bowl of a stand mixer (or a large bowl if using an electric hand mixer) and mix until combined. Pour in half of the dry ingredients and mix until fully incorporated. Add the water and mix until combined. Add the remaining dry ingredients and mix until fully incorporated.
4. Evenly spread the batter (it will be thick) in the prepared pans. Bake for 25 minutes, or until a toothpick inserted in the center of a cake comes out clean. Allow to cool completely before frosting.
5. Once the cakes are cool, remove one from the pan and place it on a serving plate. Spread one-quarter of the frosting on the top of the cake. Place a second cake layer on top of that and repeat with another one-quarter of the frosting. Add the final cake layer and spread another one-quarter of the frosting over the top. Spread the remaining frosting over the sides of the cake.
6. Slice and serve!

Tip: Reheat pieces in the microwave for a minute and you've got a fudgy cake to enjoy!

calories **554** | fat **49g** | protein **7g** | total carbs **16g** | dietary fiber **8g** | net carbs **8g**

| CAKE ONLY | calories **237** | fat **22g** | protein **7g** | total carbs **9g** | dietary fiber **5g** | net carbs **4g**

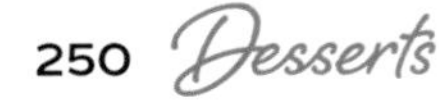

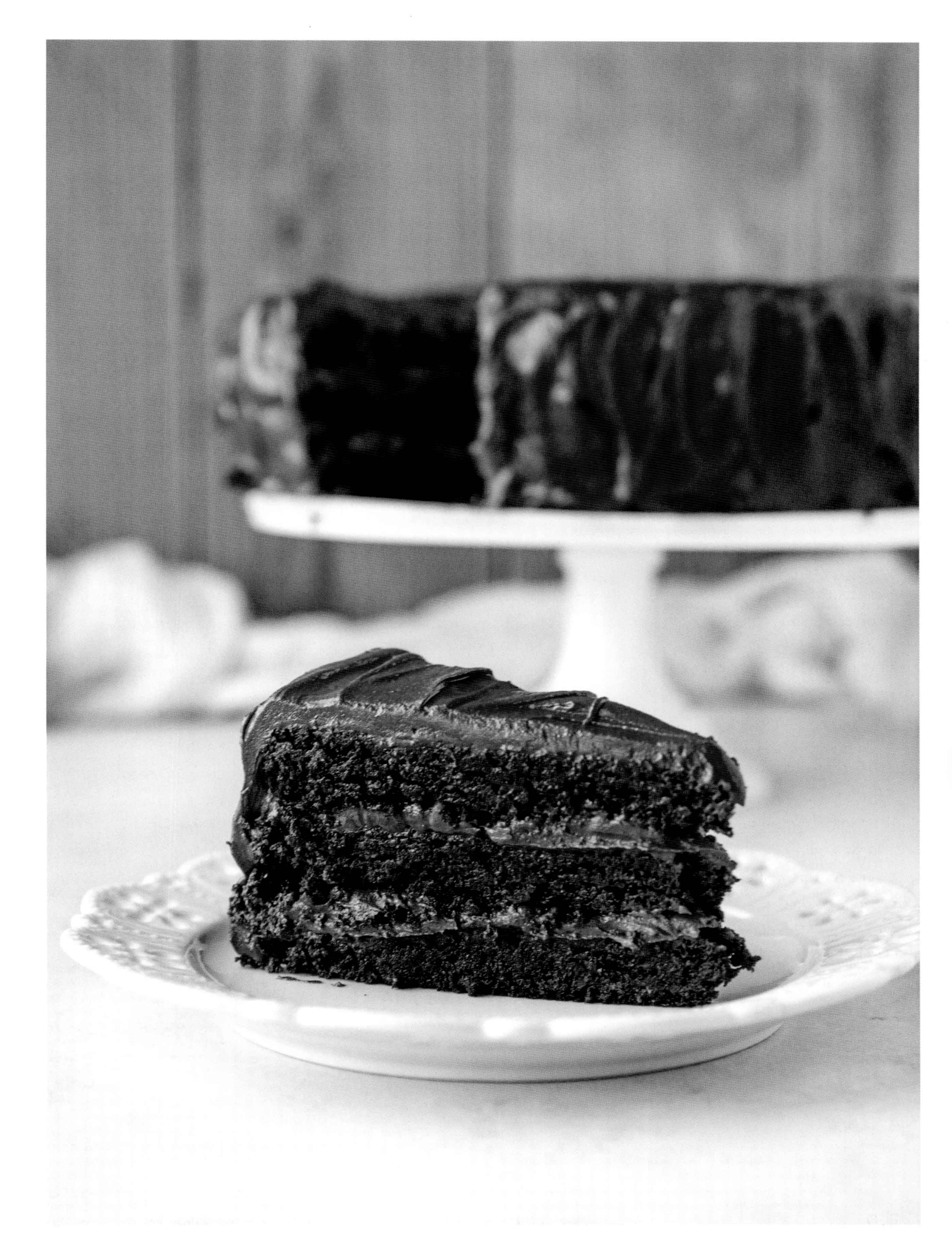

PECAN PIE

YIELD: one 9-inch pie (12 servings)

PREP TIME: 30 minutes

COOK TIME: 45 minutes

Since I don't often make recipes with nuts, I took the opportunity to create a pie that has an almond flour crust for those who might like it better than my Coconut Flour Pie Crust (page 68). My hubby adores pecan pie, and this is a recipe he loves.

FOR THE CRUST

- 2 large eggs
- 1 tablespoon extra-virgin olive oil
- 1 teaspoon vanilla extract
- 2 cups (210g) blanched almond flour
- ¼ cup (56g) Swerve granular sweetener
- ¼ teaspoon fine sea salt
- ¼ cup (½ stick) unsalted butter, cold, cubed

FOR THE FILLING

- 1 cup chopped raw pecans
- ½ cup whole raw pecans
- ½ cup sugar-free maple syrup, store-bought or homemade (page 70), or yacón syrup
- ½ cup (1 stick) unsalted butter, melted but not hot
- ⅓ cup packed Swerve brown sugar sweetener
- 2 large eggs, beaten
- 2 teaspoons maple extract
- 1 teaspoon ground cinnamon

Cover the pie with aluminum foil and store in the refrigerator for up to 4 days.

1. Preheat the oven to 325°F. Grease a 9-inch pie pan.
2. Make the crust: Place all of the crust ingredients in a food processor and pulse until crumbs form. Transfer the dough to the greased pie pan and use your fingers to press it as evenly as possible across the bottom and up the sides. Par-bake for 15 minutes.
3. While the crust is baking, prepare the filling: Place all of the filling ingredients in a large bowl and stir until the pecans are nicely coated.
4. Remove the crust from the oven and add the filling in an even layer. Cover the edges of the crust with aluminum foil and bake for an additional 30 minutes, or until a knife inserted in the center of the pie comes out clean. It shouldn't be overly jiggly when it comes out of the oven; if it is, cover the whole pie with foil and bake for another 10 minutes, or until set.
5. Slice and serve!

calories 325 | fat 32g | protein 7g | total carbs 6g | dietary fiber 3g | net carbs 3g

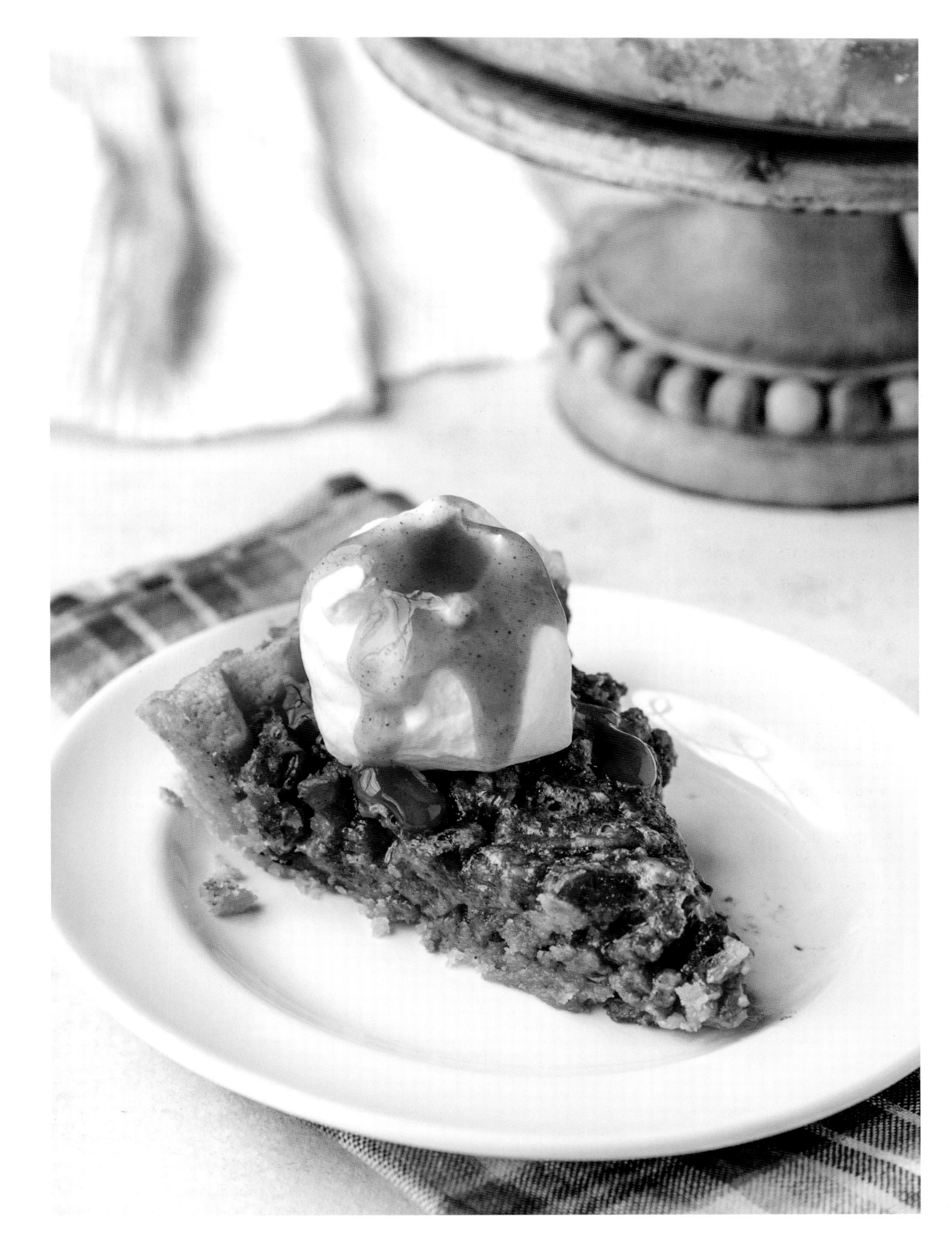

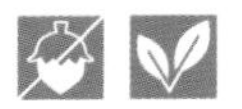

VANILLA GELATO

YIELD: 1 quart (8 servings)

PREP TIME: 45 minutes, plus at least 4 hours to chill/freeze

COOK TIME: 15 minutes

Gelato is an Italian-style ice cream. It's creamier, silkier, and denser than regular ice cream. It typically uses more milk than cream and often doesn't contain eggs. I decided to keep egg yolks in my recipe to get that creamy texture, along with a bit of xanthan gum to make it more custardlike in texture. My family loves this gelato drizzled with Hot Fudge Sauce (page 65) or on top of my Apple Crisp (page 222).

1¼ cups heavy whipping cream

1 (13½-ounce) can coconut milk

4 large egg yolks

½ cup Swerve confectioners'-style sweetener

2 tablespoons MCT oil or vodka

1 vanilla bean, scraped, or 2 teaspoons vanilla extract

½ teaspoon vanilla-flavored liquid stevia

½ teaspoon xanthan gum

Pinch of fine sea salt

SPECIAL EQUIPMENT:

Ice cream maker

Store in the freezer for up to 2 months.

1. In a medium saucepan over medium heat, bring the cream and coconut milk to a simmer, stirring constantly. Once bubbling, remove the pan from the heat and turn off the burner.

2. Whisk the egg yolks in a large bowl until lightened in color. Temper the yolks by gradually adding small amounts of the hot cream mixture until all of it is incorporated. Pour the tempered yolks into the saucepan and place the pan over low heat.

3. Whisk in the remaining ingredients and cook, stirring frequently, until the mixture thickens and coats the back of a spoon, or the temperature is between 170°F and 175°F on a candy thermometer.

4. Strain the mixture through a fine-mesh strainer to remove any lumps. Pour the mixture into another large bowl and allow to cool for 30 minutes, then refrigerate for 2 to 3 hours.

5. Pour the mixture into an ice cream maker and churn following the manufacturer's instructions. My gelato is ready in 10 minutes. Once it has the texture of soft-serve ice cream, pour it into a container, cover, and freeze for 2 hours or overnight.

6. Allow to soften on the counter for 10 to 15 minutes before serving.

calories 273 | fat 27g | protein 2g | total carbs 2g | dietary fiber 0g | net carbs 2g

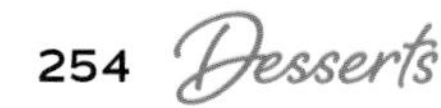

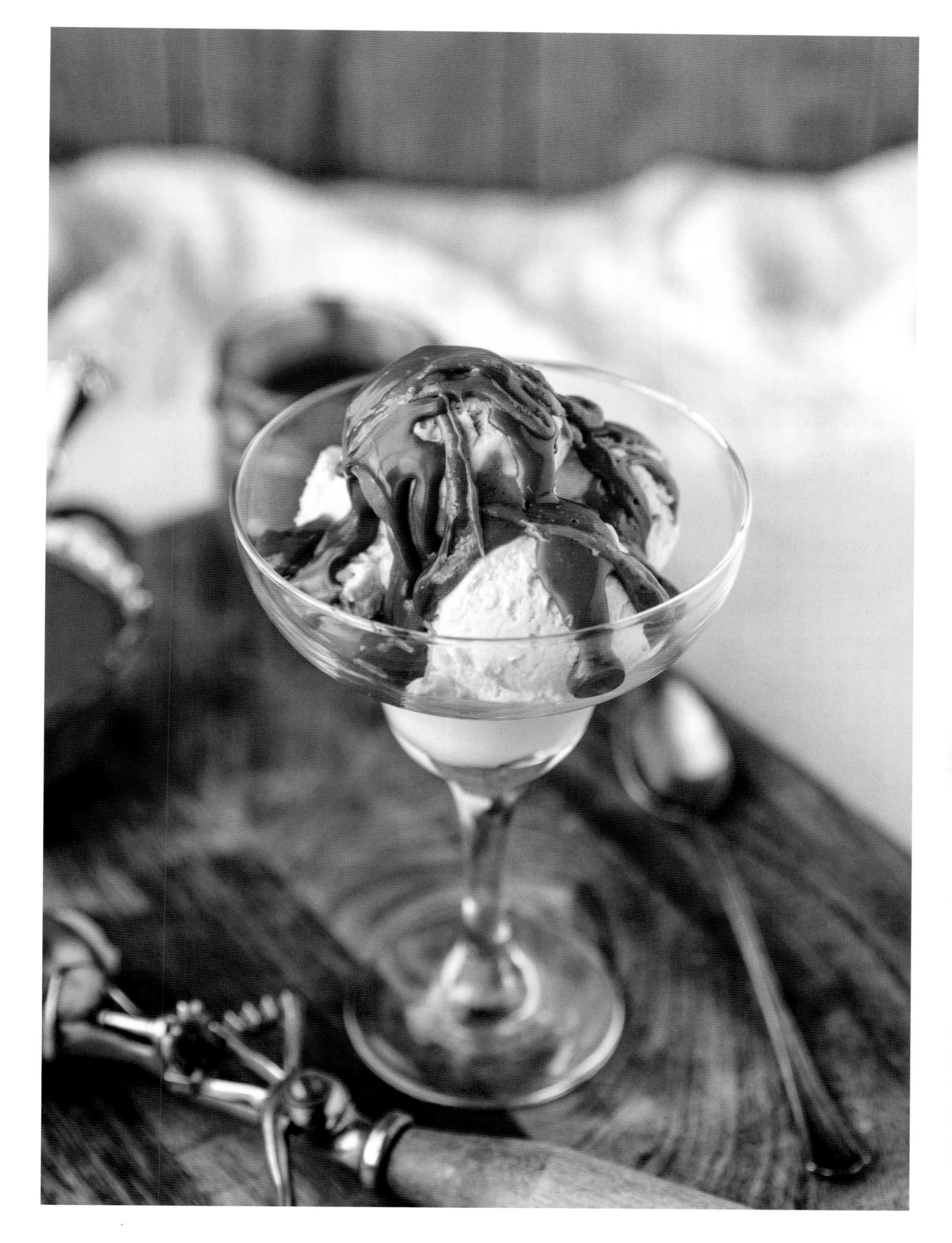

PIZZELLE

YIELD: 20 pizzelle (1 per serving)

PREP TIME: 15 minutes

COOK TIME: 10 minutes

I grew up helping my grandmother make pizzelle. Of course, the only job she let me do was to mix the batter and sprinkle on the confectioners' sugar, but still I have fond memories of baking with her. I think she'd be so proud of me if she were alive today, even if these aren't the traditional ingredients she would have used. Use this recipe to make cannoli shells! (See the variation below.)

- 3 large eggs
- ½ cup (112g) Swerve granular sweetener
- ¼ teaspoon vanilla-flavored liquid stevia
- 1½ teaspoons anise extract
- 1 teaspoon vanilla extract
- ½ cup (1 stick) salted butter, melted but not hot
- 1½ cups (180g) sesame flour
- 1 teaspoon baking soda
- Pinch of fine sea salt
- Swerve confectioners'-style sweetener, for topping

SPECIAL EQUIPMENT:

Pizzelle maker

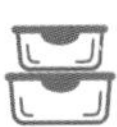

Wrap in aluminum foil and store on the counter to keep crisp for up to 3 days.

1. Lightly grease the plates of the pizzelle maker and preheat according to the manufacturer's instructions.
2. Place the eggs, sweeteners, and extracts in the bowl of a stand mixer (or a medium bowl if using an electric hand mixer) and mix to combine.
3. Slowly add the melted butter, then add the sesame flour, baking soda, and salt and stir until combined.
4. Using a greased tablespoon or cookie scoop, place a scoop of the batter in the center of each plate of the pizzelle maker. Close the lid. Once you see steam coming out the sides, check the color of the pizzelle. When they're lightly browned, they're done. Usually 3 to 5 seconds is all you need, but the time depends on the pizzelle maker, so follow the manufacturer's instructions. Some could take up to 30 seconds to lightly brown the pizzelle.
5. Remove the pizzelle with a spatula and place on a sheet pan to cool. Sprinkle with confectioners'-style sweetener. Repeat with the rest of the batter.

VARIATION: CANNOLI SHELLS. Follow Steps 1 through 4 above, then wrap the warm pizzella once around the handle of a wooden spoon or another cylinder-type handle. Place the handle with the cannoli shell seam side down on a sheet pan to hold it in place. The shell will harden within a couple minutes while you make the next pizzella. Remove the shell from the handle and repeat. If you are using these for my Cannoli recipe (page 228), you'll need only 12 shells.

calories 89 | fat 8g | protein 2g | total carbs 1g | dietary fiber 1g | net carbs 0g

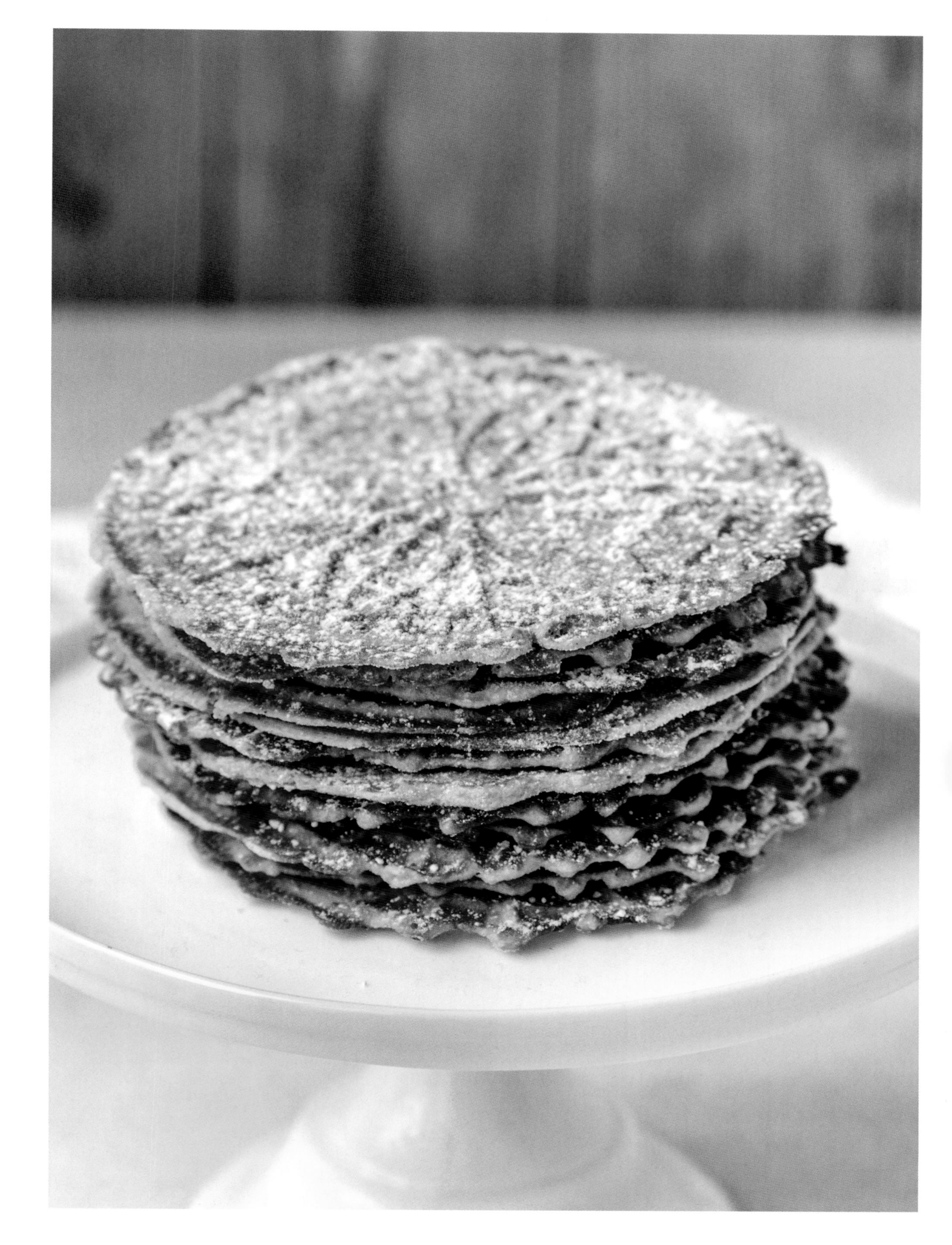

TIRAMISÙ

YIELD: 9 servings

PREP TIME: 1 hour 30 minutes, plus at least 3 hours to chill

COOK TIME: 30 minutes

When I made this dessert for my Italian father, who hails from Rome, he gave it a thumbs-up. I couldn't be happier!

FOR THE SPONGE CAKE

9 large eggs, separated

½ teaspoon cream of tartar

1 teaspoon vanilla-flavored liquid stevia

½ teaspoon vanilla extract

½ cup (65g) Swerve confectioners'-style sweetener

¼ cup (33g) coconut flour

¼ cup (25g) unflavored whey protein powder

½ teaspoon baking soda

½ teaspoon baking powder

½ teaspoon fine sea salt

¼ cup (½ stick) unsalted butter, melted but not hot

FOR THE CUSTARD

6 large egg yolks

½ cup Swerve confectioners'-style sweetener

8 ounces mascarpone cheese (1 cup)

1 teaspoon coffee extract

1 teaspoon vanilla extract

1 teaspoon vanilla-flavored liquid stevia

2 cups heavy whipping cream

FOR THE COFFEE LAYER

½ cup brewed espresso, chilled

3 tablespoons coffee liqueur or rum

2 tablespoons unsweetened cocoa powder, divided

MAKE THE SPONGE CAKE:

1. Preheat the oven to 350°F. Line a 13 by 9-inch baking dish with parchment paper.

2. Put the egg whites in a 1-cup liquid measuring cup. If you have more than 1 cup of whites, spoon off the excess. Place the 1 cup of whites in the bowl of a stand mixer (or a medium bowl if using an electric hand mixer), add the cream of tartar, and whip until stiff peaks form. Set aside.

3. Put the egg yolks, stevia, and vanilla extract in a large bowl and stir to combine. In a medium bowl, whisk together the confectioners'-style sweetener, coconut flour, protein powder, baking soda, baking powder, and salt. Gradually add half of the dry ingredients to the wet ingredients and stir until combined. Repeat with the remaining dry ingredients.

4. Fold the whipped egg whites into the batter. Drizzle in the melted butter and stir gently to combine.

5. Pour the batter into the prepared baking dish and bake for 15 to 20 minutes, or until a toothpick inserted in the center comes out clean. Allow to cool completely.

6. Wash and dry the mixer bowl.

MAKE THE CUSTARD:

1. Place the egg yolks and confectioners'-style sweetener in a medium glass or metal mixing bowl set over a pot of simmering water. Stir continually until the mixture turns yellow in color or a candy thermometer registers 170°F, about 10 minutes.

2. Add the mascarpone, extracts, and stevia and stir until the cheese is melted and the mixture is smooth. Set aside.

3. Pour the cream into the clean bowl of the stand mixer (or a clean mixing bowl if using the hand mixer) and beat until stiff peaks form, then fold the whipped cream into the custard.

calories 479 | fat 44g | protein 12g | total carbs 7g | dietary fiber 1g | net carbs 6g

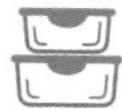

Cover tightly and store in the refrigerator for up to 4 days.

ASSEMBLE THE DESSERT:

1. Cut the cooled sponge cake horizontally to create two thin layers, then cut the layers into 16 pieces. Place eight of the pieces in a greased 9-inch square baking dish.

2. Put the espresso and coffee liqueur in a small bowl and stir to combine. Use a pastry brush to spread half of the coffee mixture on top of the sponge cake "fingers" in the baking dish.

3. Spread half of the custard mixture on the cake, then sprinkle with 1 tablespoon of the cocoa powder.

4. Lay the remaining sponge cake fingers on top of the custard layer, brush with the remaining coffee mixture, and spread the remaining custard on top of the fingers. Top with the remaining 1 tablespoon of cocoa powder.

5. Cover and refrigerate for 3 to 4 hours or overnight before slicing and serving.

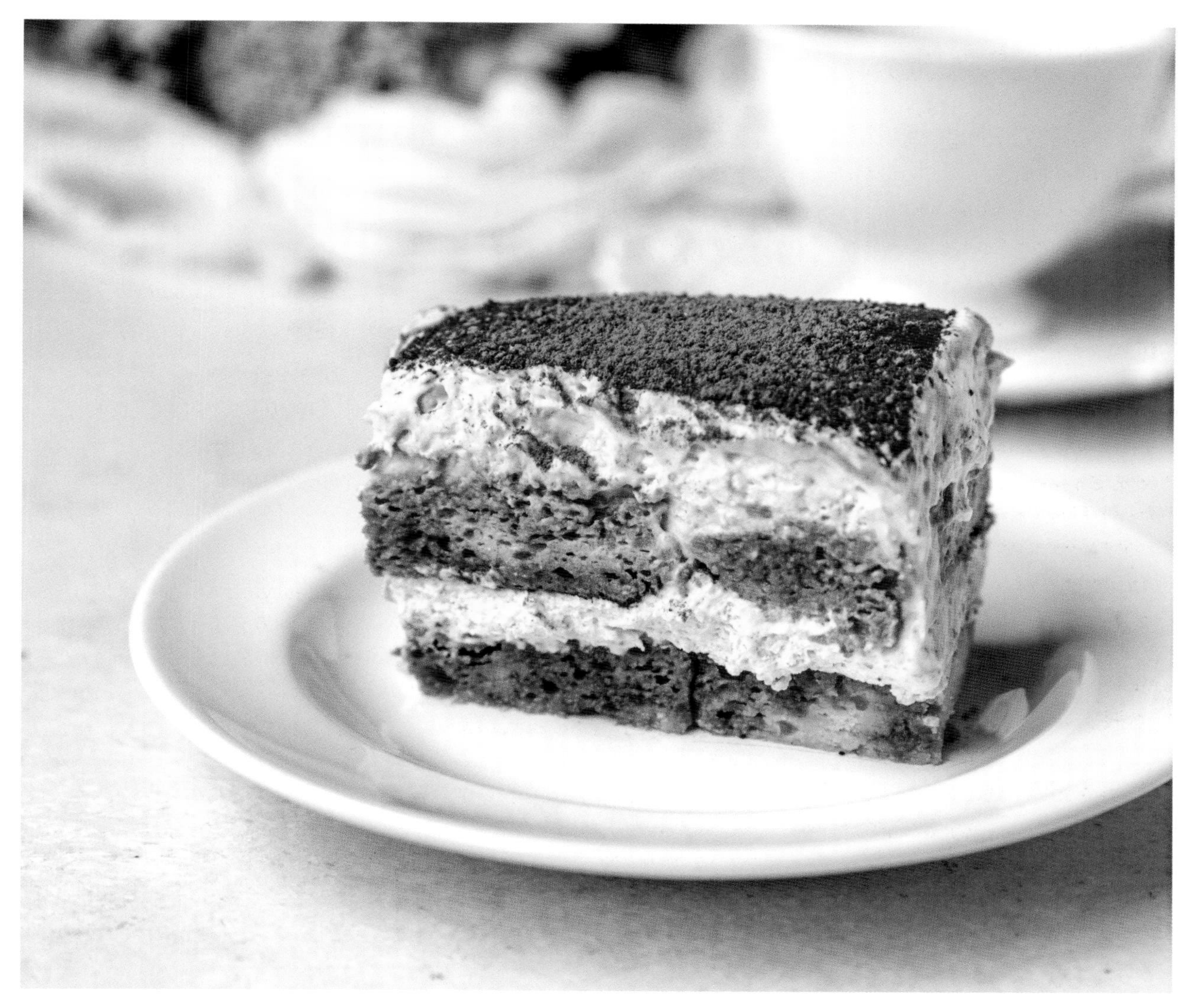

option

ICED SUGAR COOKIES

YIELD: 48 cookies (1 per serving)

PREP TIME: 20 minutes

COOK TIME: 40 minutes

A sugar-free sugar cookie—it's an oxymoron, isn't it? But when you want the traditional flavor of a beloved cookie from your childhood, you will go to any lengths to get it. These cookies have been a work in progress for years, and I can finally say that this version is much loved by my family!

1 cup (2 sticks) unsalted butter, softened

1 cup (225g) Swerve granular sweetener

1 teaspoon vanilla extract

2 large eggs

2 cups (240g) sesame flour

¼ cup (33g) coconut flour

2 tablespoons unflavored gelatin, or 1 teaspoon xanthan gum

½ teaspoon baking soda

½ teaspoon baking powder

¼ teaspoon fine sea salt

FOR THE SUGAR-FREE ICING

¾ cup Swerve confectioners'-style sweetener, divided

3 tablespoons water, divided

Natural food coloring in 2 or 3 colors

Store in an airtight container on the counter for up to 3 days or in the freezer for up to 3 months.

Note: The sprinkles shown in the photo are not keto-friendly; however, you could color unsweetened shredded coconut and use it as keto-friendly sprinkles.

1. Position one oven rack in the top third of the oven and a second rack in the bottom third. Preheat the oven to 350°F. Line four cookie sheets with parchment paper or silicone baking mats. (If you don't have four cookie sheets, you can use two and allow them to cool completely before making the second batch.)

2. Place the butter, sweetener, and vanilla extract in the bowl of a stand mixer (or a large bowl if using an electric hand mixer) and mix on high until combined. Turn the mixer to low and add the eggs one at a time, mixing after each addition.

3. In a large bowl, whisk together the flours, gelatin, baking soda, baking powder, and salt. Add half of the dry ingredients to the wet ingredients and mix on medium until combined. Repeat with the remaining dry ingredients.

4. Transfer half of the dough to a sheet of parchment paper on the counter. Cover the bowl with the rest of the dough and put it in the fridge.

5. Place another piece of parchment paper on top of the dough on the counter and roll out the dough to a ¼-inch thickness. Use cookie cutters to cut out shapes and place them on two of the lined cookie sheets. Gather up the scraps, reroll the dough, and cut out more shapes. You should have 24 cookies on the two pans.

6. Place the two pans of cookies in the oven and bake for 10 minutes, or until slightly browned on the edges. Allow to cool completely on the pans.

7. While the first batch of cookies is in the oven, repeat this process with the remaining dough, placing 24 more cookies on the other two lined cookie sheets. Bake the second batch of cookies after the first batch is done.

8. After the first batch of cookies has cooled completely, make the icing: Place ¼ cup of the sweetener in each of three small bowls. Add 1 tablespoon of water to each bowl and mix until smooth. Add food coloring for your desired colors.

9. Dip the tops of the cooled cookies into the icing and let the excess drip off, then place them back on the cookie sheets. Decorate the cookies as desired.

calories 53 | fat 4g | protein 2g | total carbs 1g | dietary fiber 0g | net carbs 1g

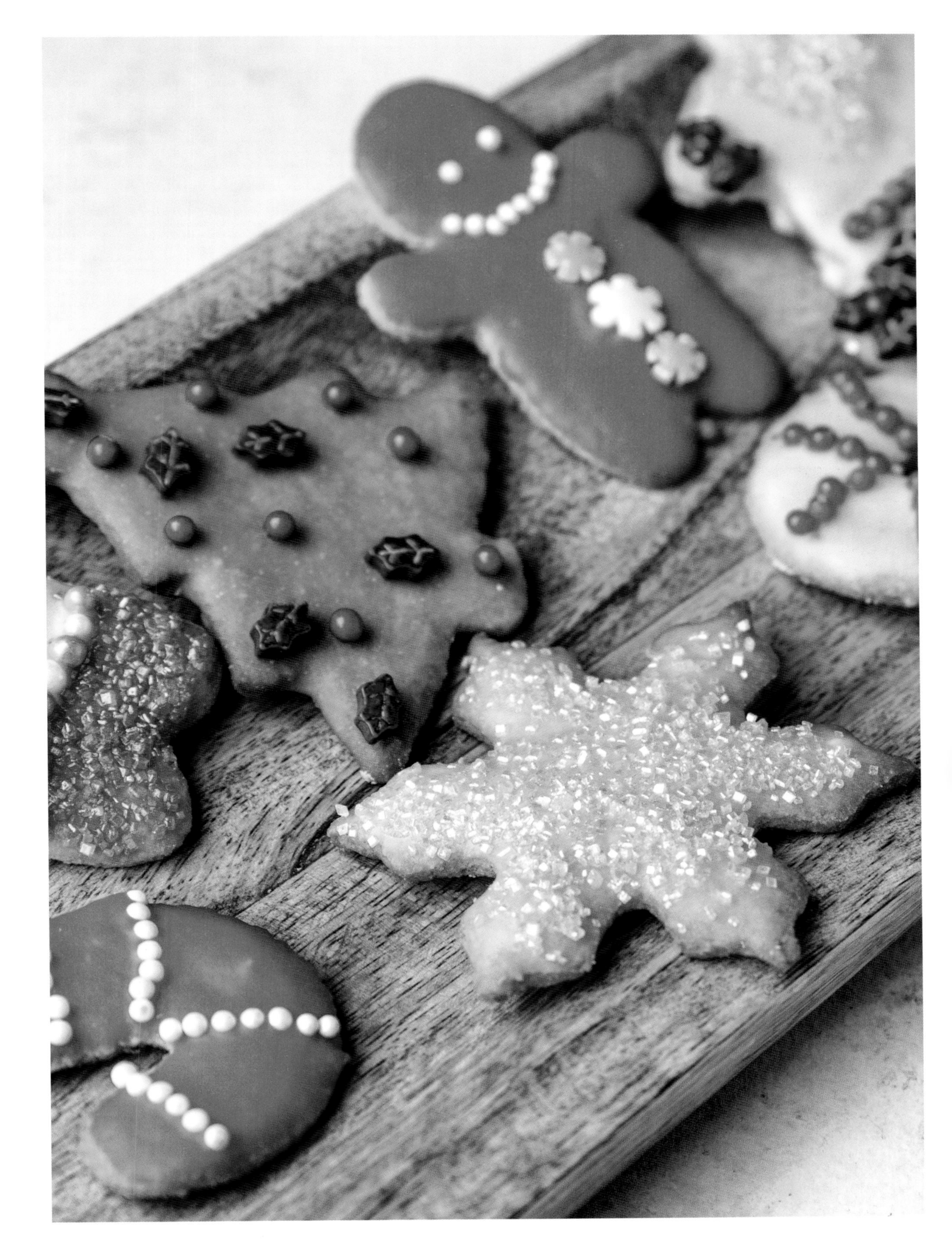

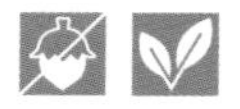

SKILLET CHOCOLATE CHIP COOKIE PIE

YIELD: one 9-inch pie (12 servings)

PREP TIME: 15 minutes

COOK TIME: 40 minutes

I created this recipe after I had made my chocolate chip cookies and thought, "Couldn't I just dump the dough into a skillet and make one big cookie?" Of course, I had to make some adaptations to my chocolate chip cookie recipe to make it denser and more pielike, but it was time well spent. I make this cookie pie for guests all the time, and everyone loves it—the non-keto crowd, too! I like to top it with Hot Fudge Sauce (page 65) and a dollop of Whipped Cream (page 73).

- 3/4 cup (1 1/2 sticks) unsalted butter, softened
- 4 ounces cream cheese (1/2 cup), softened
- 1/2 cup sour cream
- 1 cup (190g) packed Swerve brown sugar sweetener, plus more if desired
- 1/4 cup heavy whipping cream
- 1 teaspoon vanilla extract
- 1/2 teaspoon vanilla-flavored liquid stevia
- 2 large eggs
- 2 cups (240g) sesame flour
- 1 teaspoon xanthan gum
- 1 teaspoon baking powder
- 1 teaspoon fine sea salt
- 1/2 cup sugar-free chocolate chips, store-bought or homemade (page 230)

1. Preheat the oven to 350°F and grease a 9-inch cast-iron skillet.
2. Place the butter, cream cheese, and sour cream in the bowl of a stand mixer (or a large bowl if using an electric hand mixer) and mix until smooth.
3. Add the brown sugar sweetener, cream, vanilla extract, and stevia to the bowl and mix until combined. Taste and add more brown sugar sweetener, if desired.
4. Add the remaining ingredients, except the chocolate chips, and mix until incorporated. Stir in the chocolate chips by hand.
5. Spread the batter in the prepared skillet and bake for 35 to 40 minutes, or until a toothpick inserted in the center comes out clean.
6. Remove from the oven and allow to cool for 20 minutes before slicing and serving.

Cover with aluminum foil and store in the refrigerator for up to 5 days. Reheat in a preheated 350°F oven for 10 minutes or microwave individual pieces for 30 seconds.

calories 266 | fat 23g | protein 9g | total carbs 2g | dietary fiber 1g | net carbs 1g

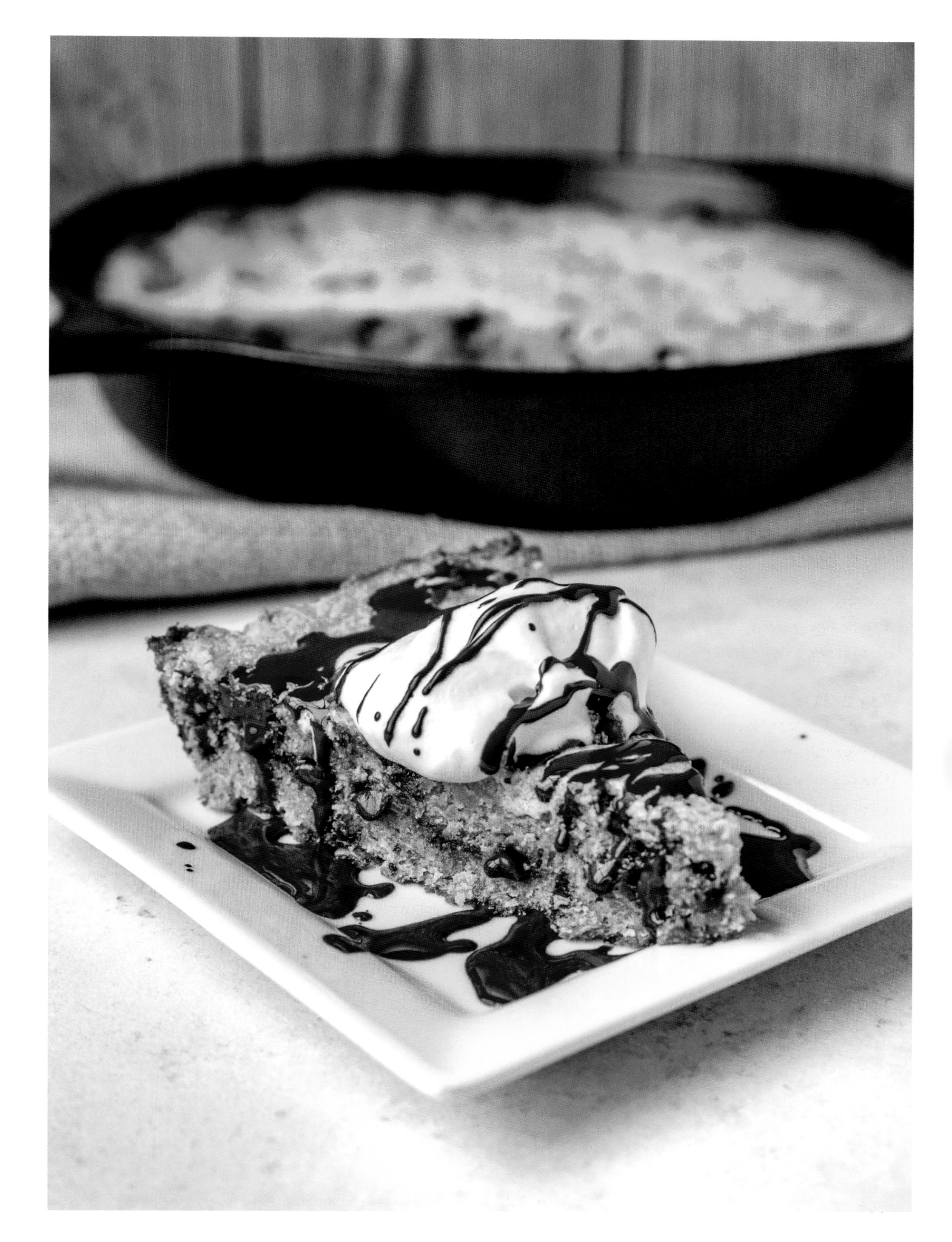

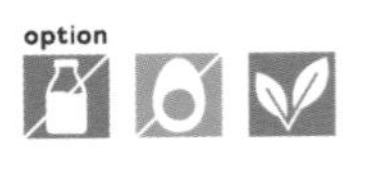

PECAN SNOWBALLS

YIELD: 24 cookies (1 per serving)

PREP TIME: 10 minutes, plus at least 30 minutes to chill

COOK TIME: 15 minutes

This recipe is near and dear to my heart. My grandmother made the traditional white flour version of these cookies all my life. When she passed, I carried on the tradition but made the cookies keto so I could enjoy them forever. My mom has declared these just as good as my grandmother's, and that is priceless!

1/2 cup (1 stick) unsalted butter, softened, or 1/2 cup ghee

1 teaspoon vanilla extract

1/2 teaspoon vanilla-flavored liquid stevia

1 1/2 cups (156g) blanched almond flour

1 cup (120g) raw pecans, chopped

1/2 cup (65g) Swerve confectioners'-style sweetener, plus more to taste if desired and for rolling

1/4 teaspoon fine sea salt

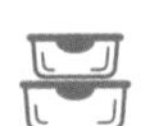
Store in an airtight container. Best if kept refrigerated or frozen; the cookies will keep for up to 2 weeks in the refrigerator or up to 1 month in the freezer.

1. Line a cookie sheet with parchment paper or a silicone baking mat.
2. Place all of the ingredients in a food processor and process until a ball of dough forms. Taste the dough and add more sweetener, if desired.
3. Using a tablespoon-sized cookie scoop, scoop up a mound of dough and roll it into a ball between your palms. Place the ball on the prepared cookie sheet and repeat with the remaining dough, spacing the cookies about 1 inch apart. You should have 24 balls.
4. Place the dough balls in the freezer for 30 minutes to 1 hour, until semi-frozen.
5. Preheat the oven to 350°F.
6. Remove the cookie sheet from the freezer. Bake the cookies for 15 minutes, or until golden around the edges. Set them aside until they are cool enough to handle but still warm.
7. Put a small amount of confectioners'-style sweetener in a small bowl. Roll each cookie in the sweetener, then place on a wire rack to cool completely before serving.

calories **112** | fat **11g** | protein **1g** | total carbs **2g** | dietary fiber **1g** | net carbs **1g**

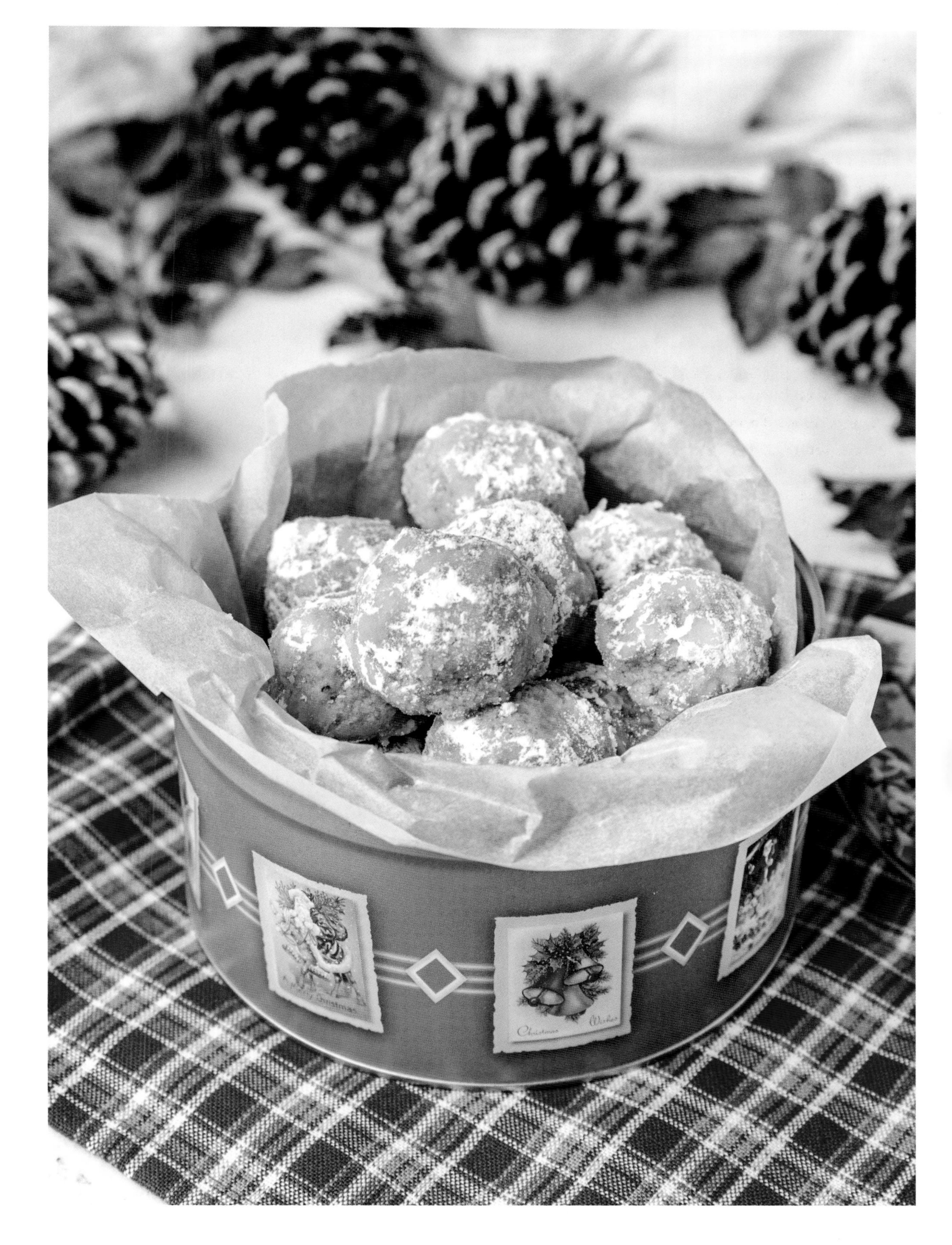
Christmas Wishes

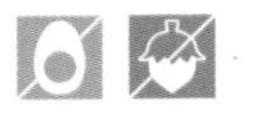

NO-BAKE COFFEE CHEESECAKE

YIELD: one 8-inch cake (12 servings)

PREP TIME: 20 minutes, plus at least 3 hours to chill

I can't deny that I'm a lover of baked keto cheesecakes, but sometimes I want a similar treat that doesn't need to be baked. For those times, this is my go-to recipe. It's always a huge hit!

FOR THE CRUST

- ¾ cup (75g) unsweetened shredded coconut
- ½ cup (80g) raw sunflower seeds
- ¼ cup (½ stick) unsalted butter, room temperature
- ¼ cup (24g) unsweetened cocoa powder
- ¼ cup Swerve confectioners'-style sweetener
- ¼ teaspoon fine sea salt

FOR THE FILLING

- ¾ cup hot strong brewed coffee (decaf or regular)
- 1 tablespoon unflavored gelatin
- 1 cup heavy whipping cream
- 2 (8-ounce) packages cream cheese, softened
- 2 teaspoons coffee extract
- 2 teaspoons vanilla extract
- 2 teaspoons vanilla-flavored liquid stevia
- ¼ teaspoon fine sea salt

FOR THE CHOCOLATE DRIZZLE

- 2 ounces dark chocolate (85% cacao), chopped
- 1 tablespoon coconut oil

SPECIAL EQUIPMENT:

8-inch springform pan

MAKE THE CRUST:

1. Place the coconut and sunflower seeds in a food processor and process until ground. Add the rest of the ingredients for the crust and process until smooth.
2. Grease an 8-inch springform pan or line it with parchment paper. Press the crust mixture into the bottom of the prepared pan. Set aside.

MAKE THE FILLING:

1. Pour the hot coffee into a medium bowl. Sprinkle in the gelatin and stir until dissolved. Set aside to come to room temperature, about 5 minutes.
2. Pour the cream into another bowl and use an electric hand mixer to whip it until stiff peaks form. Set aside.
3. Place the cream cheese in the bowl of a stand mixer (or a large bowl if using the hand mixer) and mix on high until smooth.
4. Add the cooled coffee mixture, extracts, stevia, and salt to the bowl with the cream cheese. Mix on high until incorporated. Fold in the whipped cream until well combined.
5. Pour the filling over the crust. Refrigerate for at least 3 hours or overnight.

MAKE THE CHOCOLATE DRIZZLE:

When ready to serve the cake, place the chocolate and coconut oil in a small microwave-safe bowl and microwave for 30 seconds. Stir until smooth. Remove the outer ring of the springform pan, then drizzle the chocolate over the cheesecake. Slice and serve.

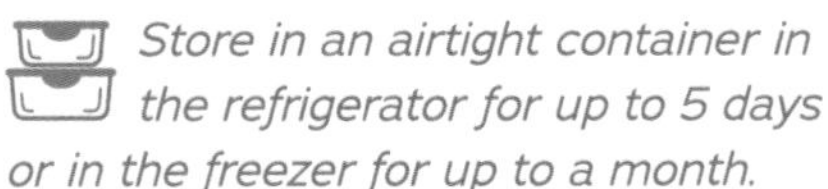

Store in an airtight container in the refrigerator for up to 5 days or in the freezer for up to a month.

calories 337 | fat 32g | protein 5g | total carbs 6g | dietary fiber 2g | net carbs 4g

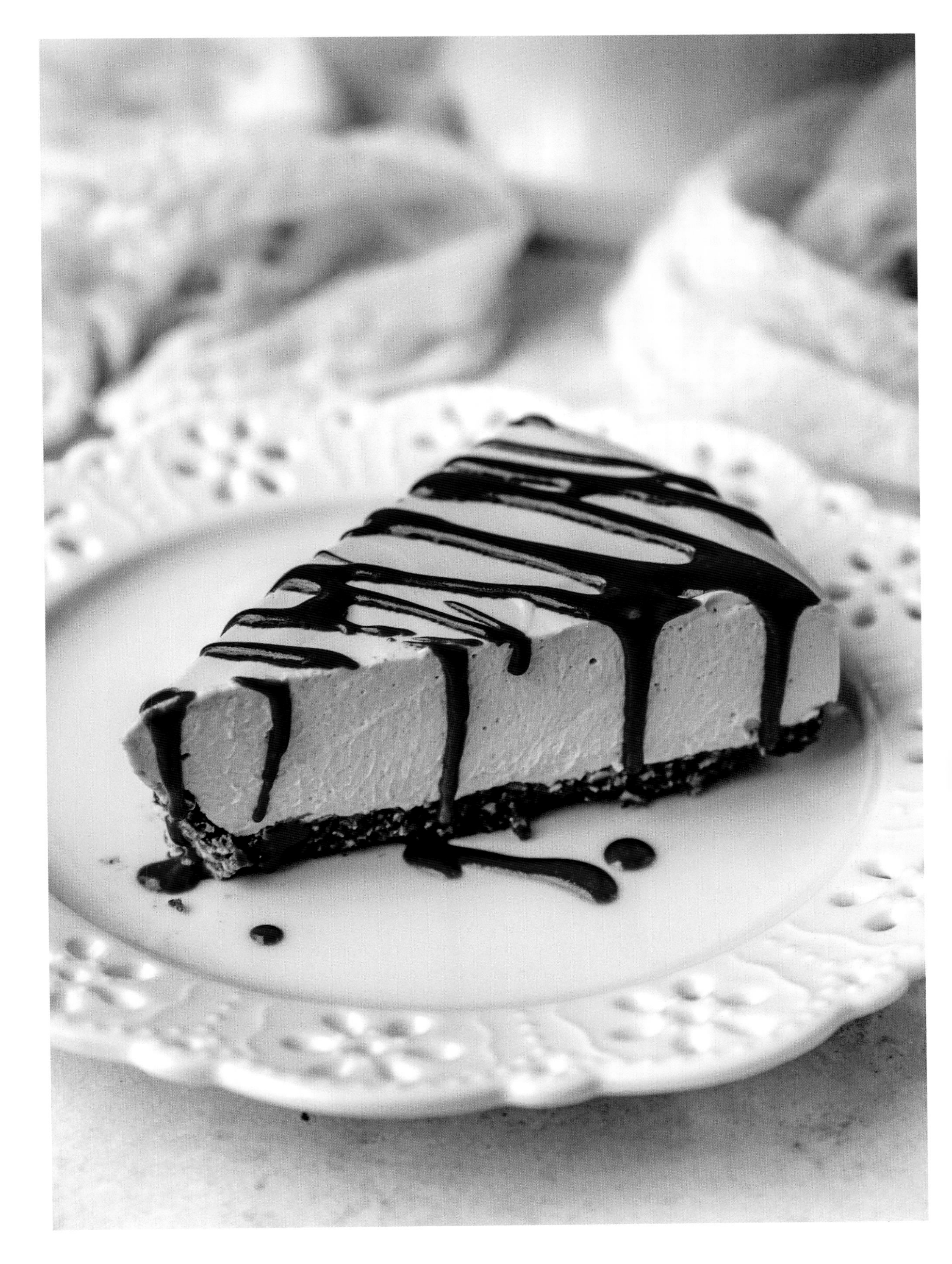

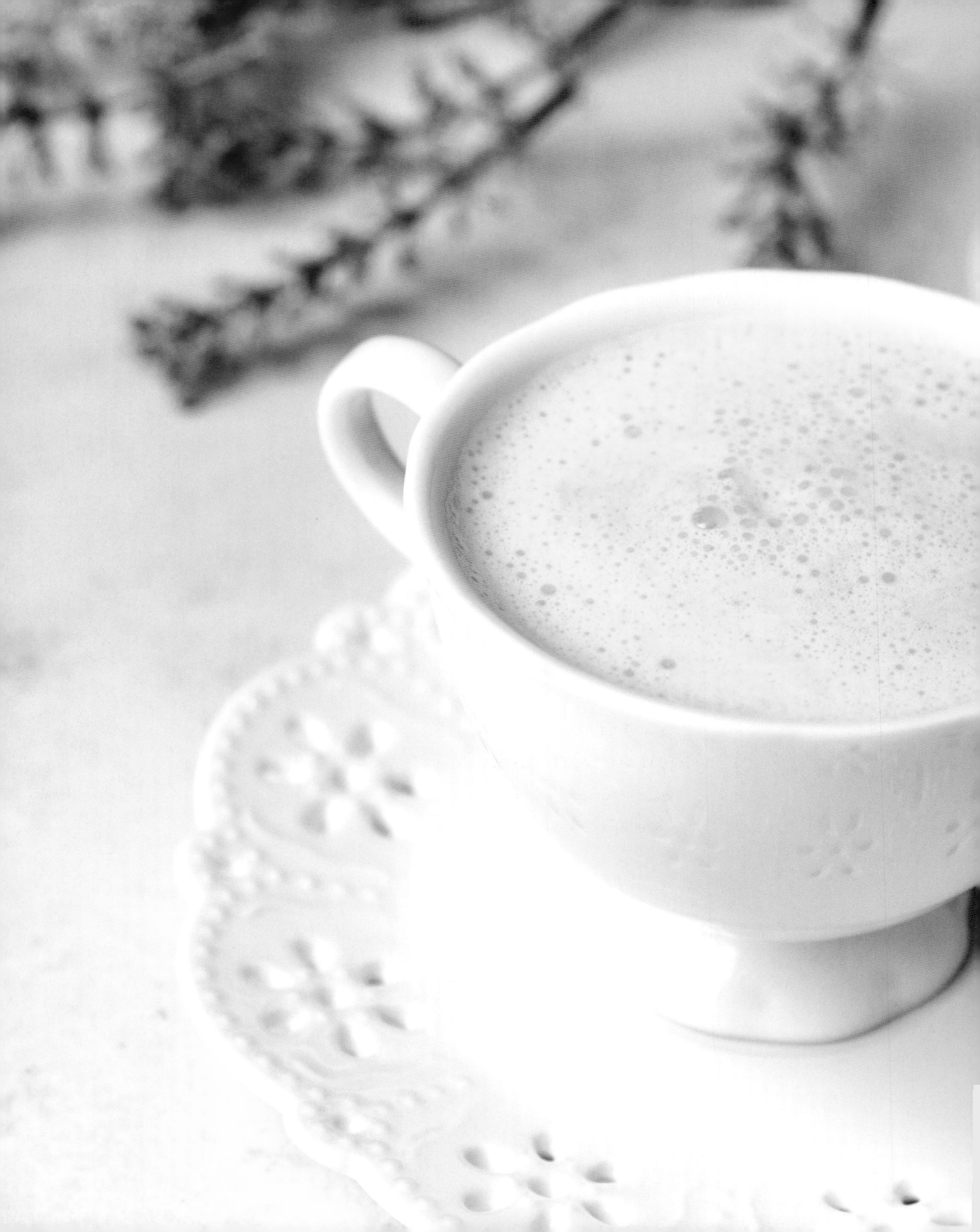

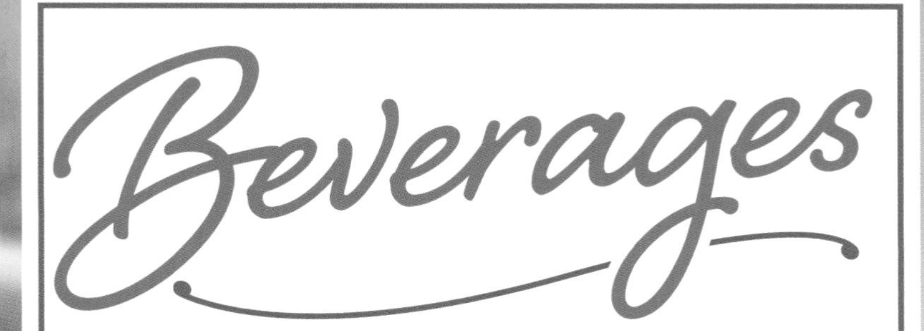

Beverages

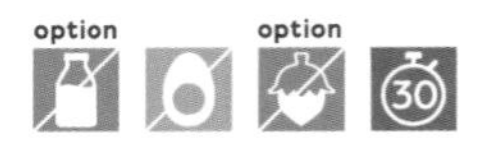

BULLETPROOF HOT CHOCOLATE

YIELD: one 12-ounce serving

PREP TIME: 5 minutes

COOK TIME: 1 minute

Here's a change of pace from coffee in the morning. The MCT oil in this chocolatey drink will give you energy, just as the caffeine in coffee would have done. Who wouldn't want to start the day with a little chocolate?

- 1½ tablespoons unsweetened cocoa powder
- 1 tablespoon collagen peptides
- 1 tablespoon MCT oil, coconut oil, unsalted butter, or ghee (see Note)
- ½ teaspoon chocolate-flavored liquid stevia or other keto sweetener of choice, plus more if desired
- ½ teaspoon ground cinnamon, plus more for topping if desired
- Pinch of fine sea salt
- 1½ cups unsweetened almond milk or coconut milk
- Whipped Cream (page 73) or Coconut Whipped Cream (page 66), for topping (optional)

Note: If you are consuming this drink in the evening, do not use MCT oil, which gives you energy; opt for coconut oil, butter, or ghee instead.

1. Place all of the ingredients except the milk in a blender. Blend on high until combined.

2. Warm the almond milk in a saucepan over low heat or in the microwave.

3. Pour the warmed almond milk into the blender and blend again until combined. Taste and add more sweetener, if desired. Pour into a 12-ounce mug, top with whipped cream and cinnamon, if desired, and enjoy immediately.

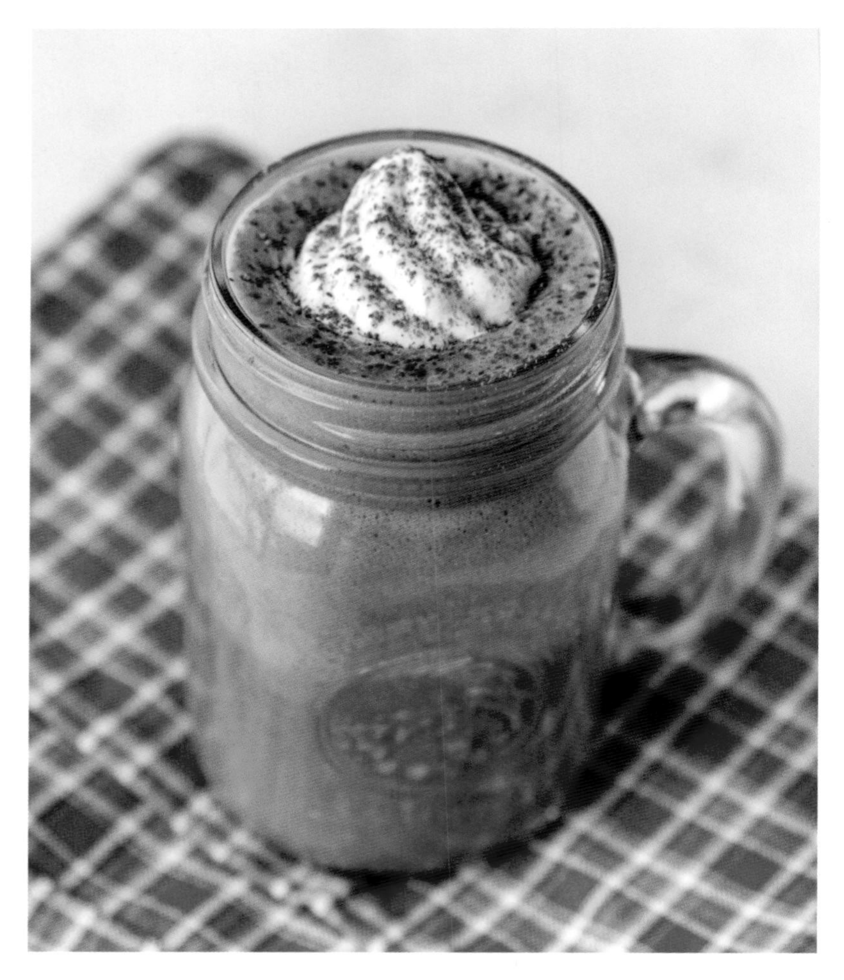

calories 193 | fat 17g | protein 6g | total carbs 7g | dietary fiber 3g | net carbs 4g

ROOT BEER ICE CREAM FLOAT

YIELD: one 12-ounce serving

PREP TIME: 1 minute, plus time for gelato to soften

I shouldn't even call this a recipe because it's so simple. As long as you have keto-friendly ice cream in the freezer and Zevia in the pantry, you can make an ice cream float whenever you want! Because Zevia is all natural with no artificial anything, you won't see any caramel color in this float, but it sure tastes like root beer. The only fat, carbs, and calories come from the ice cream you use. Obviously, I use homemade gelato, but any keto ice cream you like will work.

½ cup Vanilla Gelato (page 254) or store-bought keto vanilla ice cream

1 cup Zevia Ginger Root Beer

Allow the gelato to soften on the counter for 10 to 15 minutes, then scoop ½ cup into a 12-ounce glass. Pour the root beer over the gelato, insert a straw, and enjoy!

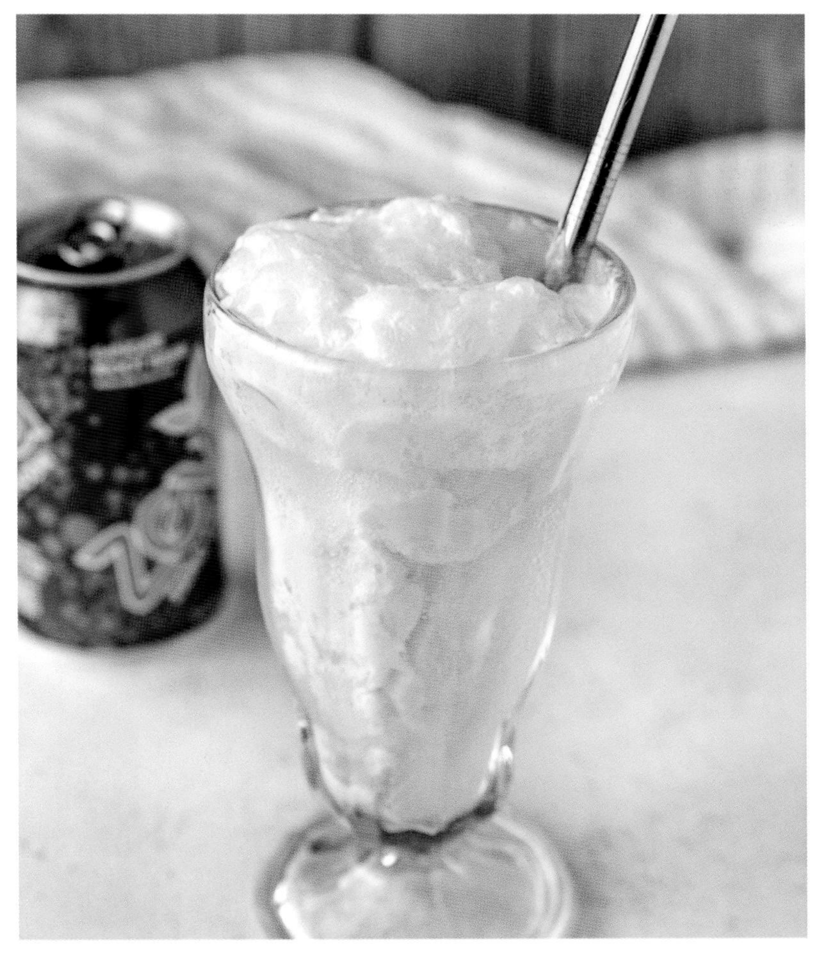

calories 273 | fat 27g | protein 2g | total carbs 2g | dietary fiber 0g | net carbs 2g

LEMON CREAM PIE SMOOTHIE

YIELD: one 14-ounce serving

PREP TIME: 5 minutes

With the amount of healthy fats and about the same amount of protein, this smoothie will keep you full for hours. And it certainly doesn't hurt that it tastes like a lemon cream pie!

- ½ cup ice
- 1 cup unsweetened almond milk
- 1 scoop vanilla-flavored whey protein powder
- 2 tablespoons heavy whipping cream or coconut cream
- 1 tablespoon hemp hearts
- 1 tablespoon coconut butter
- 2 teaspoons freshly squeezed lemon juice
- ½ teaspoon lemon-flavored liquid stevia or other keto sweetener of choice, plus more if desired
- ¼ teaspoon xanthan gum (optional, for thickening)
- Grated lemon zest, for garnish (optional)

Place all of the ingredients in a blender and blend on high until smooth. Taste and add more sweetener, if desired. Pour into a 14-ounce glass, garnish with lemon zest, if desired, and enjoy!

Make-ahead tip: Place all of the ingredients, except the ice, in a blender. Cover with the lid and store in the refrigerator. In the morning, add the ice, blend, and enjoy!

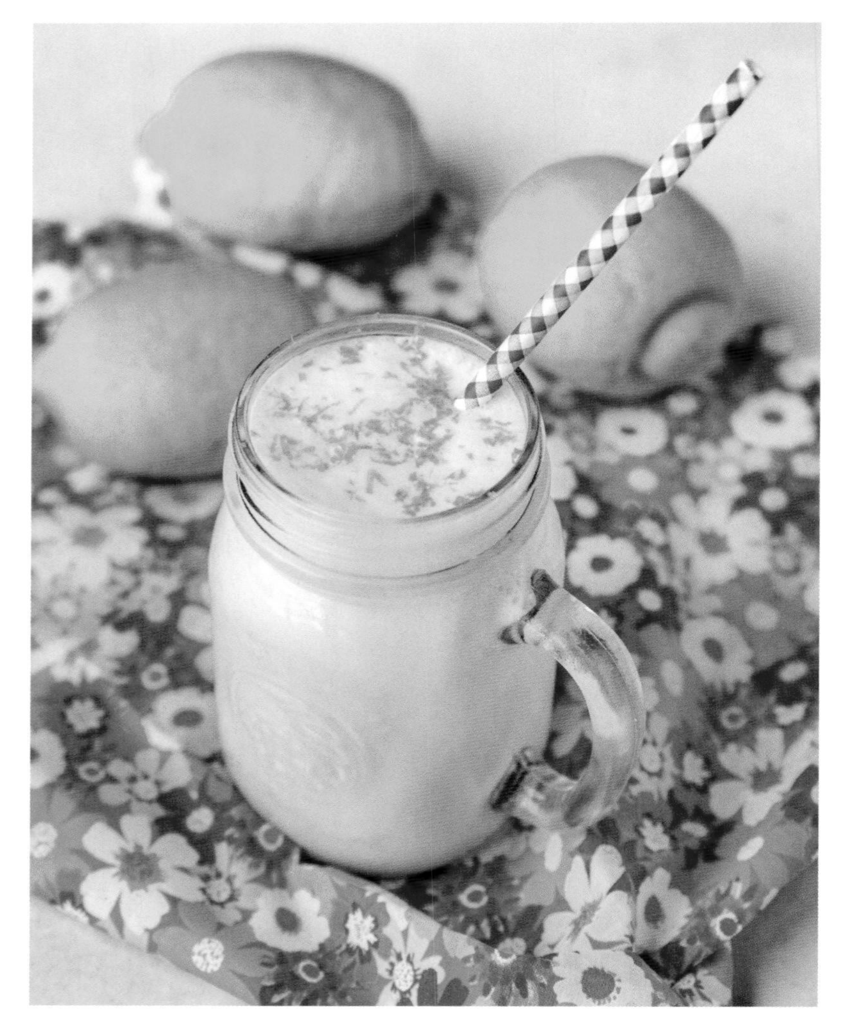

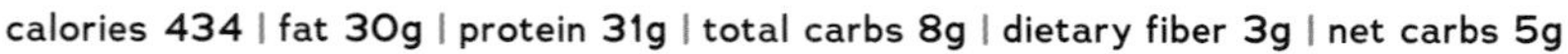

calories 434 | fat 30g | protein 31g | total carbs 8g | dietary fiber 3g | net carbs 5g

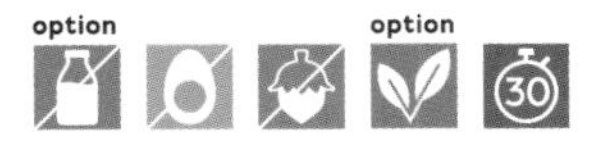

ICED BULLETPROOF MOCHA FRAPPÉ

YIELD: one 16-ounce serving

PREP TIME: 5 minutes (not including time to brew coffee)

When you want a little more kick in your coffee and a bit of chocolatey taste, too!

- 1/2 cup ice
- 1 1/2 cups brewed coffee (decaf or regular), chilled
- 2 tablespoons heavy whipping cream or coconut cream
- 1 scoop collagen peptides (optional; omit for vegetarian)
- 1 tablespoon unsweetened cocoa powder
- 1 tablespoon MCT oil or coconut oil
- 1/2 teaspoon coffee extract
- 1/2 teaspoon chocolate-flavored liquid stevia or other keto sweetener of choice, plus more if desired
- 1/4 teaspoon xanthan gum (optional, for thickening)
- 1/8 teaspoon fine sea salt

Place all of the ingredients in a blender and blend on high until smooth. Taste and add more sweetener, if desired. Pour into a 16-ounce glass or mug and enjoy!

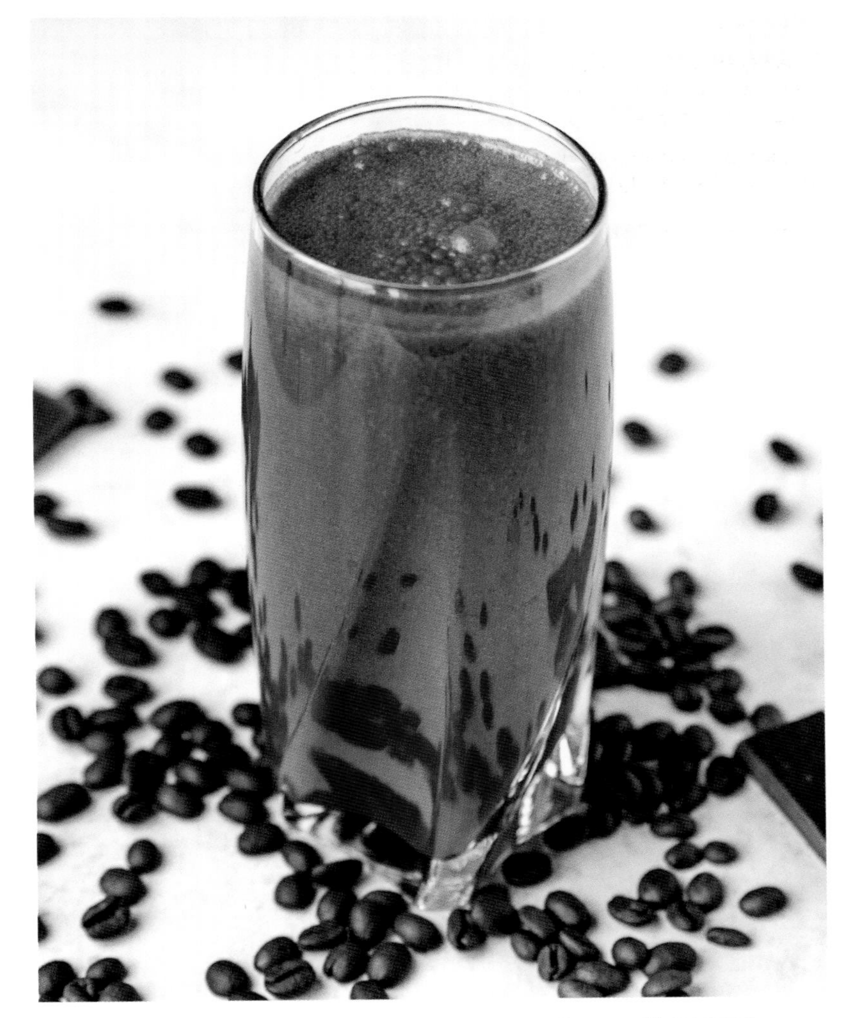

calories 239 | fat 25g | protein 1g | total carbs 3g | dietary fiber 1g | net carbs 2g

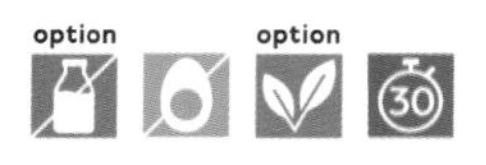

CHOCOLATE SEA SALT SMOOTHIE

YIELD: one 12-ounce serving

PREP TIME: 5 minutes

This smoothie has it all. A little bit sweet and a little bit salty, it's also creamy and smooth, with good fats in there to help keep you full!

- ½ cup ice
- 1 cup unsweetened almond milk
- 1 scoop collagen peptides or unflavored whey protein powder
- 1 tablespoon unsweetened cocoa powder
- 1 tablespoon hemp hearts
- 1 tablespoon unsweetened almond butter
- ½ teaspoon coarse sea salt
- ½ teaspoon unflavored liquid stevia or other keto sweetener of choice, plus more if desired
- ¼ teaspoon xanthan gum (optional, for thickening)
- Dark chocolate shavings, for topping (optional)

Place all of the ingredients in a blender and blend on high until smooth. Taste and add more sweetener, if desired. Pour into a 12-ounce glass, garnish with chocolate shavings, if desired, and enjoy!

Make-ahead tip: Place all of the ingredients, except the ice, in a blender. Cover with the lid and refrigerate overnight. In the morning, just add the ice and blend it up for an on-the-go breakfast!

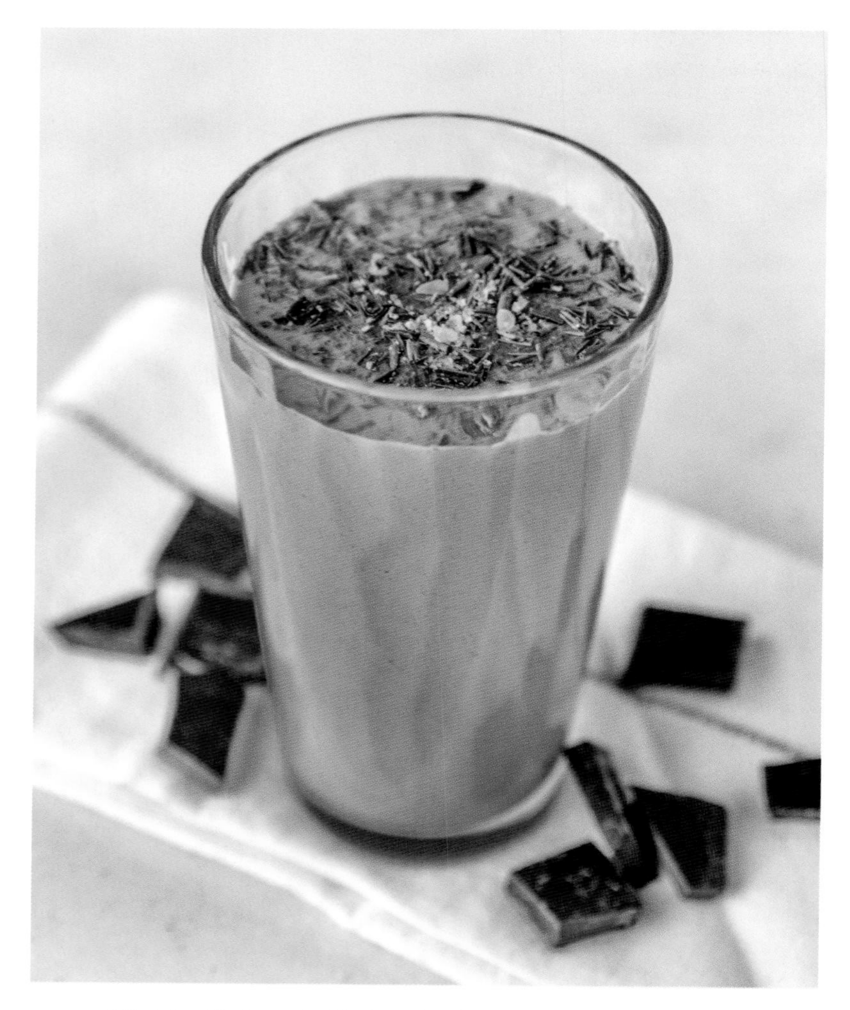

calories 254 | fat 18g | protein 19g | total carbs 8g | dietary fiber 3g | net carbs 5g

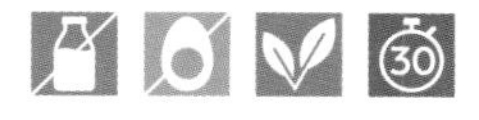

CARAMEL LATTE

YIELD: one 8-ounce serving

PREP TIME: 5 minutes (not including time to brew coffee)

When you want dessert *and* coffee, this drink will do!

1 cup hot brewed coffee (decaf or regular)

2 tablespoons sugar-free maple syrup, store-bought or homemade (page 70)

2 tablespoons unsweetened almond milk

1 tablespoon Swerve brown sugar sweetener, plus more for sprinkling if desired

1/2 teaspoon caramel extract

Coconut Whipped Cream (page 66), for topping (optional)

Place all of the ingredients except the whipped cream in a blender and blend on high until smooth. Pour into an 8-ounce mug. Top with whipped cream and a sprinkle of brown sugar sweetener, if desired.

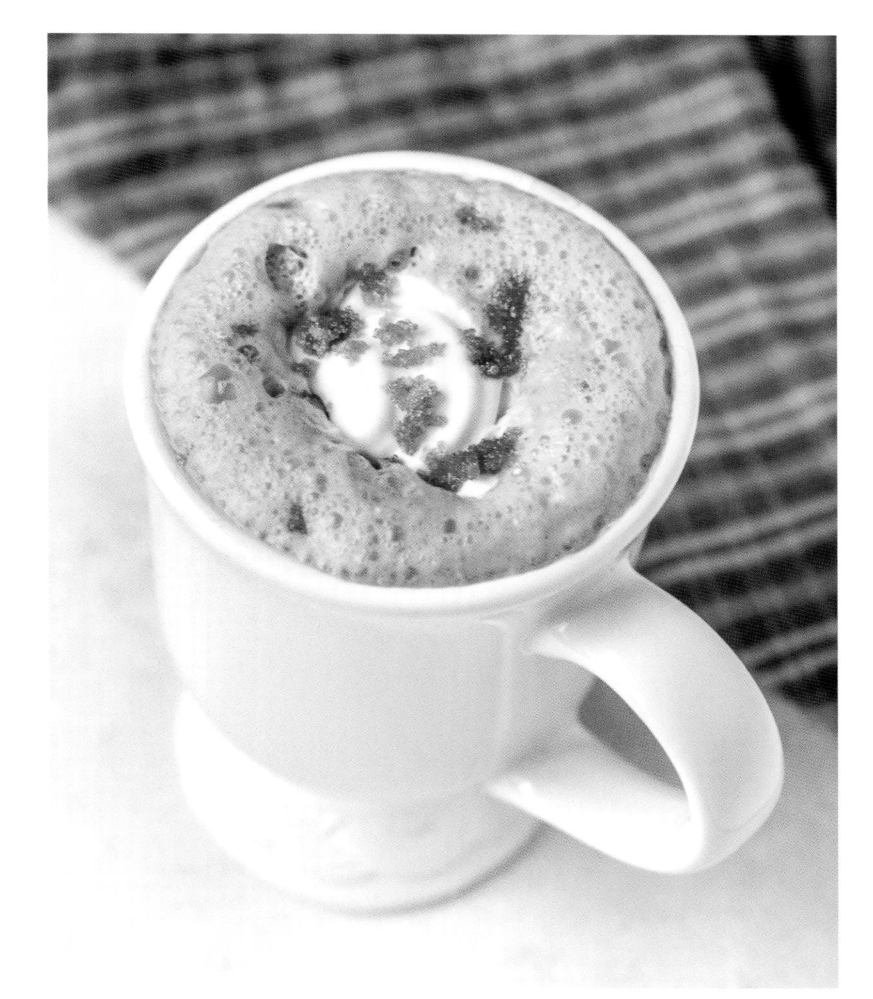

calories 21 | fat 1.4g | protein 0.2g | total carbs 1.2g | dietary fiber 0.1g | net carbs 1.1g

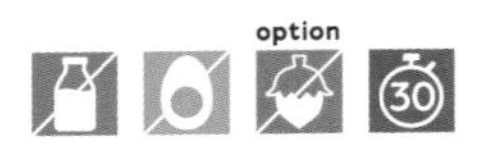

VANILLA TURMERIC GOLDEN MILK

YIELD: one 12-ounce serving

PREP TIME: 5 minutes

COOK TIME: 5 minutes

Turmeric, a flowering plant from the ginger family, has anti-inflammatory properties and strong antioxidants. Its main active ingredient is curcumin. Unfortunately, curcumin is not easily absorbed into the bloodstream, but consuming black pepper in combination with turmeric helps enhance its absorption. This warm golden milk is a soothing beverage to enjoy before bed.

1½ cups unsweetened almond milk or coconut milk

1 scoop collagen peptides

1 tablespoon ghee or coconut oil

½ teaspoon turmeric powder (see Note)

½ teaspoon vanilla extract

¼ teaspoon vanilla-flavored liquid stevia (optional)

¼ teaspoon ginger powder

⅛ teaspoon freshly ground black pepper

Pinch of fine sea salt

Note: Wash the saucepan and blender immediately after using them for this recipe. Turmeric can stain!

Place all of the ingredients in a small saucepan over medium heat. Stir and bring to a simmer, then remove from the heat. Use an immersion blender or transfer the mixture to a countertop blender and blend. Pour into a 12-ounce mug and enjoy!

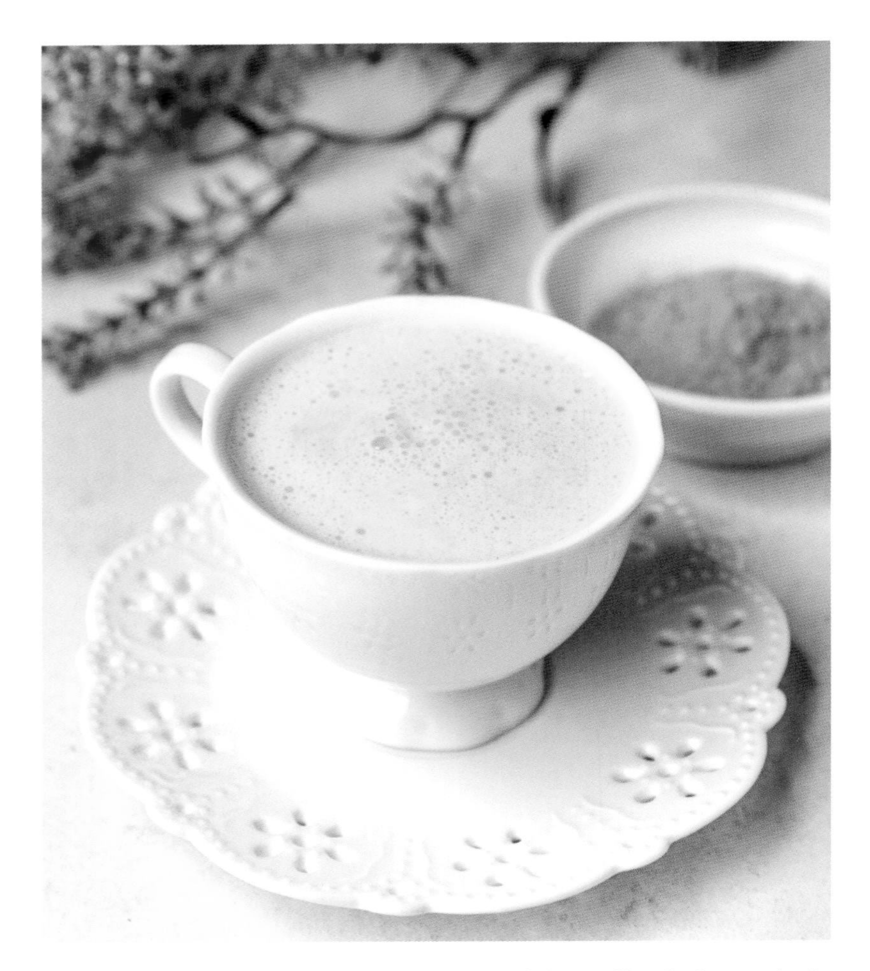

calories 214 | fat 18g | protein 9g | total carbs 2g | dietary fiber 0g | net carbs 2g

ICED COFFEE VANILLA FRAPPÉ

YIELD: one 18-ounce serving

PREP TIME: 2 minutes (not including time to brew coffee)

This is just a simple creamy vanilla coffee frappé, especially delicious in the summer!

- 1/2 cup ice
- 1 1/2 cups brewed coffee (decaf or regular), chilled
- 1/4 cup unsweetened almond milk
- 1/4 cup heavy whipping cream or coconut cream
- 1 teaspoon vanilla extract
- 1/4 teaspoon vanilla-flavored liquid stevia or other keto sweetener of choice, plus more if desired
- Whipped Cream (page 73) or Coconut Whipped Cream (page 66), for topping (optional)

Place all of the ingredients in a blender and blend on high until smooth. Taste and add more sweetener, if desired. Pour into a large glass or mug, top with whipped cream, if desired, and enjoy!

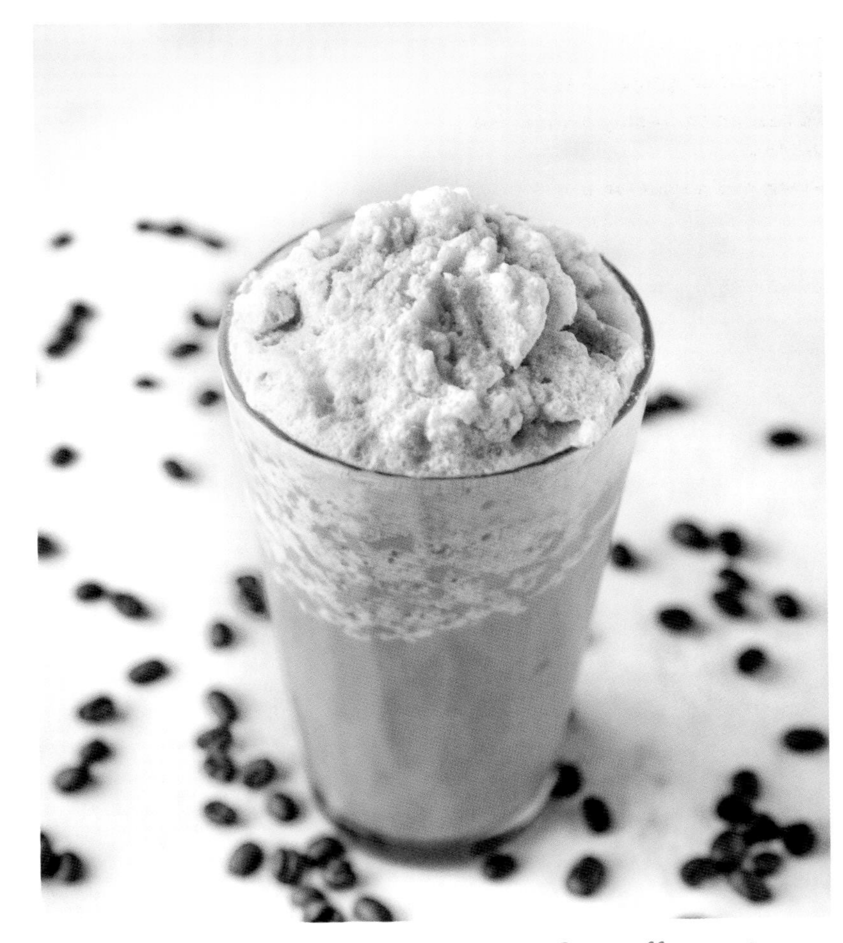

calories 221 | fat 20g | protein 0g | total carbs 1g | dietary fiber 0g | net carbs 1g

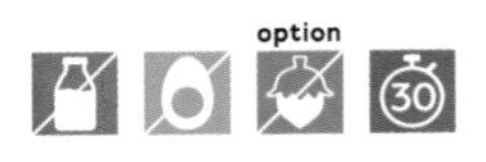

CREAMY PB&J SMOOTHIE

YIELD: one 8-ounce serving

PREP TIME: 5 minutes

A fat bomb in smoothie form—quick, tasty, and filling!

1 cup unsweetened almond milk or coconut milk

2 ounces frozen strawberries (see Tip)

1 scoop collagen peptides

1 tablespoon unsweetened smooth peanut butter or sunflower seed butter, plus more for topping if desired

Keto sweetener of choice, to taste (optional)

Coconut Whipped Cream (page 66), for topping (optional)

Tip: Using frozen strawberries gives you a nice cold smoothie without watering it down with ice. If you don't have frozen strawberries on hand, use fresh and add ½ cup ice.

Place the milk, strawberries, collagen peptides, and peanut butter in a blender and blend on high until smooth. Taste and add sweetener, if desired. Pour into an 8-ounce glass, top with whipped cream and additional peanut butter, if desired, and enjoy!

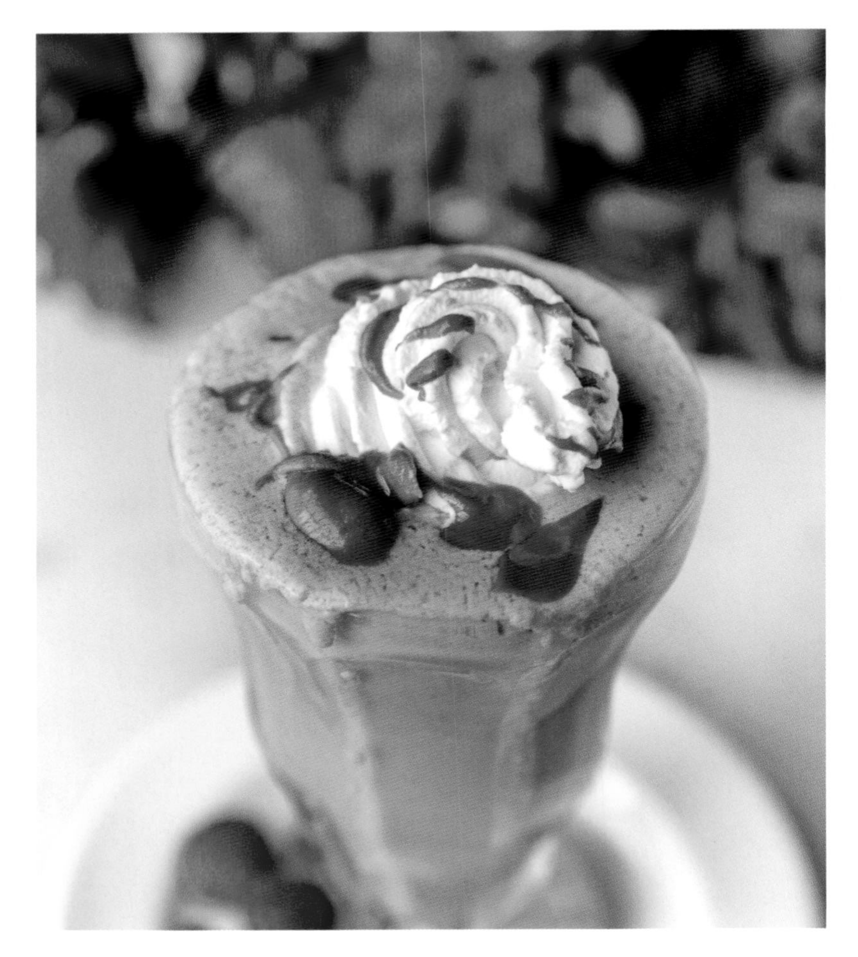

calories 143 | fat 10g | protein 4g | total carbs 8g | dietary fiber 2g | net carbs 6g

VANILLA SPICE DESSERT TEA

YIELD: one 8-ounce serving

PREP TIME: 5 minutes

COOK TIME: 3 minutes

This recipe is for all of the tea lovers! If you choose to enjoy this tea in the morning rather than in the evening, swap the heavy whipping cream with some MCT oil for an added energy boost.

1 cup boiling water

1 vanilla spice tea bag

1 tablespoon salted butter or ghee

1 tablespoon heavy whipping cream or coconut cream

¼ teaspoon vanilla-flavored liquid stevia, plus more if desired

¼ teaspoon ground cardamom

¼ teaspoon ground cinnamon

Pinch of fine sea salt

1. Pour the boiling water into an 8-ounce mug. Insert the tea bag and let it steep for 3 minutes, then remove and discard the bag.

2. Place the tea and the remaining ingredients in a blender and blend until combined. Taste and add more sweetener, if desired. Pour back into the mug and enjoy!

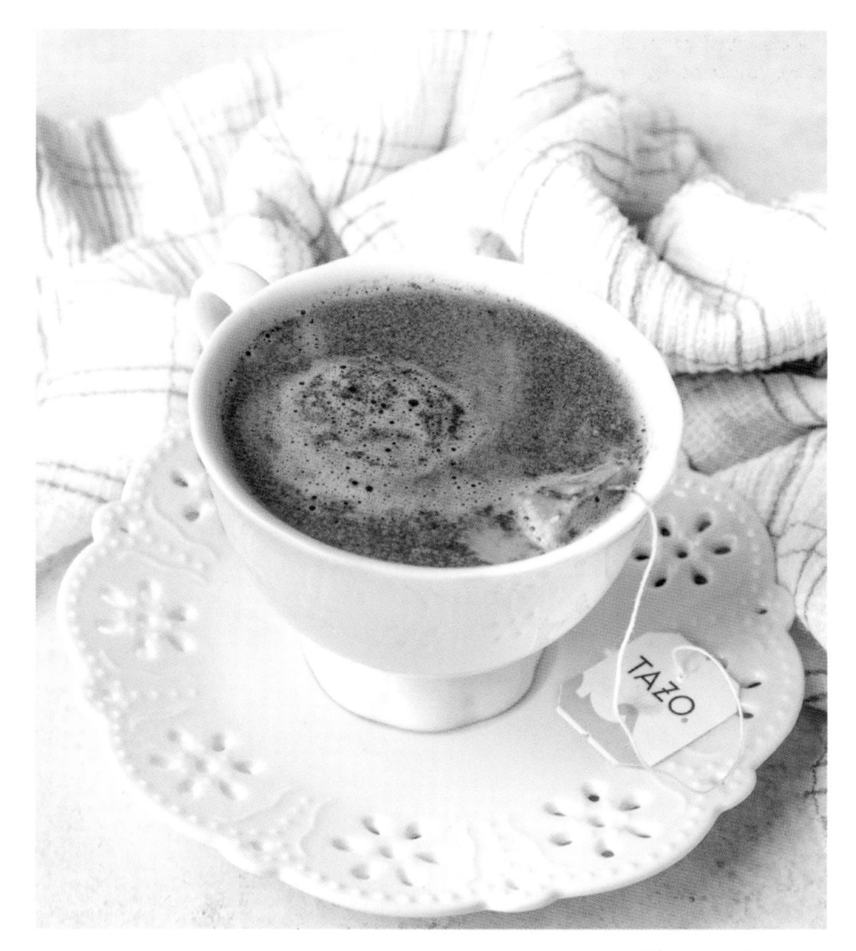

calories 155 | fat 16g | protein 0g | total carbs 1g | dietary fiber 0g | net carbs 1g

Part 3

MEAL PLANS AND SHOPPING LISTS

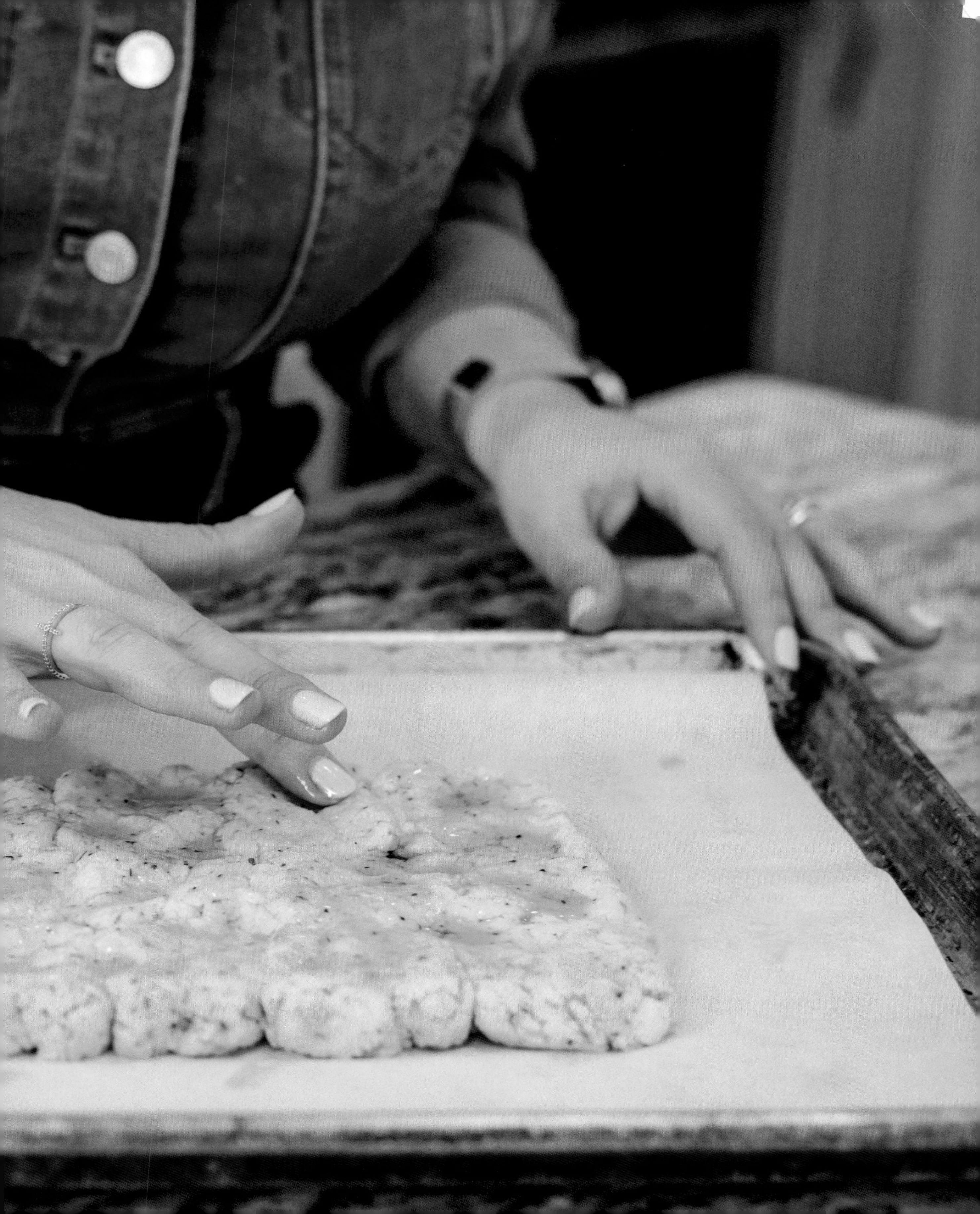

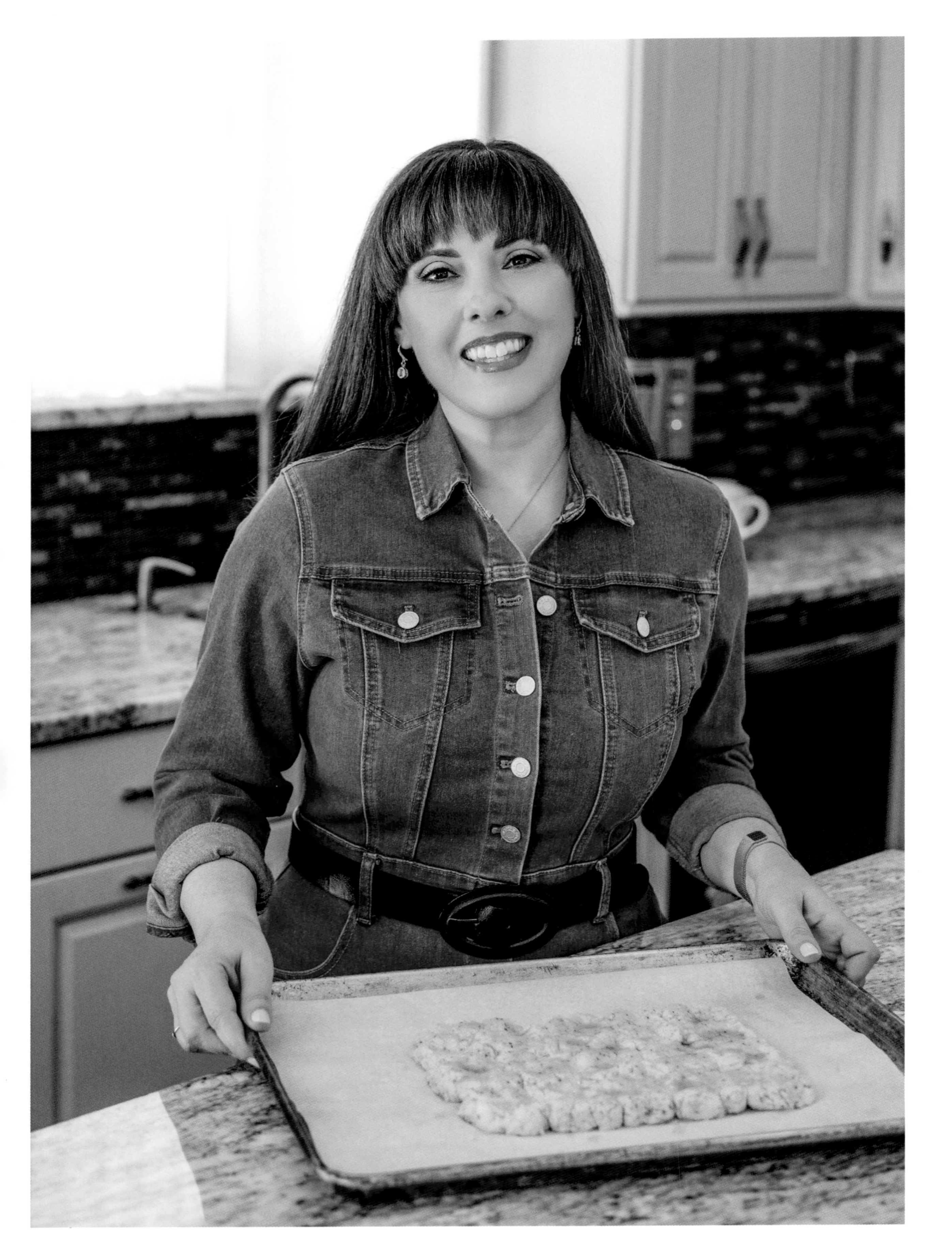

MEAL PLANS

Meal planning makes life a whole lot easier and less stressful, especially if you have children to feed. The four weekly meal plans that follow are based on the assumption you are feeding yourself breakfast and lunch and then feeding a family of four for dinner each night, with leftovers to use for lunches the next day. Most of the dinner recipes make eight servings, with the exception of the Bacon Cheeseburger Sloppy Joes, which serves ten, and the Instant Pot (or Slow Cooker) Chili, which serves twelve. If your family isn't big on leftovers, I suggest freezing soups and casseroles to use later in the month. Recipes that can be frozen are indicated in the storage instructions. Breakfast and lunches are meant for serving just yourself, but like I said, there should be enough leftovers to feed your spouse and/or children, too.

These meals are family-friendly and make following this way of eating more sustainable, especially if you are the only one on a keto diet. When you don't have to cook two different meals for yourself and your family, that's a win in my book!

Dessert is optional; include it or omit it as you see fit. If you feel that dessert will just trigger you to eat too much and not the suggested serving size, then skip it. Making the desserts on the weekend for the week ahead ensures that you will have something to enjoy when a craving hits. Also, you will notice after the first week, dessert is not included every night. Refraining from a sweet treat or the expectation of a sweet treat, even a keto one, every night is a good habit to break free from. Feel free to enjoy one of my nighttime beverages, like my Vanilla Turmeric Golden Milk or Vanilla Spice Dessert Tea, instead of the desserts listed. Please note, though, that all nutrition information is calculated with exactly what is listed for the day, including desserts.

In the first two weeks of meal plans, net carbs are no more than 25 grams, but the last two weeks transition to counting total carbs instead of net carbs, which may help you be more successful with your goals. Since dairy can be a major problem for some people, causing stalls, Week 4 is dairy-free.

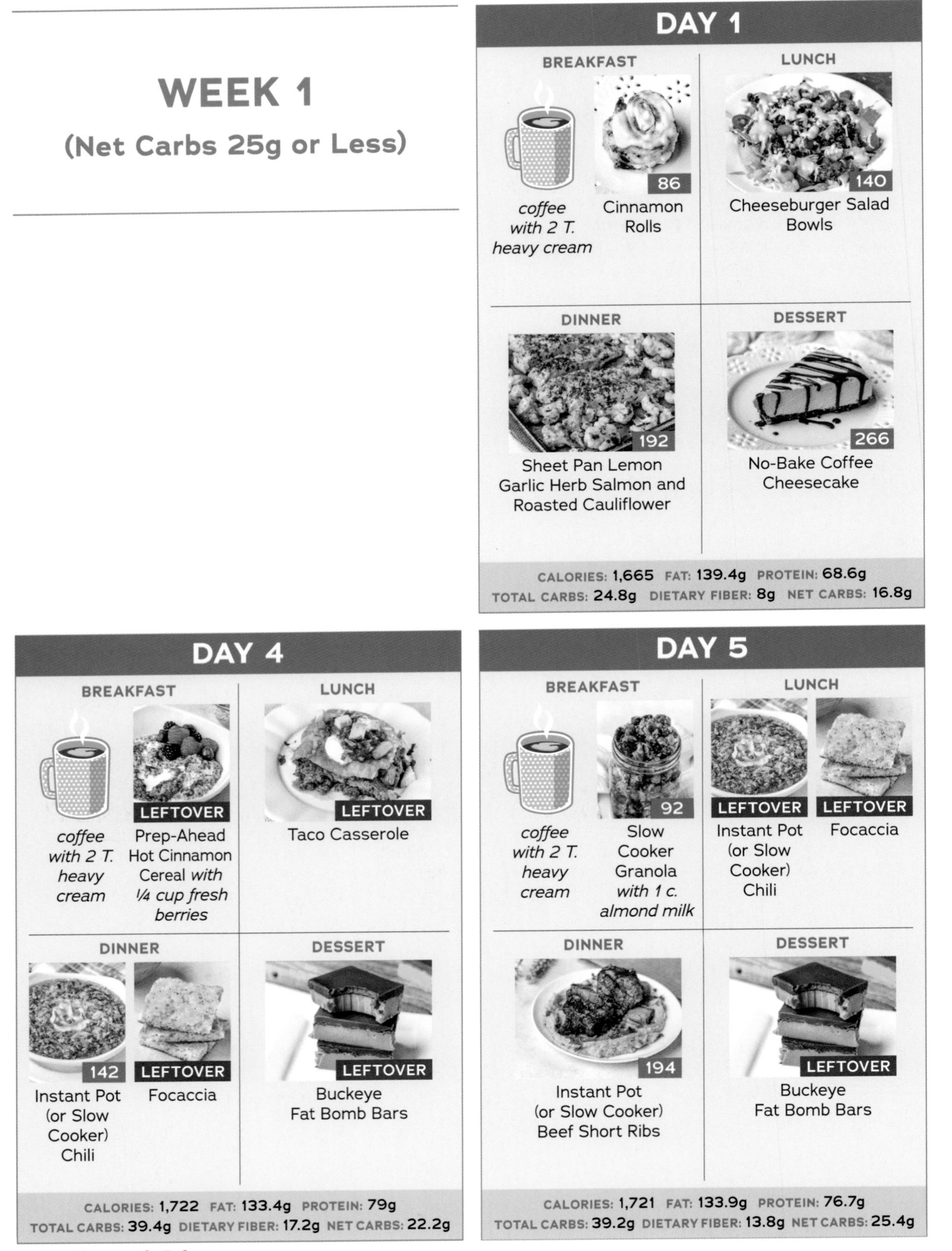

WEEK 1

(Net Carbs 25g or Less)

DAY 1

BREAKFAST

coffee with 2 T. heavy cream

86 — Cinnamon Rolls

LUNCH

140 — Cheeseburger Salad Bowls

DINNER

192 — Sheet Pan Lemon Garlic Herb Salmon and Roasted Cauliflower

DESSERT

266 — No-Bake Coffee Cheesecake

CALORIES: 1,665 **FAT:** 139.4g **PROTEIN:** 68.6g
TOTAL CARBS: 24.8g **DIETARY FIBER:** 8g **NET CARBS:** 16.8g

DAY 4

BREAKFAST

coffee with 2 T. heavy cream

LEFTOVER — Prep-Ahead Hot Cinnamon Cereal *with ¼ cup fresh berries*

LUNCH

LEFTOVER — Taco Casserole

DINNER

142 — Instant Pot (or Slow Cooker) Chili

LEFTOVER — Focaccia

DESSERT

LEFTOVER — Buckeye Fat Bomb Bars

CALORIES: 1,722 **FAT:** 133.4g **PROTEIN:** 79g
TOTAL CARBS: 39.4g **DIETARY FIBER:** 17.2g **NET CARBS:** 22.2g

DAY 5

BREAKFAST

coffee with 2 T. heavy cream

92 — Slow Cooker Granola *with 1 c. almond milk*

LUNCH

LEFTOVER — Instant Pot (or Slow Cooker) Chili

LEFTOVER — Focaccia

DINNER

194 — Instant Pot (or Slow Cooker) Beef Short Ribs

DESSERT

LEFTOVER — Buckeye Fat Bomb Bars

CALORIES: 1,721 **FAT:** 133.9g **PROTEIN:** 76.7g
TOTAL CARBS: 39.2g **DIETARY FIBER:** 13.8g **NET CARBS:** 25.4g

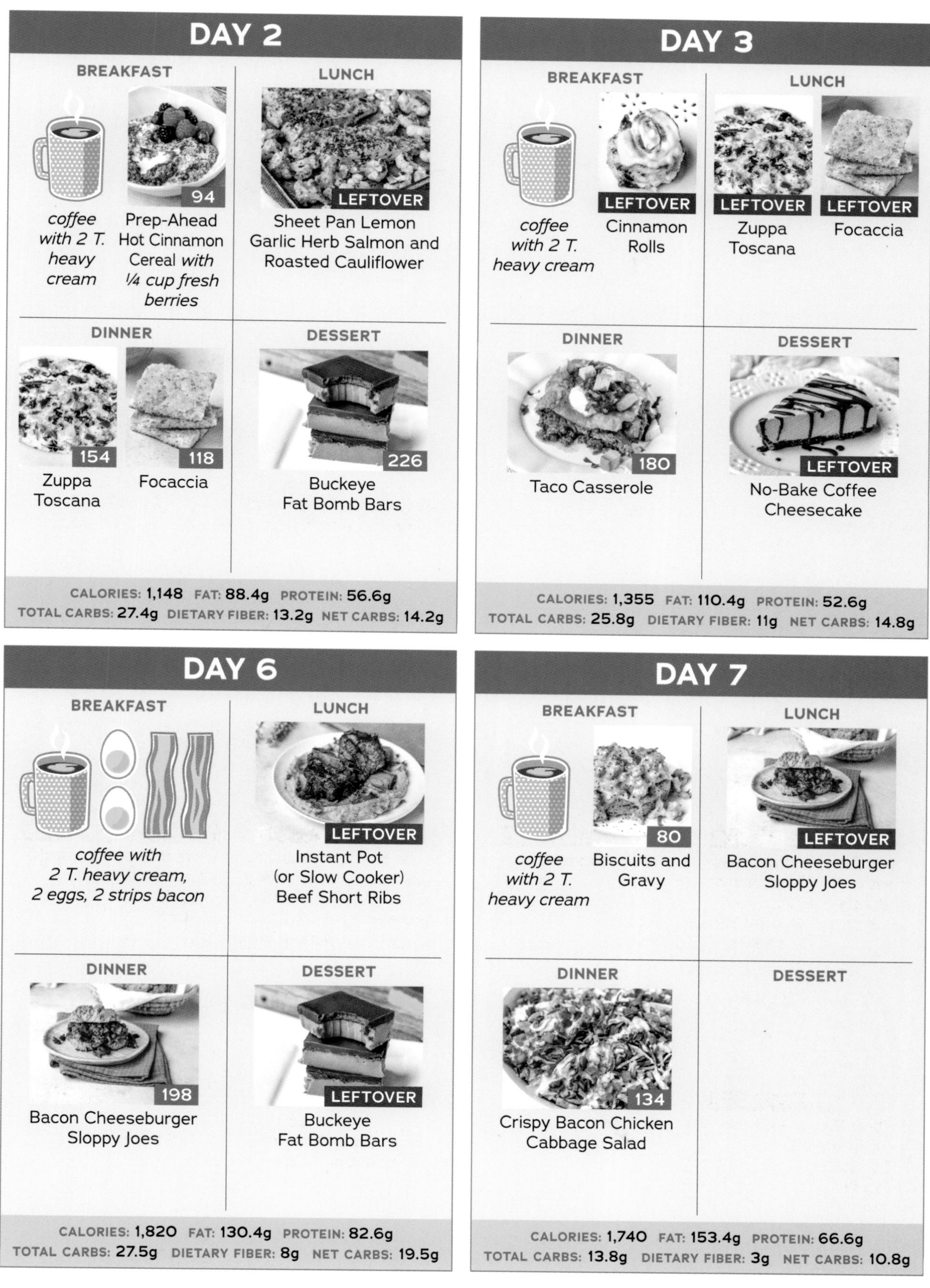
DAY 2
BREAKFAST
94
coffee with 2 T. heavy cream
Prep-Ahead Hot Cinnamon Cereal with 1/4 cup fresh berries
LUNCH
LEFTOVER
Sheet Pan Lemon Garlic Herb Salmon and Roasted Cauliflower
DINNER
154
118
Zuppa Toscana
Focaccia
DESSERT
226
Buckeye Fat Bomb Bars
CALORIES: 1,148 FAT: 88.4g PROTEIN: 56.6g
TOTAL CARBS: 27.4g DIETARY FIBER: 13.2g NET CARBS: 14.2g
DAY 3
BREAKFAST
LEFTOVER
coffee with 2 T. heavy cream
Cinnamon Rolls
LUNCH
LEFTOVER
LEFTOVER
Zuppa Toscana
Focaccia
DINNER
180
Taco Casserole
DESSERT
LEFTOVER
No-Bake Coffee Cheesecake
CALORIES: 1,355 FAT: 110.4g PROTEIN: 52.6g
TOTAL CARBS: 25.8g DIETARY FIBER: 11g NET CARBS: 14.8g
DAY 6
BREAKFAST
coffee with 2 T. heavy cream, 2 eggs, 2 strips bacon
LUNCH
LEFTOVER
Instant Pot (or Slow Cooker) Beef Short Ribs
DINNER
198
Bacon Cheeseburger Sloppy Joes
DESSERT
LEFTOVER
Buckeye Fat Bomb Bars
CALORIES: 1,820 FAT: 130.4g PROTEIN: 82.6g
TOTAL CARBS: 27.5g DIETARY FIBER: 8g NET CARBS: 19.5g
DAY 7
BREAKFAST
80
coffee with 2 T. heavy cream
Biscuits and Gravy
LUNCH
LEFTOVER
Bacon Cheeseburger Sloppy Joes
DINNER
134
Crispy Bacon Chicken Cabbage Salad
DESSERT
CALORIES: 1,740 FAT: 153.4g PROTEIN: 66.6g
TOTAL CARBS: 13.8g DIETARY FIBER: 3g NET CARBS: 10.8g

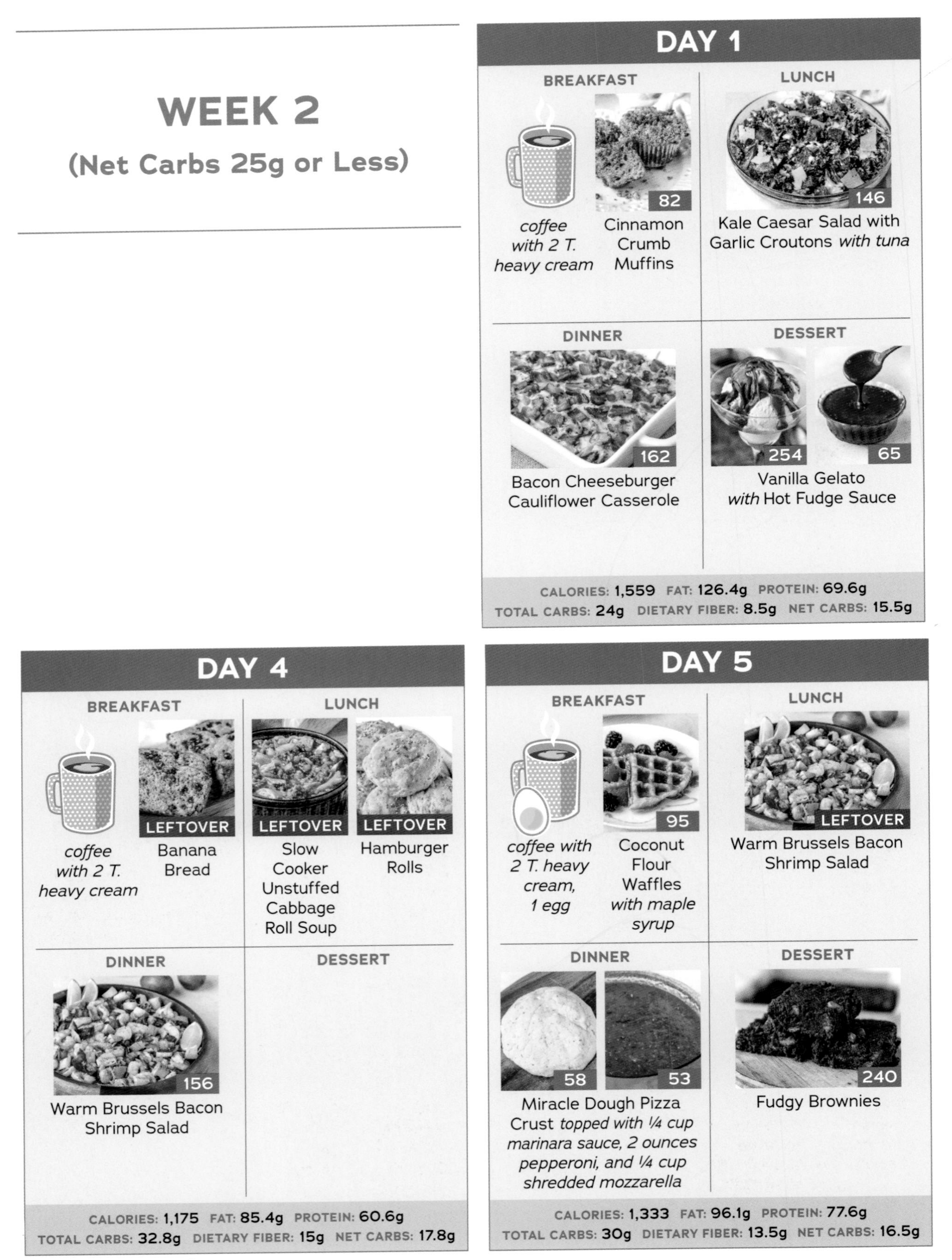

WEEK 2

(Net Carbs 25g or Less)

DAY 1

BREAKFAST

coffee with 2 T. heavy cream

82 Cinnamon Crumb Muffins

LUNCH

146 Kale Caesar Salad with Garlic Croutons *with tuna*

DINNER

162 Bacon Cheeseburger Cauliflower Casserole

DESSERT

254 Vanilla Gelato *with* 65 Hot Fudge Sauce

CALORIES: 1,559 FAT: 126.4g PROTEIN: 69.6g
TOTAL CARBS: 24g DIETARY FIBER: 8.5g NET CARBS: 15.5g

DAY 4

BREAKFAST

coffee with 2 T. heavy cream

LEFTOVER Banana Bread

LUNCH

LEFTOVER Slow Cooker Unstuffed Cabbage Roll Soup

LEFTOVER Hamburger Rolls

DINNER

156 Warm Brussels Bacon Shrimp Salad

DESSERT

CALORIES: 1,175 FAT: 85.4g PROTEIN: 60.6g
TOTAL CARBS: 32.8g DIETARY FIBER: 15g NET CARBS: 17.8g

DAY 5

BREAKFAST

coffee with 2 T. heavy cream, 1 egg

95 Coconut Flour Waffles *with maple syrup*

LUNCH

LEFTOVER Warm Brussels Bacon Shrimp Salad

DINNER

58 Miracle Dough Pizza Crust *topped with ¼ cup* 53 *marinara sauce, 2 ounces pepperoni, and ¼ cup shredded mozzarella*

DESSERT

240 Fudgy Brownies

CALORIES: 1,333 FAT: 96.1g PROTEIN: 77.6g
TOTAL CARBS: 30g DIETARY FIBER: 13.5g NET CARBS: 16.5g

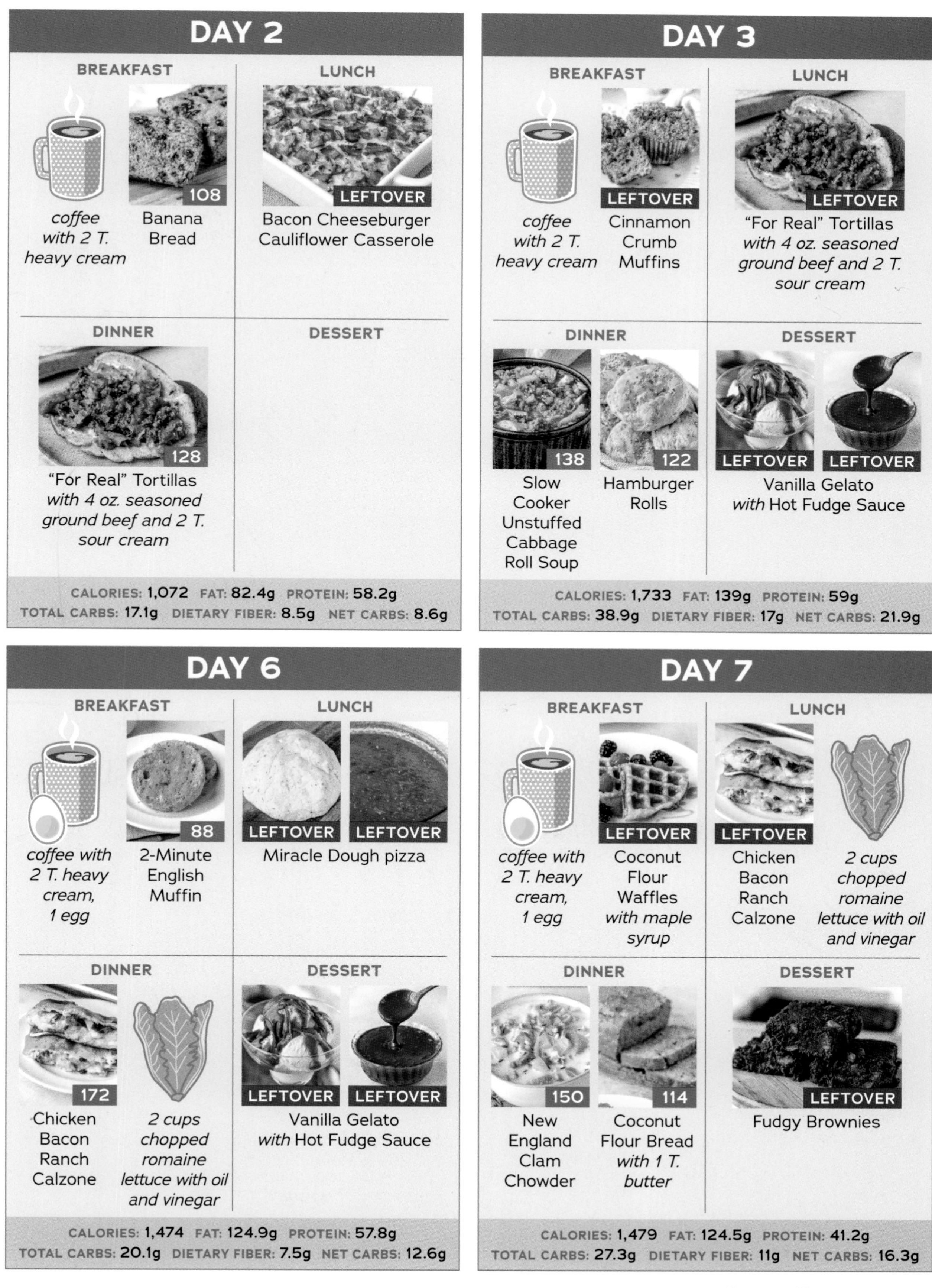
DAY 2
BREAKFAST
coffee with 2 T. heavy cream
108
Banana Bread
LUNCH
LEFTOVER
Bacon Cheeseburger Cauliflower Casserole
DINNER
128
"For Real" Tortillas with 4 oz. seasoned ground beef and 2 T. sour cream
DESSERT
CALORIES: 1,072 FAT: 82.4g PROTEIN: 58.2g
TOTAL CARBS: 17.1g DIETARY FIBER: 8.5g NET CARBS: 8.6g
DAY 3
BREAKFAST
coffee with 2 T. heavy cream
LEFTOVER
Cinnamon Crumb Muffins
LUNCH
LEFTOVER
"For Real" Tortillas with 4 oz. seasoned ground beef and 2 T. sour cream
DINNER
138
Slow Cooker Unstuffed Cabbage Roll Soup
122
Hamburger Rolls
DESSERT
LEFTOVER
LEFTOVER
Vanilla Gelato with Hot Fudge Sauce
CALORIES: 1,733 FAT: 139g PROTEIN: 59g
TOTAL CARBS: 38.9g DIETARY FIBER: 17g NET CARBS: 21.9g
DAY 6
BREAKFAST
coffee with 2 T. heavy cream, 1 egg
88
2-Minute English Muffin
LUNCH
LEFTOVER
LEFTOVER
Miracle Dough pizza
DINNER
172
Chicken Bacon Ranch Calzone
2 cups chopped romaine lettuce with oil and vinegar
DESSERT
LEFTOVER
LEFTOVER
Vanilla Gelato with Hot Fudge Sauce
CALORIES: 1,474 FAT: 124.9g PROTEIN: 57.8g
TOTAL CARBS: 20.1g DIETARY FIBER: 7.5g NET CARBS: 12.6g
DAY 7
BREAKFAST
coffee with 2 T. heavy cream, 1 egg
LEFTOVER
Coconut Flour Waffles with maple syrup
LUNCH
LEFTOVER
Chicken Bacon Ranch Calzone
2 cups chopped romaine lettuce with oil and vinegar
DINNER
150
New England Clam Chowder
114
Coconut Flour Bread with 1 T. butter
DESSERT
LEFTOVER
Fudgy Brownies
CALORIES: 1,479 FAT: 124.5g PROTEIN: 41.2g
TOTAL CARBS: 27.3g DIETARY FIBER: 11g NET CARBS: 16.3g

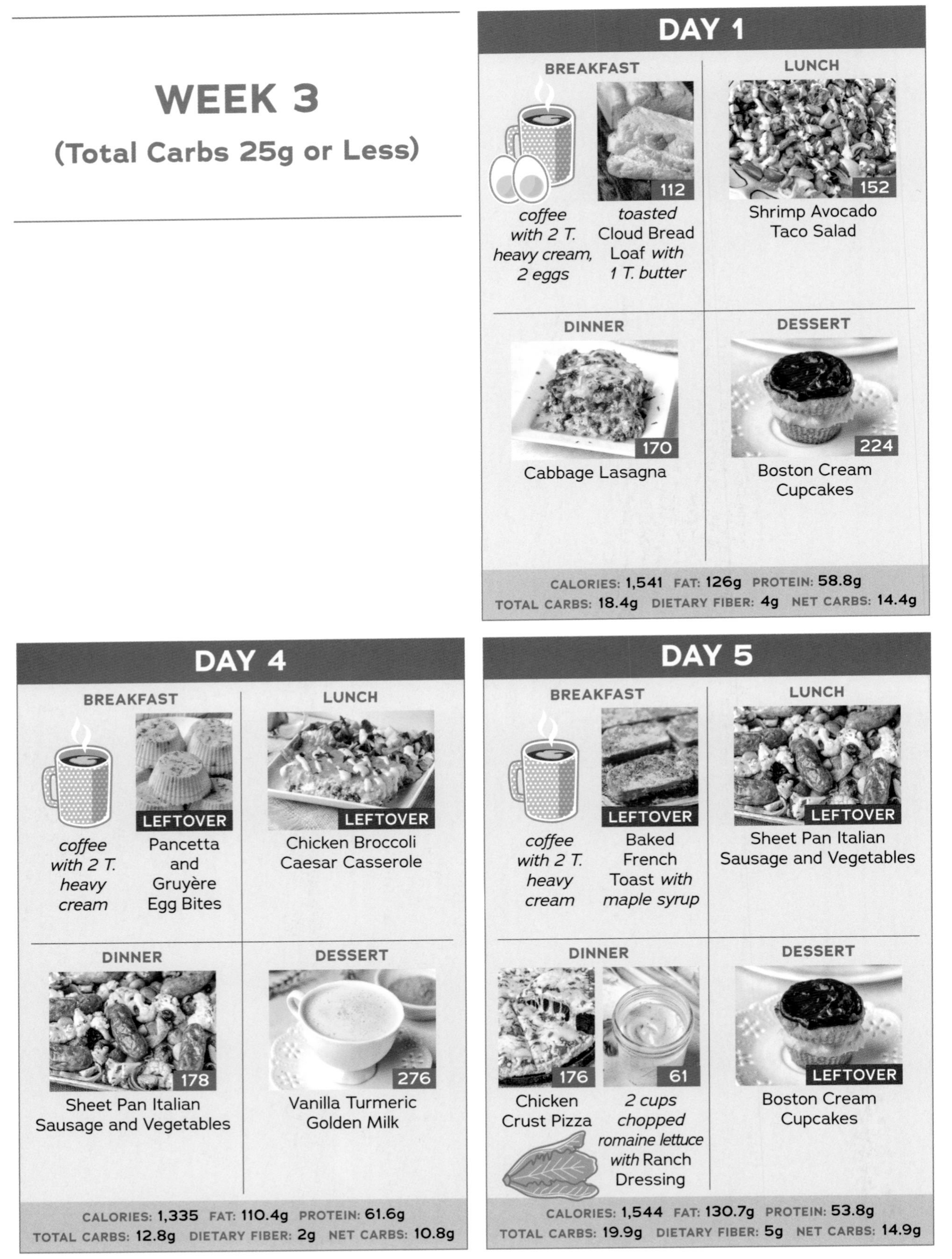

WEEK 3

(Total Carbs 25g or Less)

DAY 1

BREAKFAST

coffee with 2 T. heavy cream, 2 eggs

112 — *toasted* Cloud Bread Loaf *with 1 T. butter*

LUNCH

152 — Shrimp Avocado Taco Salad

DINNER

170 — Cabbage Lasagna

DESSERT

224 — Boston Cream Cupcakes

CALORIES: 1,541 FAT: 126g PROTEIN: 58.8g
TOTAL CARBS: 18.4g DIETARY FIBER: 4g NET CARBS: 14.4g

DAY 4

BREAKFAST

coffee with 2 T. heavy cream

LEFTOVER — Pancetta and Gruyère Egg Bites

LUNCH

LEFTOVER — Chicken Broccoli Caesar Casserole

DINNER

178 — Sheet Pan Italian Sausage and Vegetables

DESSERT

276 — Vanilla Turmeric Golden Milk

CALORIES: 1,335 FAT: 110.4g PROTEIN: 61.6g
TOTAL CARBS: 12.8g DIETARY FIBER: 2g NET CARBS: 10.8g

DAY 5

BREAKFAST

coffee with 2 T. heavy cream

LEFTOVER — Baked French Toast *with maple syrup*

LUNCH

LEFTOVER — Sheet Pan Italian Sausage and Vegetables

DINNER

176 — Chicken Crust Pizza

61 — *2 cups chopped romaine lettuce with* Ranch Dressing

DESSERT

LEFTOVER — Boston Cream Cupcakes

CALORIES: 1,544 FAT: 130.7g PROTEIN: 53.8g
TOTAL CARBS: 19.9g DIETARY FIBER: 5g NET CARBS: 14.9g

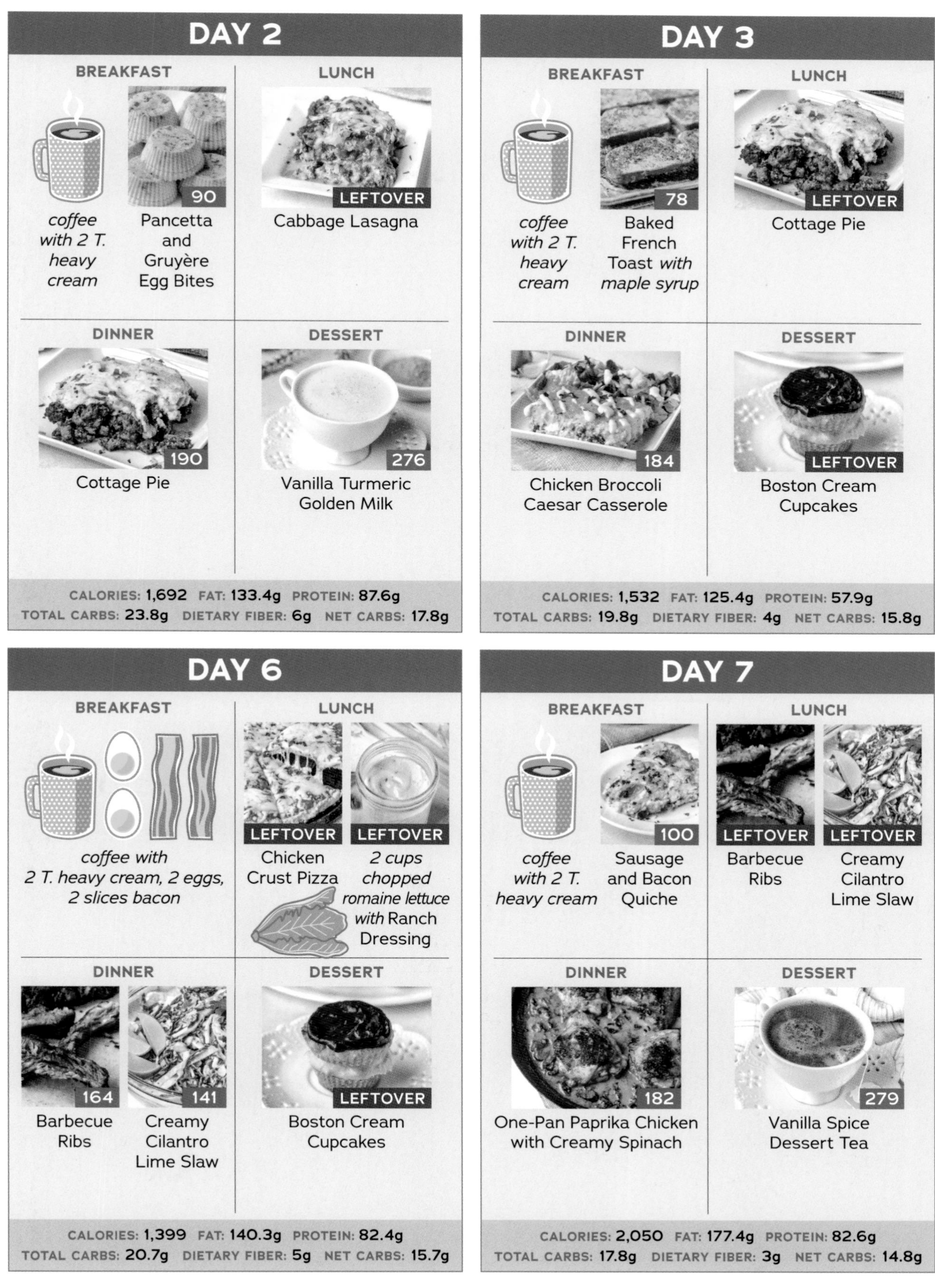
DAY 2
BREAKFAST
coffee with 2 T. heavy cream
90
Pancetta and Gruyère Egg Bites
LUNCH
LEFTOVER
Cabbage Lasagna
DINNER
190
Cottage Pie
DESSERT
276
Vanilla Turmeric Golden Milk
CALORIES: 1,692 FAT: 133.4g PROTEIN: 87.6g
TOTAL CARBS: 23.8g DIETARY FIBER: 6g NET CARBS: 17.8g
DAY 3
BREAKFAST
coffee with 2 T. heavy cream
78
Baked French Toast with maple syrup
LUNCH
LEFTOVER
Cottage Pie
DINNER
184
Chicken Broccoli Caesar Casserole
DESSERT
LEFTOVER
Boston Cream Cupcakes
CALORIES: 1,532 FAT: 125.4g PROTEIN: 57.9g
TOTAL CARBS: 19.8g DIETARY FIBER: 4g NET CARBS: 15.8g
DAY 6
BREAKFAST
coffee with 2 T. heavy cream, 2 eggs, 2 slices bacon
LUNCH
LEFTOVER
Chicken Crust Pizza
LEFTOVER
2 cups chopped romaine lettuce with Ranch Dressing
DINNER
164
Barbecue Ribs
141
Creamy Cilantro Lime Slaw
DESSERT
LEFTOVER
Boston Cream Cupcakes
CALORIES: 1,399 FAT: 140.3g PROTEIN: 82.4g
TOTAL CARBS: 20.7g DIETARY FIBER: 5g NET CARBS: 15.7g
DAY 7
BREAKFAST
coffee with 2 T. heavy cream
100
Sausage and Bacon Quiche
LUNCH
LEFTOVER
Barbecue Ribs
LEFTOVER
Creamy Cilantro Lime Slaw
DINNER
182
One-Pan Paprika Chicken with Creamy Spinach
DESSERT
279
Vanilla Spice Dessert Tea
CALORIES: 2,050 FAT: 177.4g PROTEIN: 82.6g
TOTAL CARBS: 17.8g DIETARY FIBER: 3g NET CARBS: 14.8g

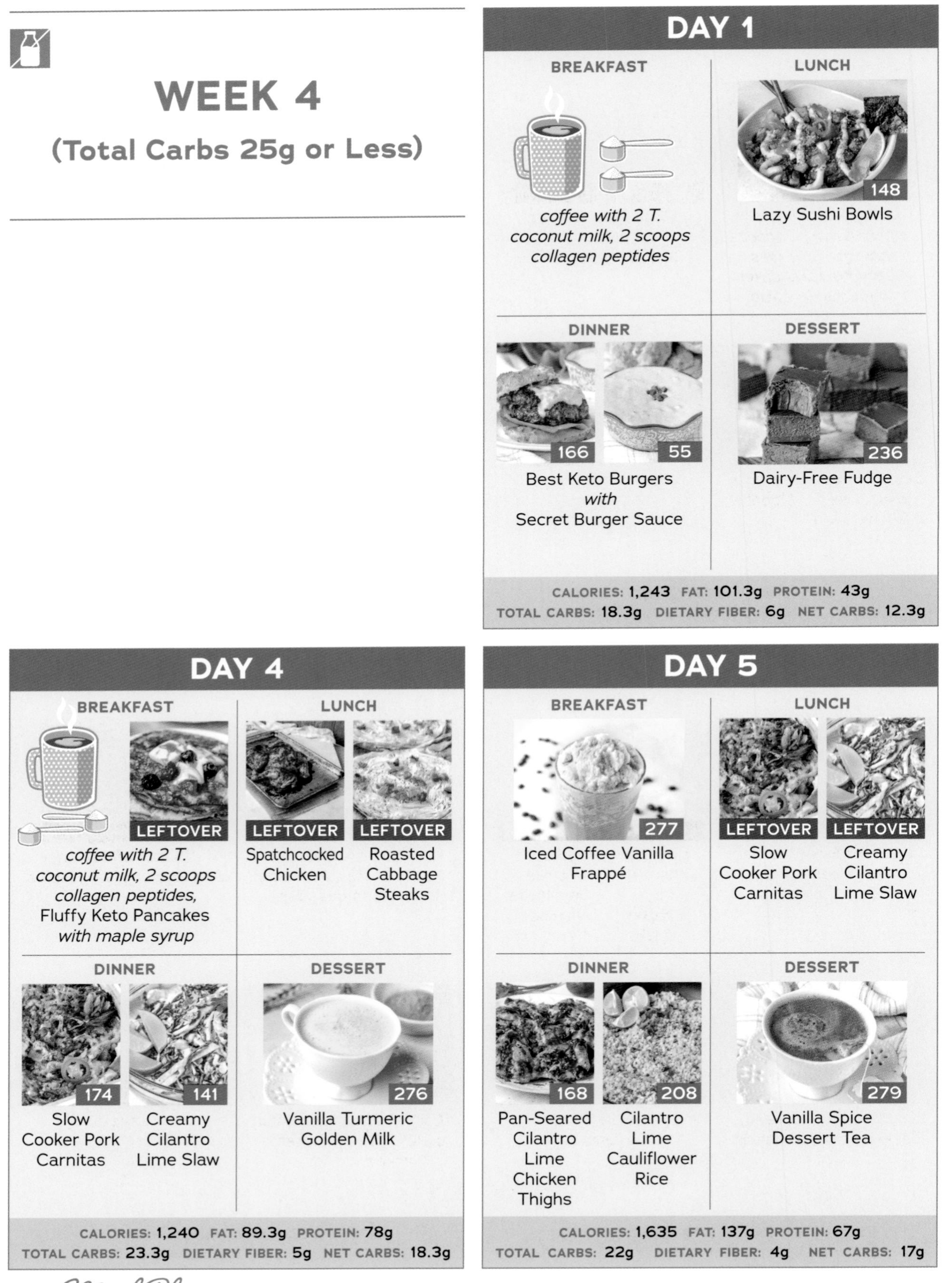

WEEK 4

(Total Carbs 25g or Less)

DAY 1

BREAKFAST

coffee with 2 T. coconut milk, 2 scoops collagen peptides

LUNCH

148

Lazy Sushi Bowls

DINNER

166 55

Best Keto Burgers *with* Secret Burger Sauce

DESSERT

236

Dairy-Free Fudge

CALORIES: 1,243 FAT: 101.3g PROTEIN: 43g
TOTAL CARBS: 18.3g DIETARY FIBER: 6g NET CARBS: 12.3g

DAY 4

BREAKFAST

LEFTOVER

coffee with 2 T. coconut milk, 2 scoops collagen peptides, Fluffy Keto Pancakes *with maple syrup*

LUNCH

LEFTOVER Spatchcocked Chicken

LEFTOVER Roasted Cabbage Steaks

DINNER

174 Slow Cooker Pork Carnitas

141 Creamy Cilantro Lime Slaw

DESSERT

276 Vanilla Turmeric Golden Milk

CALORIES: 1,240 FAT: 89.3g PROTEIN: 78g
TOTAL CARBS: 23.3g DIETARY FIBER: 5g NET CARBS: 18.3g

DAY 5

BREAKFAST

277 Iced Coffee Vanilla Frappé

LUNCH

LEFTOVER Slow Cooker Pork Carnitas

LEFTOVER Creamy Cilantro Lime Slaw

DINNER

168 Pan-Seared Cilantro Lime Chicken Thighs

208 Cilantro Lime Cauliflower Rice

DESSERT

279 Vanilla Spice Dessert Tea

CALORIES: 1,635 FAT: 137g PROTEIN: 67g
TOTAL CARBS: 22g DIETARY FIBER: 4g NET CARBS: 17g

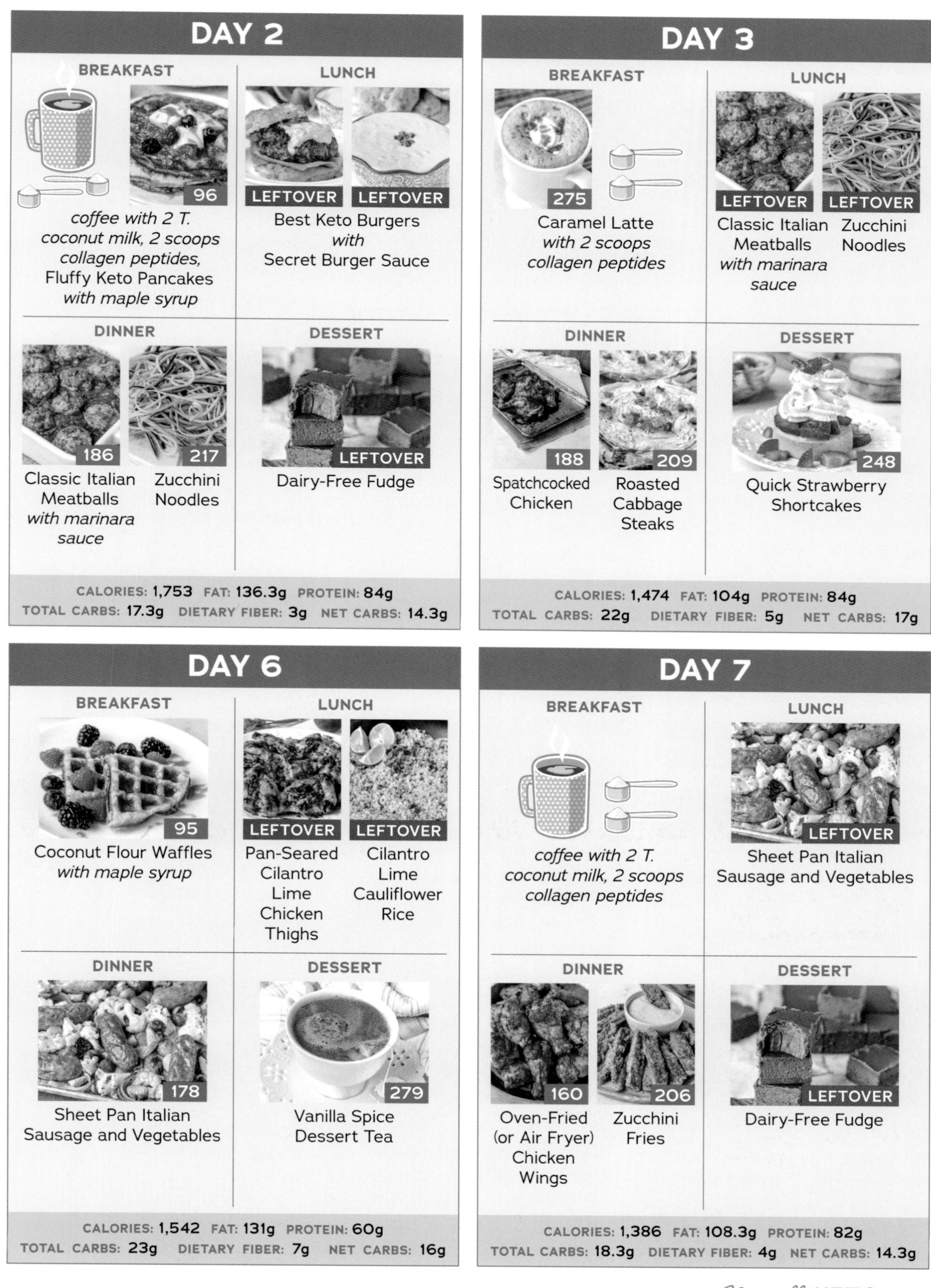

DAY 2

BREAKFAST — 96
coffee with 2 T. coconut milk, 2 scoops collagen peptides,
Fluffy Keto Pancakes *with maple syrup*

LUNCH — LEFTOVER / LEFTOVER
Best Keto Burgers *with* Secret Burger Sauce

DINNER — 186 / 217
Classic Italian Meatballs *with marinara sauce*
Zucchini Noodles

DESSERT — LEFTOVER
Dairy-Free Fudge

CALORIES: 1,753 **FAT:** 136.3g **PROTEIN:** 84g
TOTAL CARBS: 17.3g **DIETARY FIBER:** 3g **NET CARBS:** 14.3g

DAY 3

BREAKFAST — 275
Caramel Latte *with 2 scoops collagen peptides*

LUNCH — LEFTOVER / LEFTOVER
Classic Italian Meatballs *with marinara sauce*
Zucchini Noodles

DINNER — 188 / 209
Spatchcocked Chicken
Roasted Cabbage Steaks

DESSERT — 248
Quick Strawberry Shortcakes

CALORIES: 1,474 **FAT:** 104g **PROTEIN:** 84g
TOTAL CARBS: 22g **DIETARY FIBER:** 5g **NET CARBS:** 17g

DAY 6

BREAKFAST — 95
Coconut Flour Waffles *with maple syrup*

LUNCH — LEFTOVER / LEFTOVER
Pan-Seared Cilantro Lime Chicken Thighs
Cilantro Lime Cauliflower Rice

DINNER — 178
Sheet Pan Italian Sausage and Vegetables

DESSERT — 279
Vanilla Spice Dessert Tea

CALORIES: 1,542 **FAT:** 131g **PROTEIN:** 60g
TOTAL CARBS: 23g **DIETARY FIBER:** 7g **NET CARBS:** 16g

DAY 7

BREAKFAST
coffee with 2 T. coconut milk, 2 scoops collagen peptides

LUNCH — LEFTOVER
Sheet Pan Italian Sausage and Vegetables

DINNER — 160 / 206
Oven-Fried (or Air Fryer) Chicken Wings
Zucchini Fries

DESSERT — LEFTOVER
Dairy-Free Fudge

CALORIES: 1,386 **FAT:** 108.3g **PROTEIN:** 82g
TOTAL CARBS: 18.3g **DIETARY FIBER:** 4g **NET CARBS:** 14.3g

SHOPPING LIST week 1

PRODUCE

avocados, 2

bell pepper, 1

blueberries or raspberries, 1/2 cup

cauliflower, 1 medium head + 1 large head

cherry tomatoes, 1/4 cup halved

cilantro, 1 bunch

curly kale, 4 ounces

daikon radishes, 1 1/2 cups diced

garlic, 27 cloves

green cabbage, 1 small head

green onions, 1 bunch

jalapeño peppers, 3

lemons, 2

parsley, 1 bunch

red cabbage, 1 small head

red onion, 1 small

romaine lettuce, 1 head

white onions, 4

DAIRY

butter, salted, 1 1/2 sticks (6 ounces)

butter, unsalted, 2 sticks (8 ounces)

cheddar cheese, 5 1/2 cups shredded

cream cheese, 3 (8-ounce) packages

heavy whipping cream, 5 cups

mozzarella cheese, 4 cups shredded

sour cream, 1 cup

PROTEIN

bacon, 1 1/2 pounds

beef short ribs, 5 pounds

breakfast sausage, bulk, 1 pound

eggs, large, 20

ground beef, grass-fed, 8 pounds

Italian sausage, bulk, 2 pounds

pancetta, 8 ounces

rotisserie chicken, 1 whole

salmon fillets, skinless, 6 (2 pounds)

GROCERY

almond milk, unsweetened, 1 1/3 cups

almonds, raw, 1/2 cup sliced

chia seeds, 3 tablespoons

coconut, unsweetened shredded, 1 3/4 cups

diced tomatoes with green chilies, 1 (14 1/2-ounce) can

dill pickles, 1/2 cup chopped

hazelnuts, raw, 1/2 cup chopped

hemp hearts, 1 cup

marinara sauce, 3 1/2 cups (if making homemade, see page 53 for ingredients)

pecans, raw, 1/2 cup chopped

pumpkin seeds, raw, 1 cup

salsa, 1 cup

sunflower seeds, raw, 1 1/2 cups

tomato paste, 6 tablespoons

walnuts, raw, 1/2 cup

PANTRY, REFRIGERATOR, OR FREEZER

almond flour, blanched, 1 1/2 cups

apple cider vinegar, 6 1/2 teaspoons

avocado oil, 1/4 cup

avocado oil mayonnaise, 2 cups (if making homemade egg-free mayo, see page 48 for ingredients)

baking powder, 6 tablespoons

baking soda, 4 teaspoons

beef bone broth, 6 1/3 cups

chicken bone broth, 4 cups

chocolate chips, sugar-free, 6 ounces (if making homemade, see page 230 for ingredients)

cocoa powder, unsweetened, 6 tablespoons

coconut flour, 2 1/2 cups

coconut oil, 1/3 cup + 1 tablespoon

coffee

coffee extract, 2 teaspoons

dark chocolate (85% cacao), 2 ounces

dill pickle relish, 5 tablespoons

distilled vinegar, 2 tablespoons

extra-virgin olive oil, 2 cups

ground flaxseed, 2 cups

ketchup, sugar-free, 1 cup (if making homemade, see page 50 for ingredients)

peanut butter, unsweetened smooth, 1 1/4 cups

prepared yellow mustard, 1/3 cup

sesame flour, 1/2 cup

Swerve brown sugar, 1/3 cup

Swerve confectioners'-style sweetener, 9 1/2 tablespoons

Swerve granular sweetener, 1/2 cup + 1 1/2 teaspoons

unflavored gelatin, 1 tablespoon

vanilla extract, 5 1/2 teaspoons

vanilla-flavored liquid stevia, 1 1/2 tablespoons

Worcestershire sauce, 2 tablespoons

xanthan gum, 7 teaspoons

DRIED HERBS AND SPICES

black pepper

celery seed

chili powder

fine sea salt

garlic powder

granulated onion

ground cinnamon

ground cumin

Italian seasoning

mustard powder

onion powder

oregano leaves

smoked paprika

SHOPPING LIST week 2

PRODUCE

avocado, 1

Brussels sprouts, 1 pound

cauliflower, $1\frac{1}{2}$ large heads

celery, 1 bunch

curly kale, 8 ounces

flat-leaf parsley, 1 bunch

garlic, 1 head

green cabbage, 1 medium head

green onions, 1 bunch

lemons, 3

limes, 2

red radishes, 1 bag

romaine lettuce, 1 head

shallots, $\frac{1}{2}$ cup chopped

thyme, 1 teaspoon chopped

white onions, 2

DAIRY

butter, salted, 5 sticks (20 ounces)

butter, unsalted, 2 sticks + 2 tablespoons (9 ounces)

cheddar cheese, 8 ounces

cream cheese, 1 (8-ounce) package

heavy whipping cream, 8 cups

mozzarella cheese, $8\frac{1}{4}$ cups shredded

Parmesan cheese, $\frac{1}{3}$ cup grated

sour cream, 1 cup

GROCERY

almond milk, unsweetened, 1 tablespoon

clam juice, canned, 1 cup

marinara sauce, $2\frac{1}{4}$ cups (if making homemade, see page 53 for ingredients)

PROTEIN

bacon, 1 pound

clams, minced, 5 ($6\frac{1}{2}$-ounce) cans

eggs, large, 55

ground beef, grass-fed, $4\frac{1}{2}$ pounds

pepperoni, 2 ounces

rotisserie chicken, 1 whole

salt pork, no sugar added, 6 ounces

shrimp, raw, $1\frac{1}{2}$ pounds

tuna, 1 (5-ounce) can

PANTRY, REFRIGERATOR, OR FREEZER

almond butter, unsweetened, 2 tablespoons

almond flour, blanched, 2 tablespoons

apple cider vinegar, 1 tablespoon

avocado oil, 1 cup

avocado oil mayonnaise, 2 cups (if making homemade egg-free mayo, see page 48 for ingredients)

baking powder, $\frac{1}{2}$ cup

baking soda, 1 tablespoon

banana extract, 4 teaspoons

beef bone broth, $5\frac{1}{3}$ cups

chicken bone broth, 2 cups

chocolate chips, sugar-free, 1 cup (if making homemade, see page 230 for ingredients)

chocolate-flavored liquid stevia, $1\frac{1}{4}$ teaspoons

chocolate-flavored protein powder, $\frac{1}{3}$ cup

cocoa powder, unsweetened, $\frac{1}{4}$ cup

coconut flour, $7\frac{1}{2}$ cups

coconut milk, 2 ($13\frac{1}{2}$-ounce) cans

coffee

dark chocolate (85% cacao), 4 ounces

extra-virgin olive oil, $1\frac{2}{3}$ cups

ground flaxseed, $2\frac{3}{4}$ cups

instant espresso powder, $2\frac{1}{2}$ teaspoons

maple extract, 2 tablespoons

maple syrup, sugar-free (if making homemade, see page 70 for ingredients)

MCT oil, 2 tablespoons

prepared yellow mustard, 2 tablespoons + 2 teaspoons

red wine vinegar

sesame flour, $\frac{1}{2}$ cup

Swerve brown sugar, $3\frac{1}{4}$ cups

Swerve confectioners'-style sweetener, 1 cup

Swerve granular sweetener, $\frac{1}{2}$ cup

unflavored gelatin, $\frac{1}{4}$ cup

vanilla bean, 1

vanilla extract, 4 teaspoons

vanilla-flavored liquid stevia, $1\frac{1}{2}$ teaspoons

xanthan gum, 10 teaspoons

DRIED HERBS AND SPICES

basil

bay leaf

black pepper

fine sea salt

garlic powder

ground cinnamon

onion powder

oregano leaves

parsley

sesame seeds

white pepper

SHOPPING LIST week 3

PRODUCE

avocado, 1
baby spinach, 5 ounces
broccoli, 1 head
Brussels sprouts, 8 ounces
button mushrooms, 8 ounces
cauliflower, 2 large heads
cherry tomatoes, 4 ounces
cilantro, 1 bunch
flat-leaf parsley, 1 bunch
garlic, 14 cloves
green cabbage, 2 small heads
lemons, 2
limes, 3
radishes, 1 bag
red cabbage, 1 small head
red onion, 1 small
romaine lettuce, 1 head
white onion, 1

DAIRY

butter, salted, 1½ sticks + 2 tablespoons (7 ounces)
butter, unsalted, 1 stick (4 ounces)
cheddar cheese, 6 ounces
cream cheese, 2 (8-ounce) packages + 2 ounces
Gruyère cheese, 4 ounces
heavy whipping cream, 6½ cups
mozzarella cheese, 5½ cups shredded
Parmesan cheese, 1 cup grated
ricotta cheese, 2 cups
sour cream, ¾ cup

PROTEIN

baby back ribs, 4 pounds
bacon, 10 ounces
bulk breakfast sausage, 12 ounces
chicken thighs, boneless, skinless, 2 pounds
eggs, large, 50
ground beef, grass-fed, 4 pounds
Italian sausage links, mild or hot, 2 pounds
pancetta, 4 ounces
rotisserie chickens, 2 whole
shrimp, medium, raw, 2 pounds

GROCERY

almond milk, unsweetened, 3⅓ cups
marinara sauce, 2 cups (if making homemade, see page 53 for ingredients)
tomato paste, 1 tablespoon

PANTRY, REFRIGERATOR, OR FREEZER

almond flour, blanched, 1¼ cups
avocado oil, ¼ cup
avocado oil mayonnaise, 3 cups (if making homemade egg-free mayo, see page 48 for ingredients)
baking powder, 2 teaspoons
baking soda, 1 teaspoon
beef bone broth, 1½ cups
chicken bone broth, 1 cup
chocolate, sugar-free, 4 ounces (if making homemade, see page 230 for ingredients)
coconut flour, 2 tablespoons
coffee
collagen peptides, 2 scoops
cream of tartar, 1 teaspoon
extra-virgin olive oil, 1 cup
ghee or coconut oil, 2 tablespoons
maple syrup, sugar-free (if making homemade, see page 70 for ingredients)
prepared yellow mustard, 2 teaspoons
protein powder, whey or egg white, unflavored, 1¼ cups
red wine, ½ cup
red wine vinegar
Swerve brown sugar, ½ cup
Swerve confectioners'-style sweetener, 1 cup
unflavored gelatin
vanilla extract, 7 teaspoons
vanilla spice tea, 1 bag
vanilla-flavored liquid stevia, 3¼ teaspoons
white wine vinegar, ¼ cup
xanthan gum, 1½ teaspoons

DRIED HERBS AND SPICES

basil
black pepper
chili powder
fine sea salt
garlic powder
ginger powder
ground cardamom
ground cinnamon
ground cumin
Italian seasoning
kosher salt
onion powder
oregano leaves
paprika
parsley
red pepper flakes
smoked paprika
turmeric powder

SHOPPING LIST week 4

PRODUCE

avocados, 2 large
basil, 1 bunch
Brussels sprouts, 8 ounces
burger toppings of choice
cauliflower, 2 large heads
cilantro, 1 bunch
cucumber, 1
flat-leaf parsley, 1 bunch
garlic, 22 cloves
green cabbage, 1 large head + 1 small head
green onions, 1 bunch
lemons, 2
limes, 9
radishes, 1 bag
red cabbage, 1 small head
red onion, 1
strawberries, 1 cup sliced
white onion, 1 large
zucchini, 5 large

PROTEIN

chicken, 1 whole (5 pounds)
chicken thighs, boneless, skinless, 2 pounds
chicken wings, 3 pounds
eggs, large, 22
ground beef, grass-fed, 3 pounds
ground pork, 1 pound
Italian sausage links, mild or hot, 2 pounds
pancetta, 2 ounces
pork butt or shoulder, boneless, 4 pounds
smoked salmon, 1 pound

GROCERY

almond milk, unsweetened, 3 cups
coconut milk, unsweetened, 1 (1-L) carton
nori (dried seaweed), 2 pieces
nutritional yeast, 2/3 cup
wasabi

DRIED HERBS AND SPICES

basil
black pepper
chili powder
coarse sea salt
dried onion flakes
fennel seeds
fine sea salt
garlic powder
ginger powder
granulated onion
ground cardamom
ground cinnamon
ground cumin
Italian seasoning
mustard powder
onion powder
oregano leaves
parsley
sesame seeds
smoked paprika
turmeric powder

PANTRY, REFRIGERATOR, OR FREEZER

apple cider vinegar, 1/4 cup + 1 teaspoon
avocado oil, 1/4 cup
avocado oil mayonnaise, 3 cups (if making homemade egg-free mayo, see page 48 for ingredients)
baking powder, 5 1/2 tablespoons
baking soda, 1 teaspoon
beef bone broth, 1 cup
cacao butter, 4 ounces
caramel extract, 1/2 teaspoon
coconut aminos, 1/4 cup
coconut flour, 2 cups
coconut oil, 2 cups
coffee
collagen peptides, 11 scoops
dark chocolate (85% cacao), 8 ounces
dill pickle relish, 3 tablespoons
extra-virgin olive oil, 1 1/3 cups
ghee, 1 tablespoon
ground flaxseed, 3/4 cup
ketchup, sugar-free, 1/3 cup (if making homemade, see page 50 for ingredients)
lemon-flavored liquid stevia, 1 teaspoon
maple extract, 1 teaspoon
maple syrup, sugar-free, 2 tablespoons (if making homemade, see page 70 for ingredients)
pork rinds, 1 cup crushed
prepared yellow mustard, 1 tablespoon
protein powder, egg white, unflavored, 1 cup
Sriracha sauce, 1 teaspoon
Swerve brown sugar, 1 tablespoon
Swerve confectioners'-style sweetener, 7 tablespoons
Swerve granular sweetener, 10 tablespoons
unflavored gelatin, 2 tablespoons
vanilla extract, 4 1/2 teaspoons
vanilla spice tea, 1 bag
vanilla-flavored liquid stevia, 1 teaspoon
white wine vinegar, 1/4 cup
xanthan gum, 2 teaspoons

WITH GRATITUDE

All my Facebook and Instagram followers: you all have been the driving force behind SugarFreeMom.com. Some of you have been supporting me since 2011 at the start of my blog, and I can't thank you enough. Without all of you making and sharing my recipes, I am most certain I would not have had the opportunity to write this cookbook. I am forever grateful for your continued support, and I thank you from the bottom of my heart for being my tribe, my people, the ones I truly enjoy connecting with online every day.

Jim, my best friend, my husband, my love, and my greatest support: Without your encouragement all these years as well as sound advice and direction, I wouldn't have had the courage to pursue my dreams and make it come to reality. You are my everything and I thank God for you every single day.

Joshua, Rebekah, and Jack, my awesome children, my taste testers and honest critics: I love you all so very much. I pray each day that I have set an example of a woman who sought after God and who has been greatly blessed. I pray that I have shown you how God can turn your mess into your message, and that even your greatest challenge in life can one day be used to help others with His help.

Ricky, my tech-savvy brother: I will forever be grateful for you. Without you, there would have been no blog because I didn't even know what one was. Without your help that first year, I wouldn't have succeeded. Your continued guidance and our amazing talks continue to inspire me and help me grow every day.

Mom, always just a phone call away. Always there to encourage me. Always my cheerleader and in my corner. I learned the joy of hospitality at a young age because of you. I learned how to bless others with a warm meal or a delicious banana bread. Thank you for instilling in me the value of the written word to encourage others and reminding me to be careful with my words, knowing the legacy they would leave one day. I love you.

Dad, always my protector. You've taught me so much about honoring my Italian heritage. You've given me words of wisdom and always your honest opinion. I'm grateful for all of the sacrifices you made for the childhood I cherish to this day. I think Nonna and Nonno would be very proud of you and the family you created with Mom. I love you.

Andrea, my awesome praying friend. I thank God every day that whenever I'm in stress or struggle, you are always there with an encouraging word and a prayer for me. I surely needed those prayers through this book-writing process, and I am forever grateful to have you in my life.

Shawon, you make me feel like a celebrity each and every time you take my photos. I can't believe how far we both have come from our young homeschool days when we asked ourselves what we would do after that. You are one talented photographer, and I love you. God has certainly blessed us both!

Heather and Stasha, not only good friends, but also amazing recipe testers. I am so honored you took the time to make my recipes over and over again and tell me your honest opinions. You both have helped me to have confidence that each and every one of these recipes in this cookbook are my best work yet. I love you both!

Ann-Marie, my lifelong best friend. I don't know where I'd be had we not met in our teens. The influence your family has had on my life is pretty significant, and I know it was God who brought us together. Thank you for always being just a phone call away. No matter how much time goes by, I know I can always call you and we'll just pick up where we've left off.

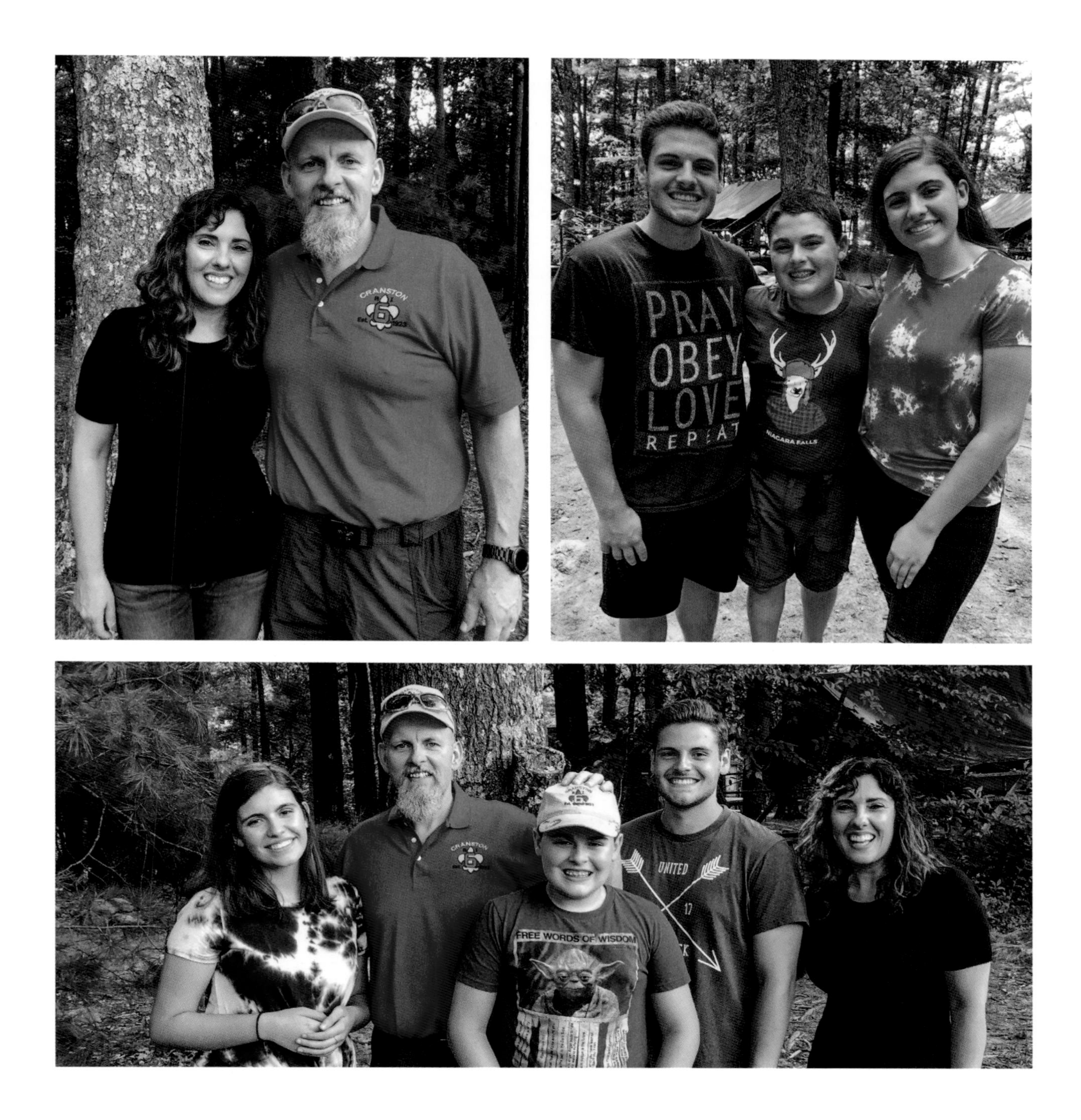

Laurie, my childhood forever friend. How amazing that we have known each other since the age of five and as life happened, reuniting eighteen years ago! It's been full circle for us, and I want you to know I have saved every card you have ever sent to me! You've always encouraged me, and I want you to know how much I appreciate and love you.

The Victory Belt team, I am forever grateful for the opportunity to write this keto cookbook. Thank you, Erich and Lance, for that very first encouraging call to me, as I was so hesitant and uncertain I could do this. Susan, Pam, Donna, Holly, Justin, thank you so much for making this book a success in every way. All of you are what make Victory Belt the best team to work with, and I thank you for this wonderful experience!

RESOURCE GUIDE

Learning all you can about how ketosis works and how to get your body to function at its best is important for living this way of life, for the rest of your life. The more information you have, the better equipped you'll be when speaking with doctors or friends who are skeptics. Knowledge is power! Learn all you can and share your own experience along the way. Your own experience may encourage and inspire others toward food and sugar freedom.

Books

- *The Art and Science of Low Carbohydrate Living* by Stephen Phinney and Jeff S. Volek
- *Cholesterol Clarity* by Jimmy Moore with Eric C. Westman, MD
- *The Complete Guide to Fasting* by Jason Fung, MD, and Jimmy Moore
- *Craveable Keto* by Kyndra D. Holley
- *The Everyday Ketogenic Kitchen* by Carolyn Ketchum
- *Keto* by Maria and Craig Emmerich
- *Keto Clarity* by Jimmy Moore with Eric C. Westman, MD
- *The Keto Diet* by Leanne Vogel
- *Simply Keto* by Suzanne Ryan

Podcasts

You can learn so much from listening to others who have years of experience on the keto diet. Here are some of my favorite podcasts:

- Fast Keto with Vanessa Spina
- The Keto Diet Podcast with Leanne Vogel
- Keto Talk with Jimmy Moore and Dr. Will Cole
- Keto for Women Show with Shawn Mynar
- Naturally Nourished Podcast with Ali Miller

Websites

- alldayidreamaboutfood.com
- dietdoctor.com
- ditchthecarbs.com
- gnom-gnom.com
- grassfedgirl.com
- ibreatheimhungry.com
- ketoadapted.com
- ketodietapp.com
- livinlavidalowcarb.com
- lowcarbmaven.com
- lowcarbsosimple.com
- mariamindbodyhealth.com
- peaceloveandlowcarb.com
- reddit.com/r/keto/
- sugarfreemom.com
- thecastawaykitchen.com

Keto Coaching

- healthfulpursuit.com
- ketogenicgirl.com
- mariamindbodyhealth.com

Products and Brands

I realize we are all busy, and making things like ketchup, salad dressings, and snacks from scratch can be too time-consuming for many. I tried my best to include easier recipes in my cookbook for that reason, but as a mom of three, I know it can be hard to keep up, especially if you have teens like I do. Having your pantry stocked with these products is a huge time-saver.

AlternaSweets: Delicious low-carb BBQ sauce and ketchup using erythritol as the sweetener. *www.alternasweets.com*

Bunker Hill Cheese: Not only do they sell fantastic raw milk cheeses, but they also have amazing crunchy cheese crisps in many different flavors, like Buffalo, Cheddar, Jalapeño, and Parmesan. *www.bunkerhill.com*

Cali'flour Foods: Cauliflower pizza crusts in different flavors like Italian, Spicy Jalapeño, and Sweet Red Pepper. *www.califlourfoods.com*

ChocZero: Flavored syrups, chocolate squares, keto bark, and soon chocolate chips, all sweetened with monk fruit. *www.choczero.com*

Chosen Foods: I use their avocado oil daily for cooking. They also have dressings, infused avocado oil sprays, and avocado oil mayo I like. *www.chosenfoods.com*

Epic: Meat strips in beef, venison, bison, chicken, boar, turkey, and smoked salmon. They also sell bacon bites, bone broth, duck fat, bison tallow, beef tallow, and pork rinds. *www.epicprovisions.com*

Keto Krate: Keto-friendly snacks delivered to your door each month. No contracts and you can cancel anytime. Prices are reasonable considering the number of items you get in a box. This allows you to try individual items to see which ones you like before purchasing a larger quantity. *www.ketokrate.com*

Lakanto: For those who dislike erythritol and stevia, Lakanto is a great alternative, as it's a monk fruit sweetener. It can be subbed one-for-one with sugar. In addition to a granular version, they now have a confectioners' style as well as a liquid sweetener. Their sugar-free maple syrup is fantastic! *www.lakanto.com*

Lily's Chocolate: Delicious chocolate bars and chips sweetened with a combination of erythritol and stevia. *www.lilyssweets.com*

Moon Cheese: My kids love these crunchy cheese balls in different flavors like Cheddar, Gouda, Mozzarella, Pepper Jack, and Sriracha. *www.mooncheese.com*

Perfect Keto: MCT oil powder, keto bars, electrolytes, but the product I love the most is the flavored collagen protein, which I put in my coffee. It comes in chocolate, vanilla, and salted caramel flavors. *www.perfectketo.com*

Swerve: The best erythritol on the market, in my opinion, and that's why I use it in my recipes. Their confectioners'-style sweetener is incredible, as is the granular, and the new brown sugar substitute is fantastic, too. *www.swervesweet.com*

Vital Proteins: I use beef gelatin to make my Egg-Free Mayo (page 48) and in desserts to get that gel-like texture and chewiness in baked goods. Vital Proteins also sells collagen peptides and now has flavored collagen creamers as well. But what I have found really helpful are the individual collagen peptide packs that you can carry in your purse or briefcase. *www.vitalproteins.com*

Zevia: Zero-calorie, zero-sugar, stevia-sweetened soda in fourteen different flavors, like black cherry, cream soda, ginger ale, and ginger root beer. I find it at my local Whole Foods, but you can also buy it on Amazon. *www.zevia.com*

ALLERGEN INDEX

RECIPE TITLE	PAGE				
Alfredo Sauce	44			✓	✓
BBQ Sauce	45	✓	✓	✓	✓
Beef Spice Rub	46	✓	✓	✓	✓
Chicken Spice Rub	47	✓	✓	✓	✓
Egg-Free Mayo	48	✓	✓	✓	
Easy Blender Ketchup	50	✓	✓	✓	✓
Lemon Aioli	51	✓	○	✓	○
Fry Sauce	52	✓	○	✓	✓
Quick Marinara Sauce	53	✓	✓	✓	✓
Pesto	54	○	✓	○	
Secret Burger Sauce	55	✓	○	✓	✓
Keto Breading	56	○	○	✓	
Olive Sauce	57	✓	✓	✓	
Miracle Dough Pizza Crust	58			✓	✓
Caesar Dressing	60		○	✓	
Ranch Dressing	61	✓	○	○	✓
Taco Seasoning	62	✓	✓	✓	✓
Caramel Sauce	63		✓	✓	✓
Blueberry Syrup	64	✓	✓	✓	✓
Hot Fudge Sauce	65		✓	✓	✓
Coconut Whipped Cream	66	✓	✓	✓	✓
Coconut Flour Pie Crust	68	○		✓	✓
Sugar-Free Maple Syrup	70	○	✓	✓	✓
Raspberry Chia Jam	72	✓	✓	✓	✓
Whipped Cream	73		✓	✓	✓
Salted Caramel Sunflower Seed Butter	74	✓	✓	✓	✓
Baked French Toast	78			✓	✓
Biscuits and Gravy	80		✓	✓	
Cinnamon Crumb Muffins	82			✓	✓
Miracle Dough Bagels	84			✓	○
Cinnamon Rolls	86			✓	✓
2-Minute English Muffins	88	○			✓
Pancetta and Gruyère Egg Bites	90			✓	
Slow Cooker Granola	92	✓	✓		✓
Prep-Ahead Hot Cinnamon Cereal	94	○	✓		✓
Coconut Flour Waffles	95	○		○	
Fluffy Keto Pancakes	96	○		○	✓
Pumpkin Donuts	98	○		✓	✓
Sausage and Bacon Quiche	100			✓	
Vanilla Bean Scones	102			✓	
Zucchini Spice Muffins	104	○		○	✓
Banana Bread	108	○		○	✓
Bunless Cheeseburger Bites	110		✓	✓	
Cloud Bread Loaf	112	○		✓	✓
Coconut Flour Bread	114	○		✓	
Burrata Pesto Caprese Stacks	116		✓	○	✓
Focaccia	118			✓	✓
Fried Halloumi Sticks	120		✓	✓	✓
Hamburger Rolls	122	✓		✓	✓
Salt and Vinegar Zucchini Chips	124	✓	✓	✓	✓
Sesame Crackers	126	✓		✓	✓
“For Real” Tortillas	128	○		✓	
Spicy Sausage-Stuffed Mushrooms	130		✓	✓	
Crispy Bacon Chicken Cabbage Salad	134	✓	○	✓	
Smoked Salmon Avocado Fennel Salad	136	✓	✓	✓	
Slow Cooker Unstuffed Cabbage Roll Soup	138	✓	✓	✓	
Cheeseburger Salad Bowls	140	○	○	✓	
Creamy Cilantro Lime Slaw	141	✓	○	✓	✓
Instant Pot (or Slow Cooker) Chili	142	✓	✓	✓	
Italian Seafood Salad	144		✓	✓	
Kale Caesar Salad with Garlic Croutons	146		○	✓	✓
Lazy Sushi Bowls	148	✓	○	✓	
New England Clam Chowder	150		✓	✓	
Shrimp Avocado Taco Salad	152	✓	○	✓	

RECIPE TITLE	PAGE				
Zuppa Toscana	154		✓	✓	
Warm Brussels Bacon Shrimp Salad	156	✓	✓	✓	
Oven-Fried (or Air Fryer) Chicken Wings	160	✓	✓	✓	
Bacon Cheeseburger Cauliflower Casserole	162		✓	✓	
Barbecue Ribs	164	✓	✓	✓	
Best Keto Burgers	166	✓	○	✓	
Pan-Seared Cilantro Lime Chicken Thighs	168	✓	✓	✓	
Cabbage Lasagna	170			✓	
Chicken Bacon Ranch Calzone	172			✓	
Slow Cooker Pork Carnitas	174	✓	✓	✓	
Chicken Crust Pizza	176			✓	
Sheet Pan Italian Sausage and Vegetables	178	✓	✓	✓	
Taco Casserole	180			✓	
One-Pan Paprika Chicken with Creamy Spinach	182		✓	✓	
Chicken Broccoli Caesar Casserole	184			✓	
Classic Italian Meatballs	186	○		✓	
Spatchcocked Chicken	188	✓	✓	✓	
Cottage Pie	190		✓	✓	
Sheet Pan Lemon Garlic Herb Salmon and Roasted Cauliflower	192	✓	✓	✓	
Instant Pot (or Slow Cooker) Beef Short Ribs	194	○	✓	✓	
Skillet Chicken Parmesan	196			✓	
Bacon Cheeseburger Sloppy Joes	198		✓	✓	
Blistered Garlic Green Beans	202	✓	✓	✓	✓
Cauliflower Hash Browns	204			✓	✓
Zucchini Fries	206	✓		✓	
Cilantro Lime Cauliflower Rice	208	✓	✓	✓	✓
Roasted Cabbage Steaks	209	✓	✓	✓	○
Creamy Kale with Pancetta	210		✓	✓	
Mashed Roasted Cauliflower	212		✓	✓	✓
Crispy Brussels Sprouts	214	✓	✓	✓	✓
Jicama Fries	216	✓	✓	✓	✓
Zucchini Noodles Without a Spiralizer	217	✓	✓	✓	✓
Zucchini Tots	218			✓	✓
Apple Crisp	222	○	✓	✓	✓
Boston Cream Cupcakes	224				✓
Buckeye Fat Bomb Bars	226		✓		✓
Cannoli	228			✓	✓
Chocolate Bars or Chocolate Chips	230		✓	✓	✓
Vanilla Buttercream Frosting	231		✓	✓	✓
Chocolate Buttercream Frosting	232		✓	✓	✓
Chocolate Chip Cookies	234	○		✓	
Dairy-Free Fudge	236	✓	✓	✓	✓
Italian Cream Puffs	238			✓	✓
Fudgy Brownies	240	○		✓	✓
Mini Crustless Blueberry Lemon Cheesecakes	242			✓	✓
Gingerbread Biscotti	244	○		✓	
Italian Amaretti	246	✓			✓
Quick Strawberry Shortcakes	248	○		✓	✓
Triple-Layer Chocolate Cake	250			✓	✓
Pecan Pie	252				✓
Vanilla Gelato	254			✓	✓
Pizzelle	256			✓	✓
Tiramisù	258			✓	✓
Iced Sugar Cookies	260			✓	○
Skillet Chocolate Chip Cookie Pie	262			✓	✓
Pecan Snowballs	264	○		✓	✓
No-Bake Coffee Cheesecake	266		✓	✓	
Bulletproof Hot Chocolate	270	○	✓	○	
Root Beer Ice Cream Float	271			✓	✓
Lemon Cream Pie Smoothie	272		✓		✓
Iced Bulletproof Mocha Frappé	273	○	✓	✓	○
Chocolate Sea Salt Smoothie	274	○	✓		○
Caramel Latte	275	✓		✓	✓
Vanilla Turmeric Golden Milk	276	✓	✓	○	
Iced Coffee Vanilla Frappé	277	○	✓		✓
Creamy PB&J Smoothie	278	✓	✓	○	
Vanilla Spice Dessert Tea	279	○	✓	✓	✓

RECIPE INDEX

Basics

Breakfast

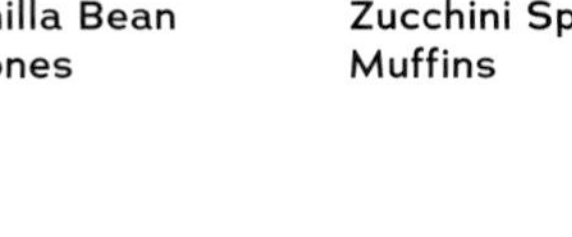
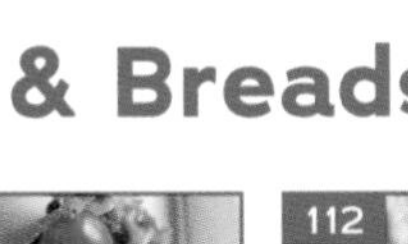

Appetizers & Breads

Soups & Salads

Mains

Sides

Desserts

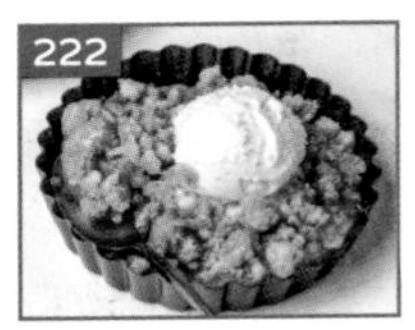
222 Apple Crisp

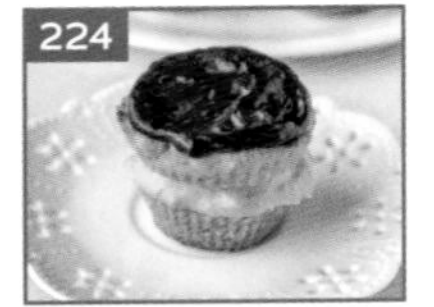
224 Boston Cream Cupcakes

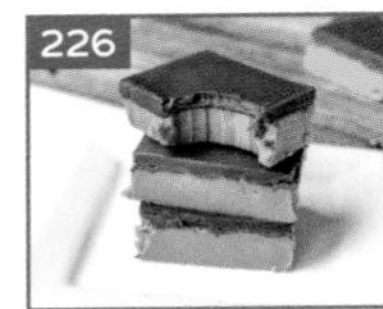
226 Buckeye Fat Bomb Bars

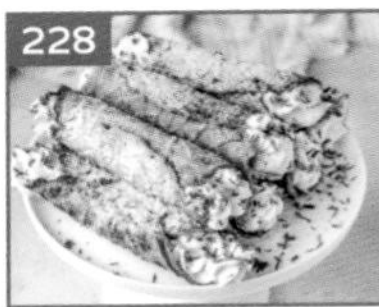
228 Cannoli

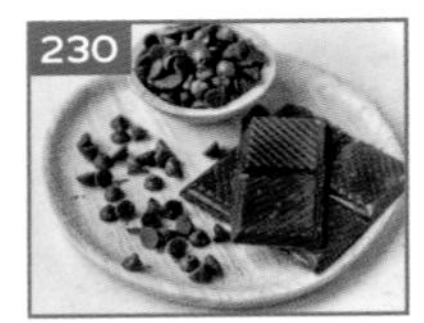
230 Chocolate Bars or Chocolate Chips

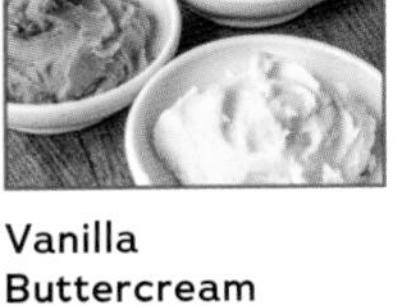
231 Vanilla Buttercream Frosting

232 Chocolate Buttercream Frosting

234 Chocolate Chip Cookies

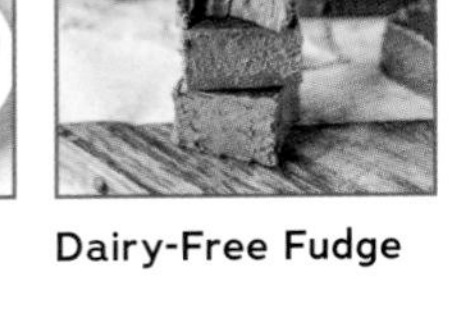
236 Dairy-Free Fudge

238 Italian Cream Puffs

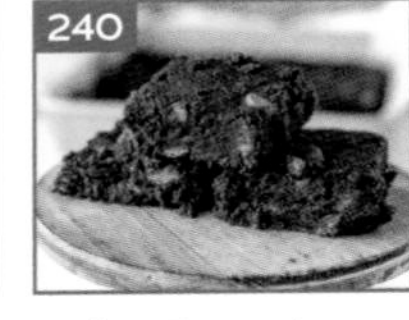
240 Fudgy Brownies

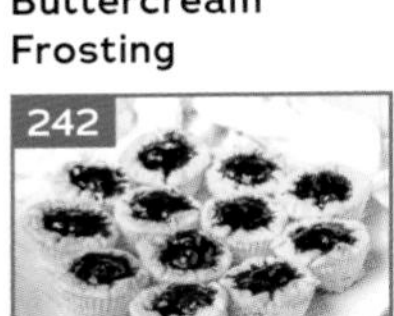
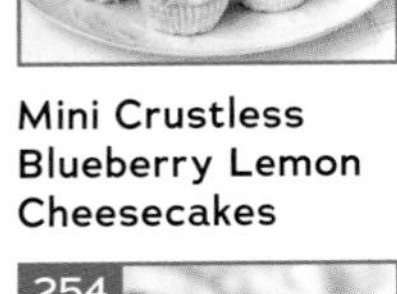
242 Mini Crustless Blueberry Lemon Cheesecakes

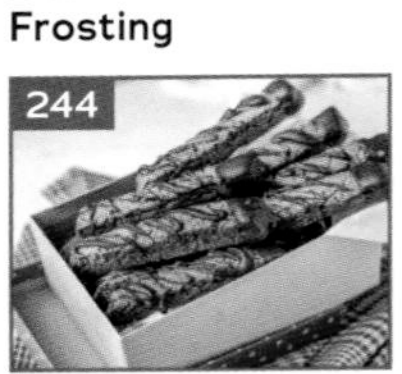
244 Gingerbread Biscotti

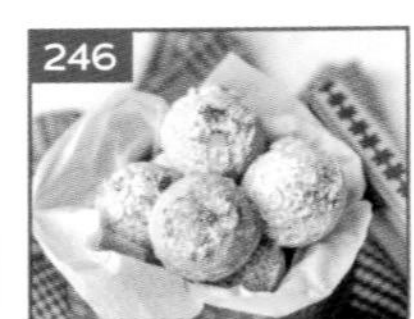
246 Italian Amaretti

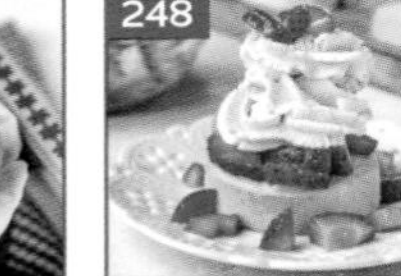
248 Quick Strawberry Shortcakes

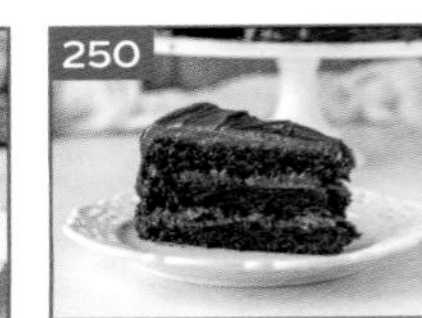
250 Triple-Layer Chocolate Cake

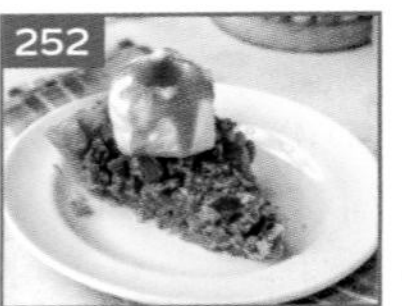
252 Pecan Pie

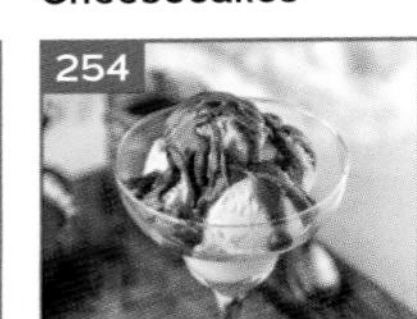
254 Vanilla Gelato

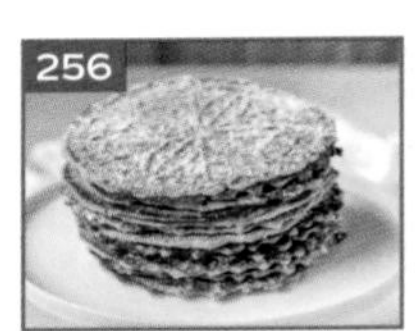
256 Pizzelle

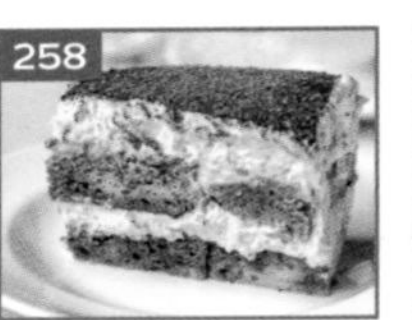
258 Tiramisù

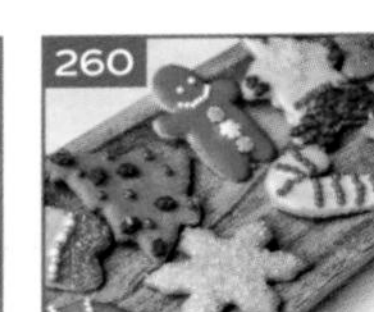
260 Iced Sugar Cookies

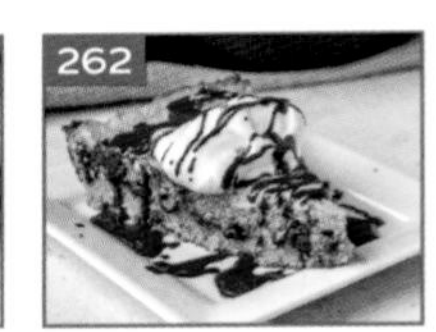
262 Skillet Chocolate Chip Cookie Pie

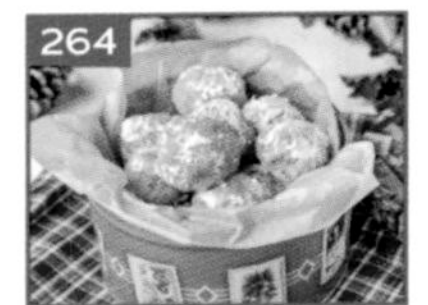
264 Pecan Snowballs

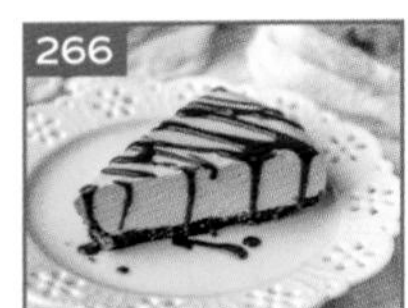
266 No-Bake Coffee Cheesecake

Beverages

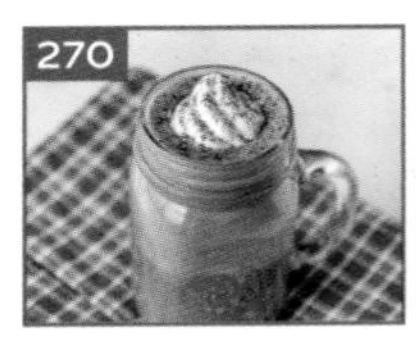
270 Bulletproof Hot Chocolate

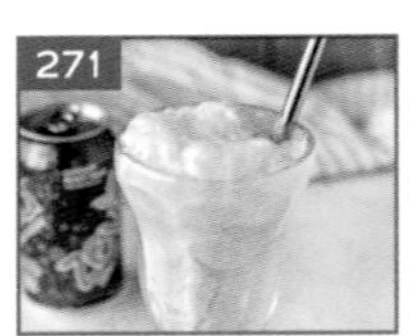
271 Root Beer Ice Cream Float

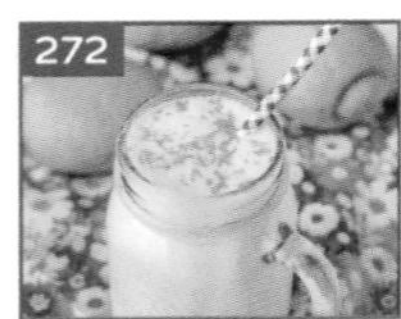
272 Lemon Cream Pie Smoothie

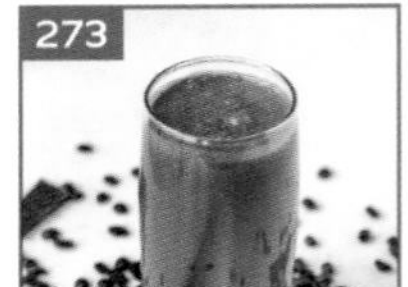
273 Iced Bulletproof Mocha Frappé

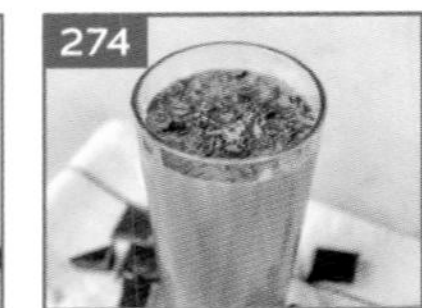
274 Chocolate Sea Salt Smoothie

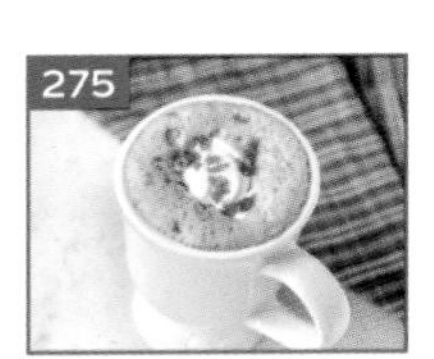
275 Caramel Latte

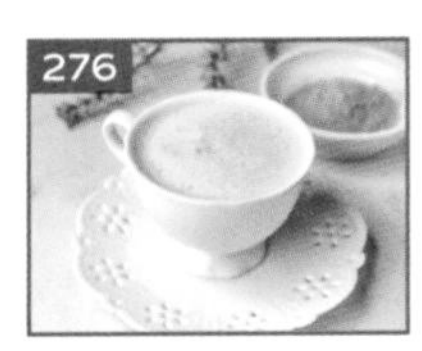
276 Vanilla Turmeric Golden Milk

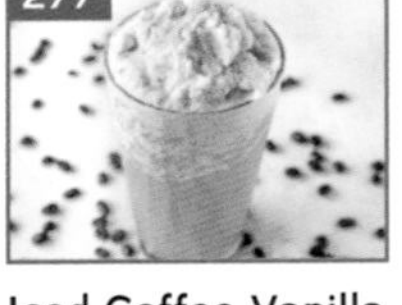
277 Iced Coffee Vanilla Frappé

278 Creamy PB&J Smoothie

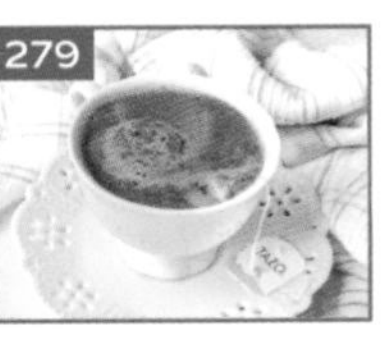
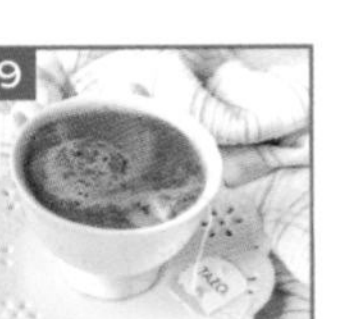
279 Vanilla Spice Dessert Tea

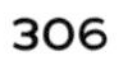

GENERAL INDEX

C

H

I

T